KT-528-752

Minor Surgery:

A TEXT AND ATLAS

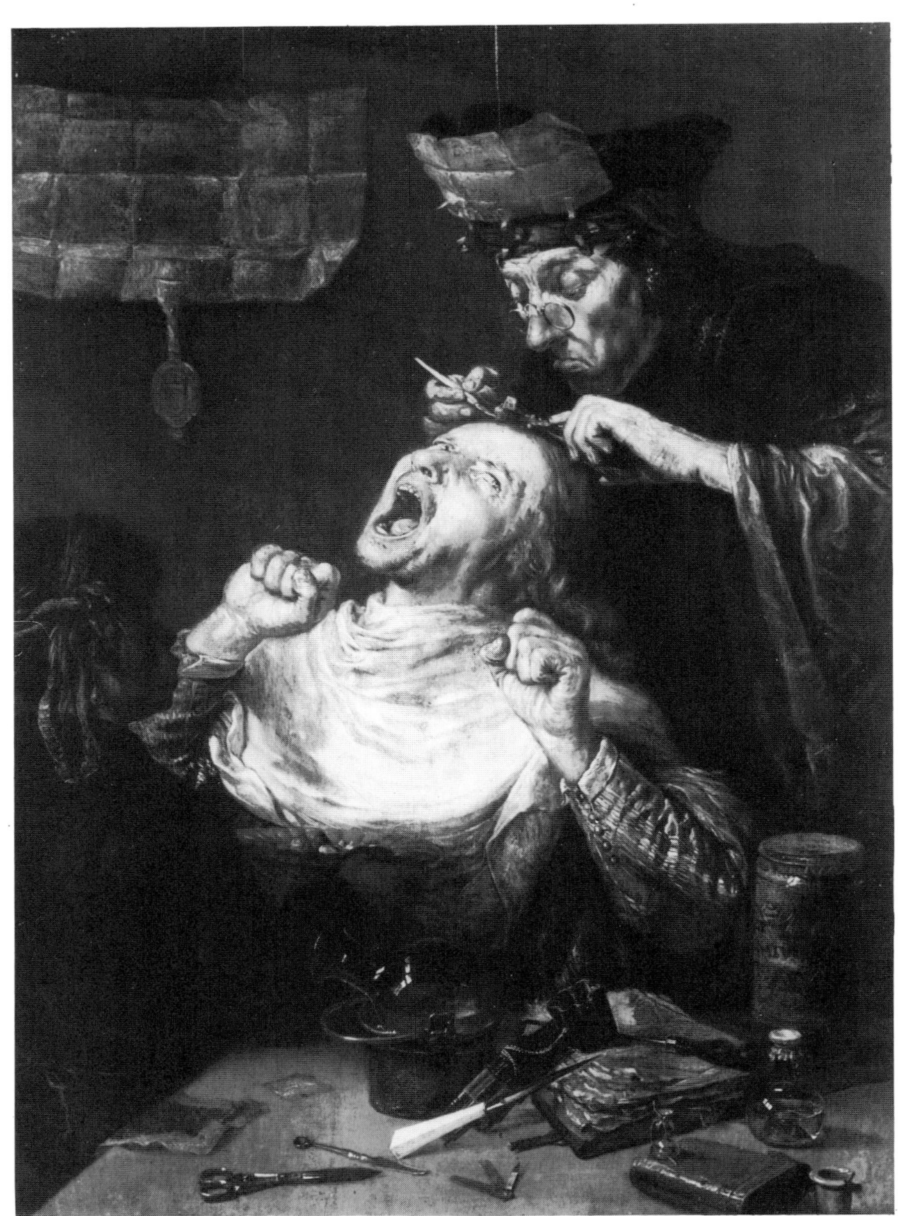

'The extraction of the stone'
Painting by Jan de Bray (17th century)
Museum Boymans-van Beuningen, Rotterdam
(Photograph: Wellcome Institute Library, London)

Minor Surgery:

A TEXT AND ATLAS

John Stuart Brown

SBStJ, MB, BS (Honours, London),
MRCS (England), LRCP (London),
MRCGP, DCH (England)
D(Obst) RCOG, AKC

General Practitioner
Thornhills Medical Group, Larkfield
Maidstone, England

LONDON
CHAPMAN AND HALL

First published in 1986 by
Chapman and Hall Ltd
11 New Fetter Lane, London EC4P 4EE

Printed in Great Britain by
Jolly & Barber Ltd, Rugby

ISBN 0 412 27190 7

British Library Cataloguing in Publication Data

Brown, John Stuart
Minor surgery: a text and atlas.
1. Surgery, Minor
I. Title
617'.024 RD111
ISBN 0-412-27190-7

To Anne

Contents

Foreword

I have been very impressed by the surgical skills of many of my House Surgeons who have later entered general practice. I have often wondered if their undoubted talents and physical dexterity are still being put to good use. Regretfully I have to doubt this. It is a pity that in this country general practitioners are hardly encouraged by anything, other than by their own enthusiasm, to carry out minor surgery. Yet, given adequate training and good equipment, general practitioners will definitely be benefiting the National Health Service as a whole and their patients in particular if they deal personally with the very wide range of procedures that come under the heading of 'minor surgery'. Hospital waiting lists for both in-patient care and out-patient appointments will be shortened, patients will be treated at much greater convenience to themselves and G.P.s' own job satisfaction will undoubtedly improve.

The long list of operations, investigations and other minor procedures in Chapter 12 of this volume will give the reader an idea of the surprising spectrum of conditions which a general practitioner will encounter each year and which are perfectly amenable to treatment in his or her own surgery.

I have read through Dr Brown's book with interest and enjoyment. Indeed, I have learned a few new tricks which I look forward to putting into practice in the near future! I have been impressed by the clear descriptions of the techniques an enthusiastic general practitioner can put into use in the safe and efficient care of his or her patients.

Hospital surgeons worth their salt would be only too happy to encourage local general practitioners in their interest in minor surgery. A period of attachment of just a few months as a clinical assistant would be a very good way of surgical revision for those who have been divorced for some time from hospital practice. I am particularly thinking of general surgical, orthopaedic, varicose vein, gynaecological, ENT and eye out-patients.

Astley Cooper was created a Baronet after his successful removal of the sebaceous cyst of the scalp of George IV. I cannot offer the readers of this volume any hope of such a reward but certainly if they put the advice in this book into practice they will soon start to collect a following of very grateful patients in the community.

HAROLD ELLIS, DM, MCh, FRCS
Surgical Unit, Westminster Hospital, London SW1

Preface

This book provides an illustrated step-by-step guide to minor surgery. It covers all minor surgical conditions and treatments encountered by the author over twenty-five years in general practice.

The selection of suitable instruments and equipment is described, followed by methods of instrument sterilization, skin preparation, choice of incisions and a comprehensive description of methods of anaesthesia, including intravenous regional anaesthesia, nerve blocks and infiltration anaesthesia.

Wound closure and the use of different suture materials are described, together with a section on the timing of suture removal to obtain the neatest scars. Follow-up and statistical analysis of the types of operation feasible in general practice are covered.

Individual minor surgical procedures are then described with illustrations. The practitioner is taken through each operation, commencing with simple injection techniques, through excision of cysts, biopsies, ingrowing toe-nails and varicose veins to more complex minor operations including decompression of the carpal tunnel, release of trigger finger and excision of ganglion.

Finally, simple diagnostic procedures such as proctoscopy, sigmoidoscopy and biopsy are described.

This volume provides a valuable reference book for all general medical practitioners, both in practice and in training.

Although all the operations described can be performed under general or local anaesthesia, the author has described local anaesthetic techniques almost exclusively.

Acknowledgements

This book is based on a series of articles on minor surgery in the *Pulse* reference section, 1984, and my grateful thanks are due to the staff of *Pulse* who gave me so much help and advice, and in particular to Cynthia Clarke for her medical illustrations and Philip Fraser Betts for his photographs.

To Mrs Vaux and Mrs Harrison, state registered chiropodists in Maidstone, my grateful thanks for their tuition on the method for treating ingrowing toe-nails.

My thanks are also due to Mr W. Keith Yeates for allowing me to use his colour transparencies illustrating vasectomy which appeared in *Update*.

I am very grateful to my partners, and to all the nurses who have worked with us at Larkfield and given so much help and advice; also to all our receptionists and staff for all their help.

I am especially grateful to Mrs Sylvia Smith, the practice manager of the Thornhills Medical Group, for all her invaluable help in typing, reading and correcting the manuscripts.

Finally, to my family, who excused me from 'household and gardening jobs' to write the book – my deep and sincere thanks!

J.S.B.

Minor Surgery:
A TEXT AND ATLAS

ONE

Introduction

'If thou examinest a man having a gaping wound in his head, penetrating to the bone, thou shouldst lay thy hand upon it and thou shouldst palpate his wound. If thou findest his skull uninjured thou shouldst say regarding him "an ailment which I will treat" '

(Edwin Smith, Surgical Papyrus, 3000–2500 BC)

All doctors have seen many minor operations performed, and as medical students, resident house-surgeons and trainee general practitioners have performed many of them personally. Before the advent of the National Health Service in the United Kingdom, most family doctors undertook their own minor surgery – lancing boils and abscesses, excising cysts, and suturing lacerations. Some had contracts with the local hospitals and performed all their own minor surgery, together with many major surgical procedures. Patients expected their family doctors to operate, and family doctors themselves expected to undertake most minor surgical procedures – including delivering babies at home, and even 'tonsillectomy on the kitchen table'!

In recent years, there has been a gradual move away from general practitioner minor surgery – family doctors in hospitals have been replaced by specialist consultant colleagues, fewer general practitioners are now undertaking their own minor surgery, preferring instead to refer the majority of their patients with such conditions to hospital. Inevitably, as this trend increased, hospital surgical waiting lists increased.

In many instances because the patient realizes his or her condition is not serious, and knows that there are long delays, he or she may not even consult the family doctor, preferring to keep the 'cyst' or 'mole' or 'veins'. In recent years however, there has been a renewed interest by general medical practitioners in minor surgery; with training now taking up to ten years, and many doctors moving into purpose-built premises complete with treatment rooms, and working with attached community nurses or practice nurses, many now feel they would like to undertake their own minor operations again. This has been welcomed by the patients, who now find they can receive treatment for their minor lesions promptly, in familiar surroundings, and done by a doctor they know well, with follow up by the nurses they know already.

Because of the great variety of minor surgical procedures, there is a good chance that doctors will never have seen some actually performed, and if they wish to learn the techniques they may have to refer to twelve or more specialized textbooks of surgery. For example a GP would need to consult a surgical instrument catalogue for the choice of instruments, equipment firms for sterilizers, tables and lights, textbooks on general surgery for the excision of sebaceous cysts, and reference books on ophthalmic surgery for the treatment of meibomian cysts.

Removal of intradermal naevi might be found in a textbook of dermatology or general surgery, whereas intra-articular steroid injections

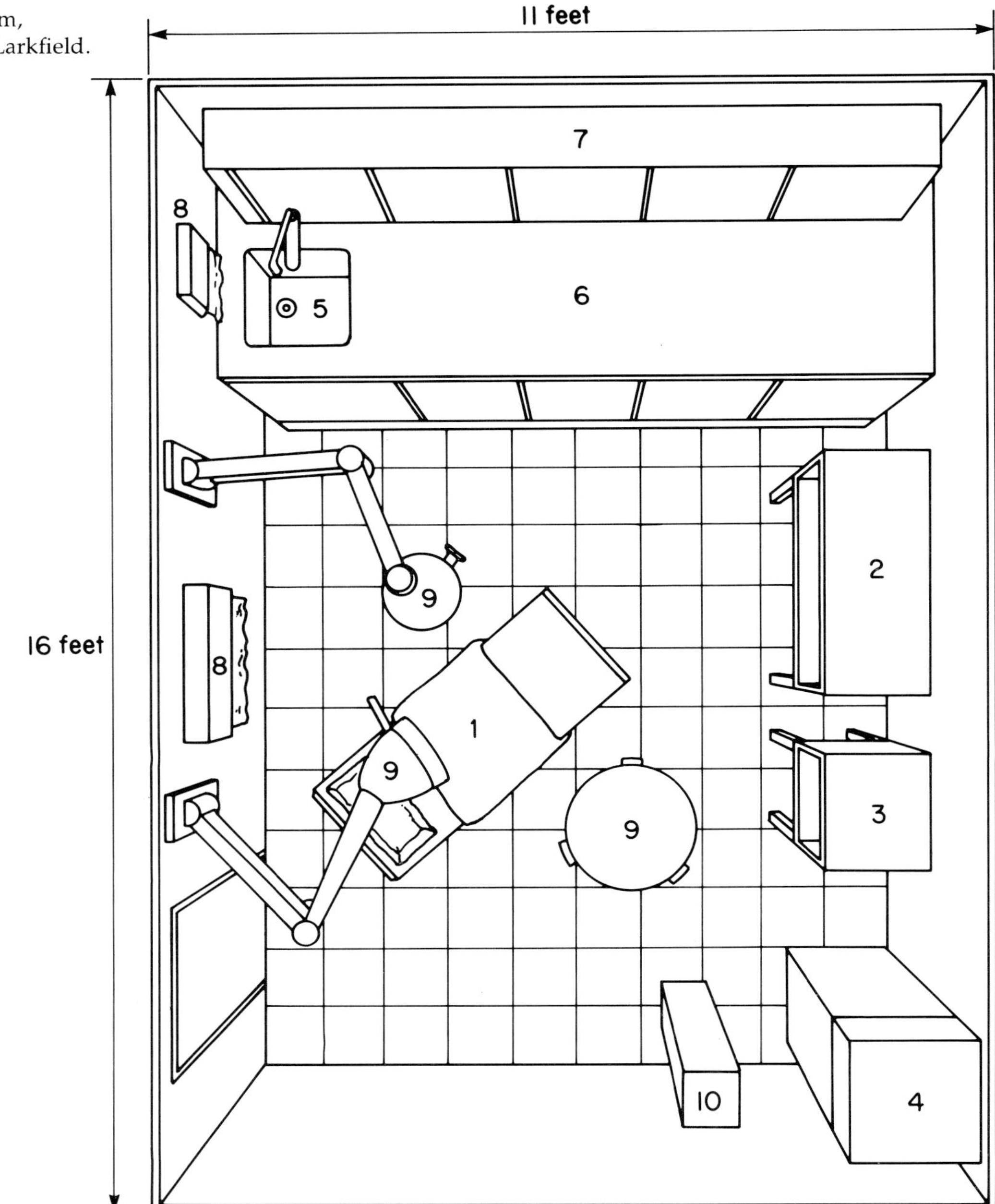

Fig. 1.1 The treatment room, Thornhills Medical Group, Larkfield. Key:

1. Operating theatre table
2. Dressing trolley
3. Dressing trolley
4. Instrument cupboard
5. Hand wash-basin
6. Work surface
7. Storage cupboards
8. Paper towel dispenser
9. Lights
10. Waste bin.

might be found in books on rheumatology, general medicine or orthopaedics. Proctoscopy, sigmoidoscopy and the injection of haemorrhoids could be covered in three separate textbooks, while the treatment of ingrowing toe-nails might be included in books of general surgery, orthopaedics, dermatology and chiropody! Skin tumours and their management would be found in specialist books on oncology, dermatology, general surgery, plastic surgery and even lasers in medicine. Decompression of the carpal tunnel might come under orthopaedics or general surgery, while injection of the carpal tunnel would be included in

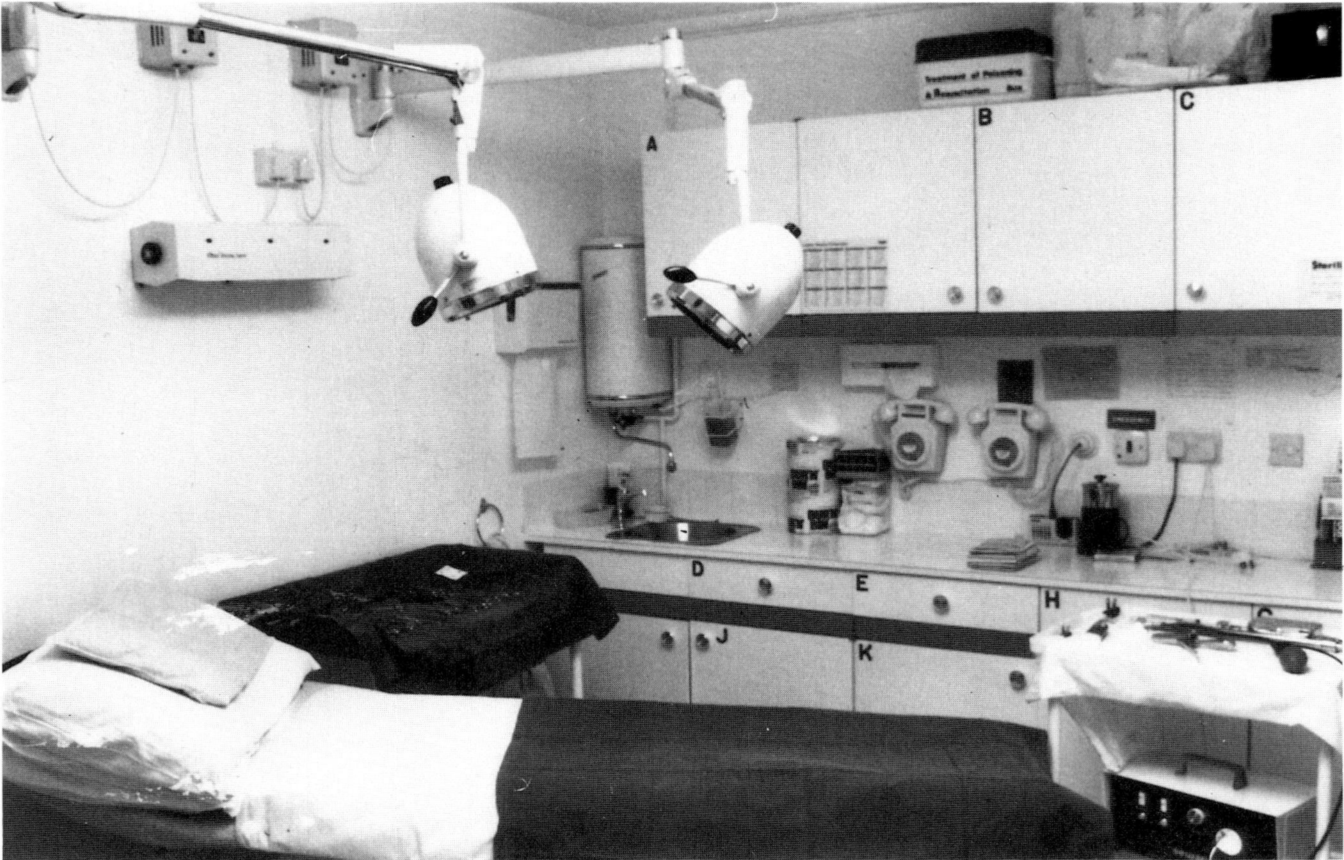

Fig. 1.2 The treatment room, Thornhills Medical Group, Larkfield, Kent.

books on rheumatology, neurology, physical medicine or general surgery. Practitioners wishing to learn the technique of cryotherapy might have difficulty knowing which specialized textbook to consult, as they would if they wished to sterilize instruments or equipment. Thus, although each procedure may correctly be classified as minor surgery, nevertheless the term embraces many different specialities, and hence the reason for this book: it is an attempt to bring together under one cover all the minor operations and practical surgical procedures that general practitioners might wish to perform themselves.

With a few exceptions, all the minor operations described can be performed single-handed by the practitioner or with the assistance of an 'unscrubbed' nurse. The techniques described and the instruments used are those which the author has found most suitable over twenty-five years performing more than 5000 minor operations personally. The choice of firms supplying instruments and equipment is always difficult as there are many excellent firms both in the United Kingdom and America; thus only a representative sample has been included in the book, mainly of suppliers the author has used himself.

1.1 SCOPE AND LIMITATIONS OF MINOR SURGERY

All the minor operations described in this book are well within the capability of any general medical practitioner, house-surgeon, casualty officer or trainee general practitioner as well as the specialist. Some require

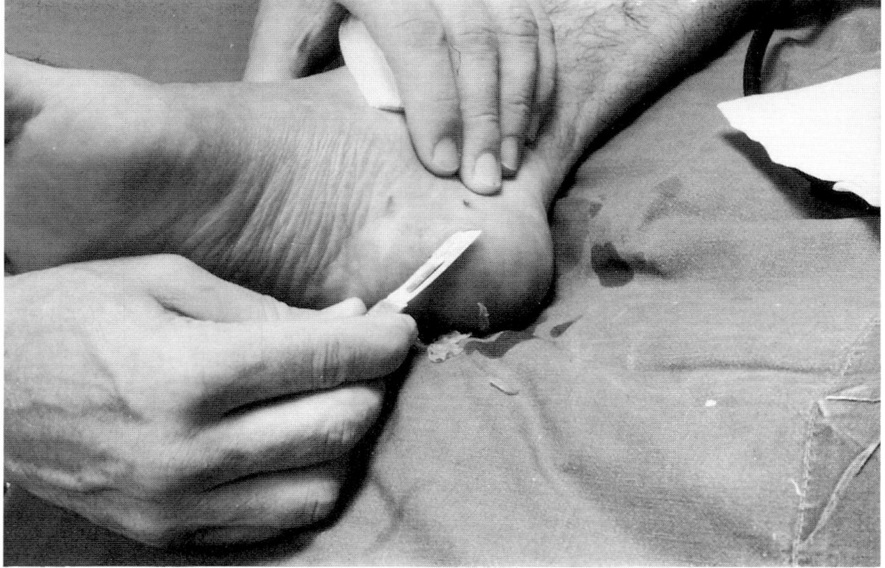

Fig. 1.3 For many minor surgical procedures it is not necessary to use sterile gloves or gowns.

the purchase of a special item of equipment such as an electrocautery, others require a special instrument, for example chalazion ring forceps for meibomian cysts. Above all, practitioners must satisfy themselves that they can safely carry out *any* particular surgical procedure *before* attempting it. Thus it may be helpful, as well as referring to texts and photographs, to watch a procedure being performed by a colleague and obtain expert tuition before embarking on it.

As experience grows, so the number and variety of minor operations attempted will increase, and the final decision of what to attempt, and what not to attempt will rest entirely with the doctor. A single-handed practitioner will be inadvised to attempt any operation involving intravenous regional anaesthesia, where an assistant is mandatory, and although the majority of operations described can safely be performed

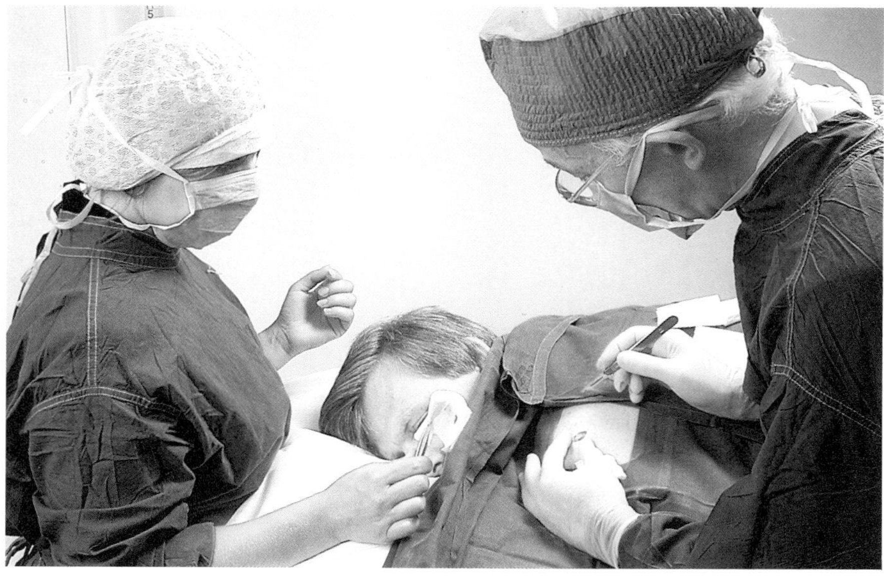

Fig. 1.4 For others, such as decompression of the carpal tunnel, opening joints, and excision of lipomata, sterile gloves and gowns may be used, together with masks.

Table 1.1 Advantages of GP minor surgery

1.	Staff already known to patient
2.	Saving of time for patient and hospital
3.	Financial savings to local hospital
4.	Continuity of care
5.	Less infection
6.	Greater job satisfaction
7.	Greater efficiency
8.	Offering a better service
9.	Rapid biopsy and histology results
10.	Greater patient satisfaction

single handed, nevertheless, if an assistant such as a nurse or colleague can be available, it helps considerably both the patient and operator. For this reason, if the doctor contemplates undertaking minor surgery to any extent, it is a good idea at the outset to reserve a time for an operating session or 'list'; this may be daily, weekly, or once a month depending on numbers and circumstances. General anaesthesia has not been included in this book as it was assumed most general practitioners would not have adequate recovery beds and facilities in the average GP surgery. However, all the procedures described can easily be performed very safely and comfortably using local anaesthetic techniques.

Where the patient can have a short rest afterwards and transport can be arranged, there are very few minor operations which cannot readily be performed in the general practitioner's consulting or treatment room. Where the patient is too ill (e.g. malignant ascites) or too handicapped (e.g. confined entirely to bed) it may be preferable to bring the equipment and instruments to the patient's home rather than bringing the patient to the doctor's premises, and in this respect, minor surgery lends itself admirably.

1.2 ADVANTAGES AND DISADVANTAGES

There are considerable advantages where the patient's doctor undertakes minor surgery (see Table 1.1). First, the patient and doctor are already well known to each other, and this immediately allays much anxiety, particularly with very young patients. Secondly, there is saving of time both for the patient and the hospital; the patient can generally choose a convenient time and the hospital, by not seeing the patient, can offer the time saved to another patient. Thirdly, there are considerable financial savings, particularly to the hospital budget. It has been shown that one general practitioner performing only a few minor operations per week can save the local hospital a significant amount [1, 2] and that on average, it is fifteen times cheaper to perform the same operation in general practice compared with hospital. Fourthly, there is a continuity of care; the doctor performing the operation is the same doctor who initially saw the patient – the nurse assisting at the operation is likewise already known to the patient, and is the same nurse who will remove any sutures and undertake any further follow-up, and, when the patient is ready to return to school or work, it is the very same doctor who will check all is well and discharge the patient.

Table 1.2 Disadvantages of GP minor surgery

1. Lack of suitable training
2. Lack of suitable equipment and premises
3. The risk of missing serious pathology
4. Allocating sufficient time
5. Worry should complications occur
6. Financial disincentives

Cross-infection outside hospital is much less of a problem than inside hospital, commonly less than 1 or 2%. Among other advantages could be included greater job satisfaction, greater efficiency, offering a better service, rapid biopsy and histology results, and greater patient satisfaction.

Offset against these many advantages are a few disadvantages (Table 1.2). One of the most commonly voiced worries is lack of suitable training, lack of suitable equipment and premises, the risk of missing serious pathology, the expense, setting aside enough time, the worry should complications occur, and, in the UK, the financial disincentives for doctors to undertake their own minor surgery within the terms of the National Health Service. Generally, however, the advantages greatly outweigh any disadvantages, and rarely does one find a doctor who has started to undertake surgery thinking of abandoning it.

1.3 ORGANIZATION WITHIN THE PRACTICE

Some procedures such as injection of tennis elbow, golfer's elbow, carpal tunnel and the like, take so little time that it is usually preferable to perform these at the time of the initial consultation. Similarly, if the electrocautery and an ampoule of local anaesthetic are available easily, small skin tags, papillomata and warts and naevi may all be dealt with in less than five minutes.

Where any number are to be done, or where it is likely to take longer than the initial consultation appointment time, it is easier and preferable to set aside a certain time each week, and to make a minor operations 'list' at which the practice nurse and/or an assistant can help. With a little experience the doctor will soon know how long each procedure takes, and will be able to offer appropriate appointments accordingly.

Accurate records of all operations performed should be kept, together with any drugs used, and types of sutures and dressings; a register of operations enables the doctor to analyse his or her work and produce an annual breakdown of the type of work being done (see Chapter 12).

Many 'elementary' procedures are described in this book, and lists of instruments are often repeated throughout the book. This is a deliberate policy to avoid the reader having to refer back to several previous sections.

TWO

Instruments

'When thou meetest a tumour that has attacked a vessel . . . say "I will treat the disease with the knife, poultice it with fat, and burn it with fire so that it bleeds not too much".'

(Ebers Papyrus, 1500 BC)

Every doctor has a favourite selection of instruments; what suits one surgeon does not always suit another. One practitioner may prefer small, fine toothed delicate instruments whereas another is happier with larger instruments. However, certain basic sets of instruments seem to be generally popular, and the following are included as being the most commonly used by the author (Fig. 2.1).

1 size 3 scalpel handle
scalpel blades 15, 10, 11
5″ toothed dissecting forceps (Treves) (12.7 cm)
5″ standard (sharp/sharp) stitch scissors (12.7 cm)
5″ straight artery forceps (Halstead) (12.7 cm)
1 $5\frac{1}{4}$″ Kilner needle holder (13.3 cm)

These five instruments plus scalpel blades form the nucleus of most minor operating sets; they can be used for simple suturing of lacerations and excision of most dermal lesions. Where the practitioner intends building up various instrument packs to be sterilized by the CSSD (Central Sterile Supplies Department) several such basic packs should be made up.

The next most useful instruments are the sharp-spoon Volkmann curette and electrocautery, which between them enable the practitioner to remove most warts, verrucae, papillomata, granulomas, keratoses, and similar intradermal lesions. The curette is generally easy to choose, depending on

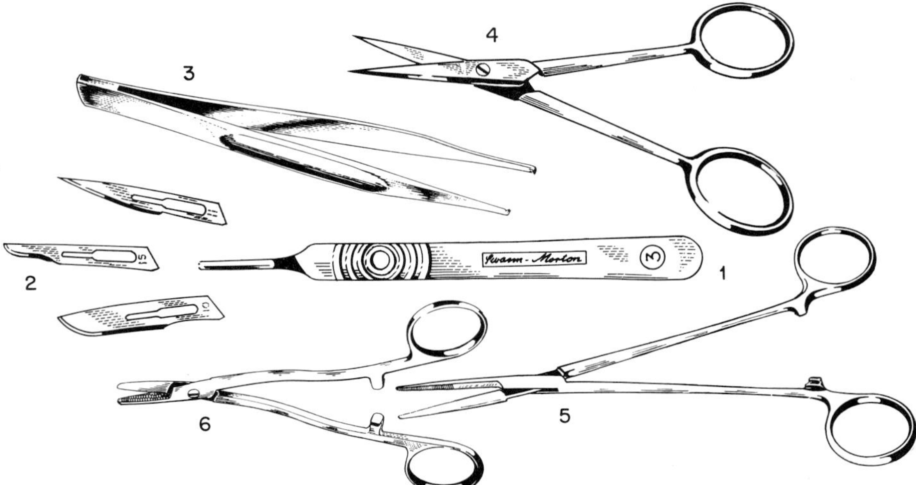

Fig. 2.1 A basic instrument pack.
1. Scalpel handle, size 3
2. Scalpel blades, sizes 10, 11 and 15
3. 5″ (12.7 cm) toothed dissecting forceps
4. 5″ (12.7 cm) standard stitch scissors, pointed
5. 5″ (12.7 cm) straight artery forceps (Halstead's)
6. $5\frac{1}{4}$″ (13.3 cm) Kilner needle holder.

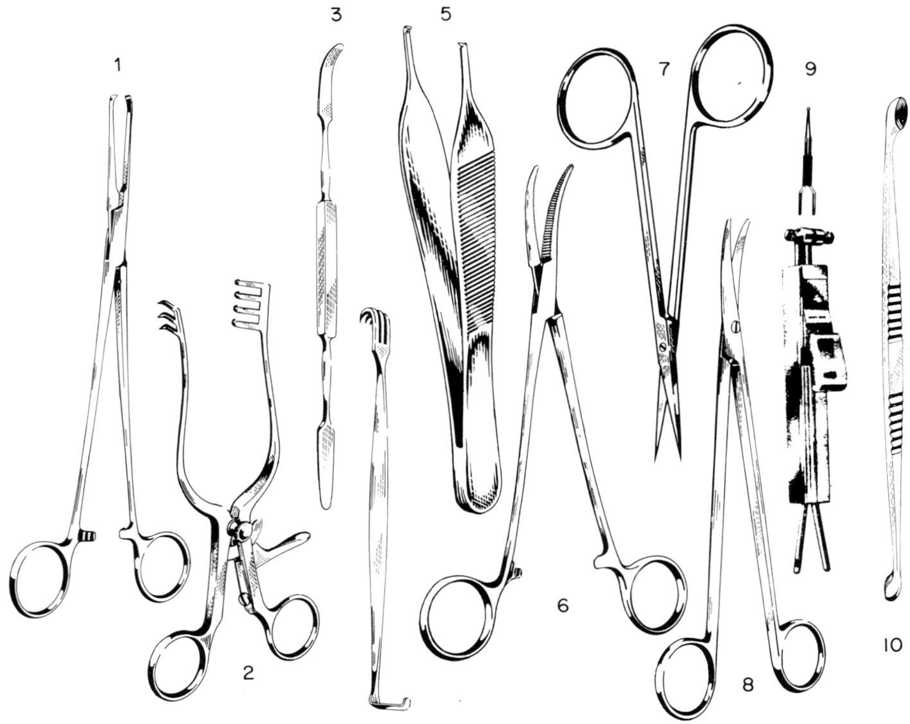

Fig. 2.2 Some of the most commonly used instruments in addition to the 'basic set'.

1. Allis tissue forceps 3 × 4 teeth 6″ (15.2 cm)
2. Self-retaining retractor (Kocher's thyroid or equivalent)
3. McDonald's double-ended dissector $7\frac{1}{2}$″ (19 cm)
4. Retractor: double-ended Kilner Senn Miller 6″ (15.2 cm) (so-called cat's paw retractor)
5. Adson's toothed dissecting forceps $4\frac{3}{4}$″ (12 cm)
6. 5″ (12.7 cm) curved fine artery forceps (Halstead's mosquito)
7. Iris scissors, straight, $4\frac{1}{2}$″ (11.4 cm)
8. Curved 7″ (17.8 cm) McIndoe's scissors
9. Electrocautery burner and handle (Mark Hovell's)
10. Volkmann double-ended sharp-spoon curette

the doctor's preference, but selection of an electrocautery can be difficult as there are many excellent models on the market (see Chapter 3).

Where smaller instruments are required for fine surgery, Adson's $4\frac{3}{4}$″ (12 cm) toothed dissecting forceps are ideal, together with a pair of Iris scissors, fine $4\frac{1}{2}$″ (11.4 cm) straight or curved. Similarly, the fine 5″ (12.7 cm) Halstead mosquito forceps, curved or straight are most useful instruments.

Sebaceous cysts and lipomata can be nicely dissected using a pair of curved 7″ (17.8 cm) McIndoe scissors which may also double up for cutting the threads of intra-uterine contraceptive devices after they have been inserted (Fig. 2.2).

At some stage, the practitioner will need some small retractors: these may be either self-retaining such as the Kocher's thyroid retractor, West Weitlaner $5\frac{1}{2}$″ (14 cm), or the baby Kilner/Dickson Wright spring self-retaining retractor, or single/double retractors which will need to be held by an assistant. Of these, the Gillies skin hooks $6\frac{1}{2}$″ (16.5 cm) are popular, as are the double-ended Kilner Senn Miller 6″ (15.2 cm) (so called cat's paw retractors).

To complete the list of small general instruments is the McDonald's double-ended $7\frac{1}{2}$″ (19 cm) dissector, extremely useful for operations on the carpal tunnel and 'trigger' fingers. All general practitioners regularly see patients suffering from meibomian cysts; normally such patients need to be referred to an ophthalmic surgeon, but the treatment of incision and curettage is so simple and quick that it can be one of the most rewarding conditions to treat, provided the practitioner has the necessary instruments. These comprise a pair of chalazion ring forceps, a small chalazion curette, no. 3 scalpel handle with the pointed no. 11 blade together with syringe and needle for administering local anaesthetic (Fig. 2.3).

Another valuable instrument, although not used as frequently as the

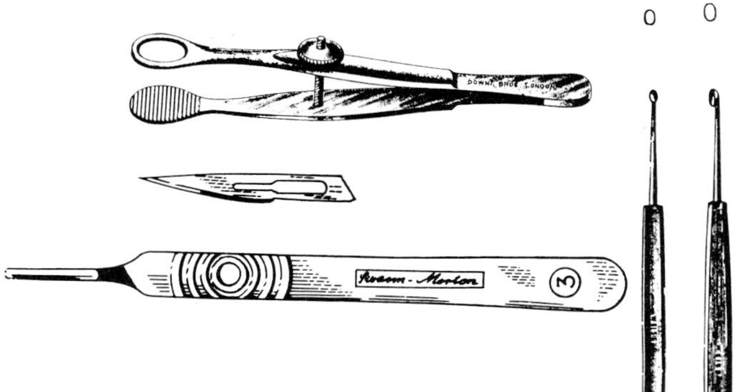

Fig. 2.3 Instruments required for incision and curette of meibomian cyst (chalazion).

above is the abdominal trocar and cannula for draining abdominal ascites (Fig. 2.4).

In general practice, the commonest cause of ascites is inoperable malignant disease, and great relief, albeit temporary, can be offered by the judicious tapping of ascitic fluid when symptoms of pressure become distressing.

As the treatment of haemorrhoids is included in the textbook, a choice of proctoscope, sigmoidoscope and haemorrhoid injection syringe should be considered. There are many different sigmoidoscopes and proctoscopes on the market with a variety of methods of illumination and magnification, some disposable, some non-disposable, and costs vary considerably. Where a practitioner is considering purchasing such instruments, it is often helpful to ask the advice of the local general surgeon and ask for a demonstration.

The Lloyd Davies stainless steel sigmoidoscope has been in use for many years and is a popular, virtually indestructable instrument. Illumination can be by fibre-optic cable, or filament bulb, tungsten or quartz halogen lamp; they are rigid, reasonably priced and interchangeable (Fig. 2.5). More recently, flexible, fibre-optic sigmoidoscopes have been marketed, but the cost is still high, and probably outside the price range of the average practitioner. However, the illumination and view are excellent and more of the sigmoid colon can be visualized than with the rigid instrument.

Naunton Morgan's proctoscope is ideal for the general practitioner. As with the sigmoidoscope, illumination may be from either a fibre-optic cable or filament bulb. It is an excellent instrument to use if the practitioner contemplates injecting haemorrhoids. For this latter procedure, a Gabriel's haemorrhoid syringe is used. It has the advantage of good finger control, although many simpler disposable haemorrhoid syringes have now been introduced with Luer-lock fittings to prevent the needle being expelled under pressure (Fig. 2.6).

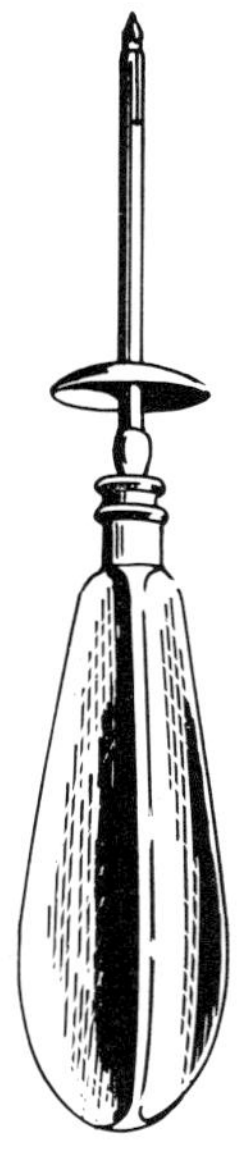

Fig. 2.4 Trocar and cannula used for draining abdominal ascites.

As all the operations described in this book are performed under local anaesthesia, it is important that this be made as discomfort-free as possible. To this end, the finest possible needle should be used for infiltration anaesthesia, and there is no better needle to use than the 30 SWG (0.3 mm) needle mounted on a dental syringe loaded with a cartridge of local anaesthetic. If the injection is given slowly and gently, it can be virtually painless; a point greatly appreciated by the younger patients! (Fig. 2.7).

Where larger volumes of local anaesthetic need to be injected, the initial

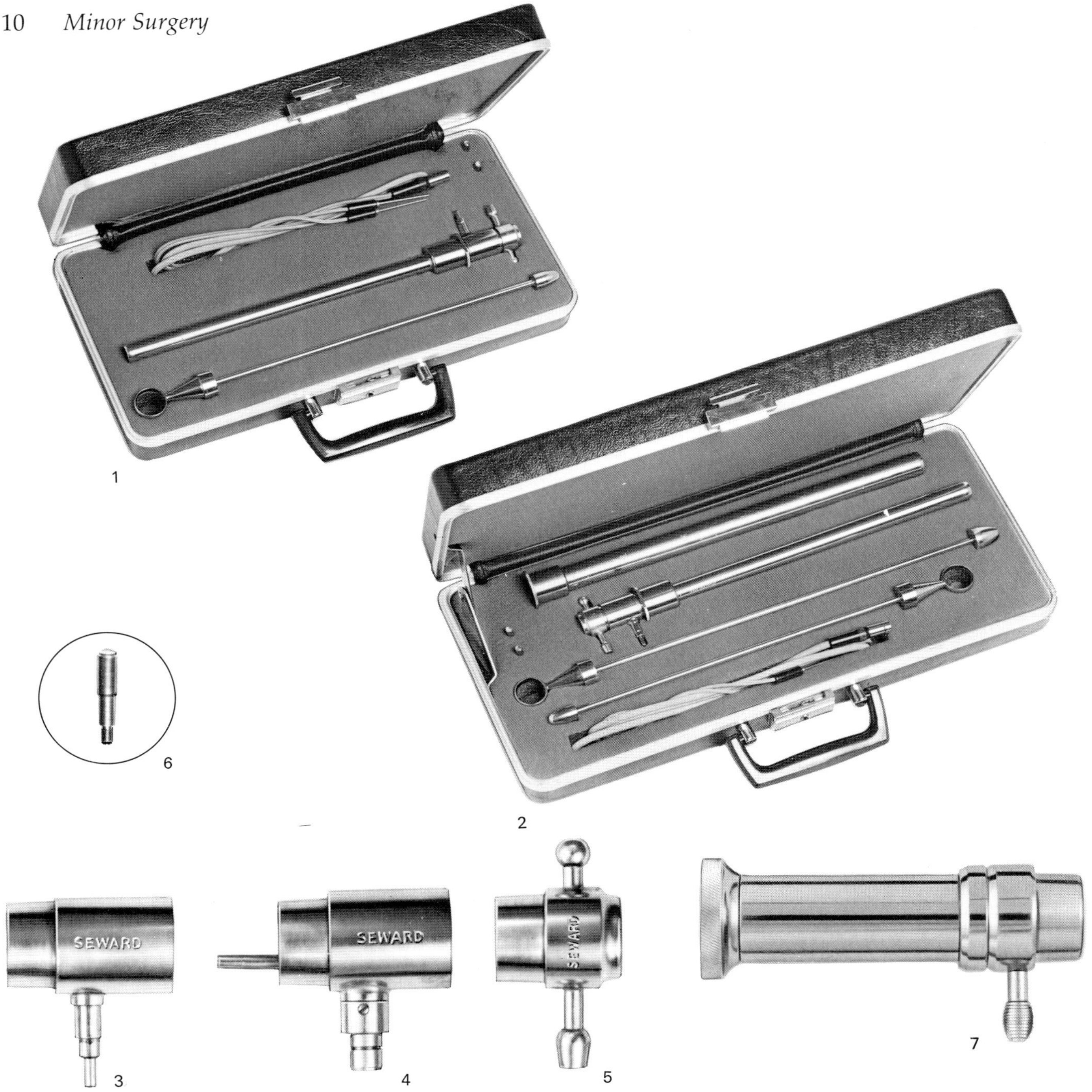

Fig. 2.5 The Lloyd-Davies stainless steel rigid sigmoidoscope.
1. Adult size 250 mm × 15 mm
2. Adult size 300 mm × 20 mm
3. 3.5 V lighting chamber
4. Fibre-optic lighting chamber
5. Inflation window
6. 3.5 V tungsten-filament bulb
7. Telescopic attachment (× 1.5 magnification) (Seward Medical, London).

'bleb' or 'weal' can still be raised with the dental syringe and needle. Larger needles merely traumatize the tissues, cause unnecessary pain, delay healing and increase the risks of infection.

Finally, before leaving this section on the choice of instruments, mention must be made of two invaluable instruments in the surgical treatment of ingrowing toe-nails, these are the nail chisel and the Thwaites nail nipper (Figs 2.8 and 2.9). With these two instruments plus a pair of straight artery forceps the practitioner can offer a treatment for ingrowing toe-nails which carries a 99% cure rate! (See Chapter 26.)

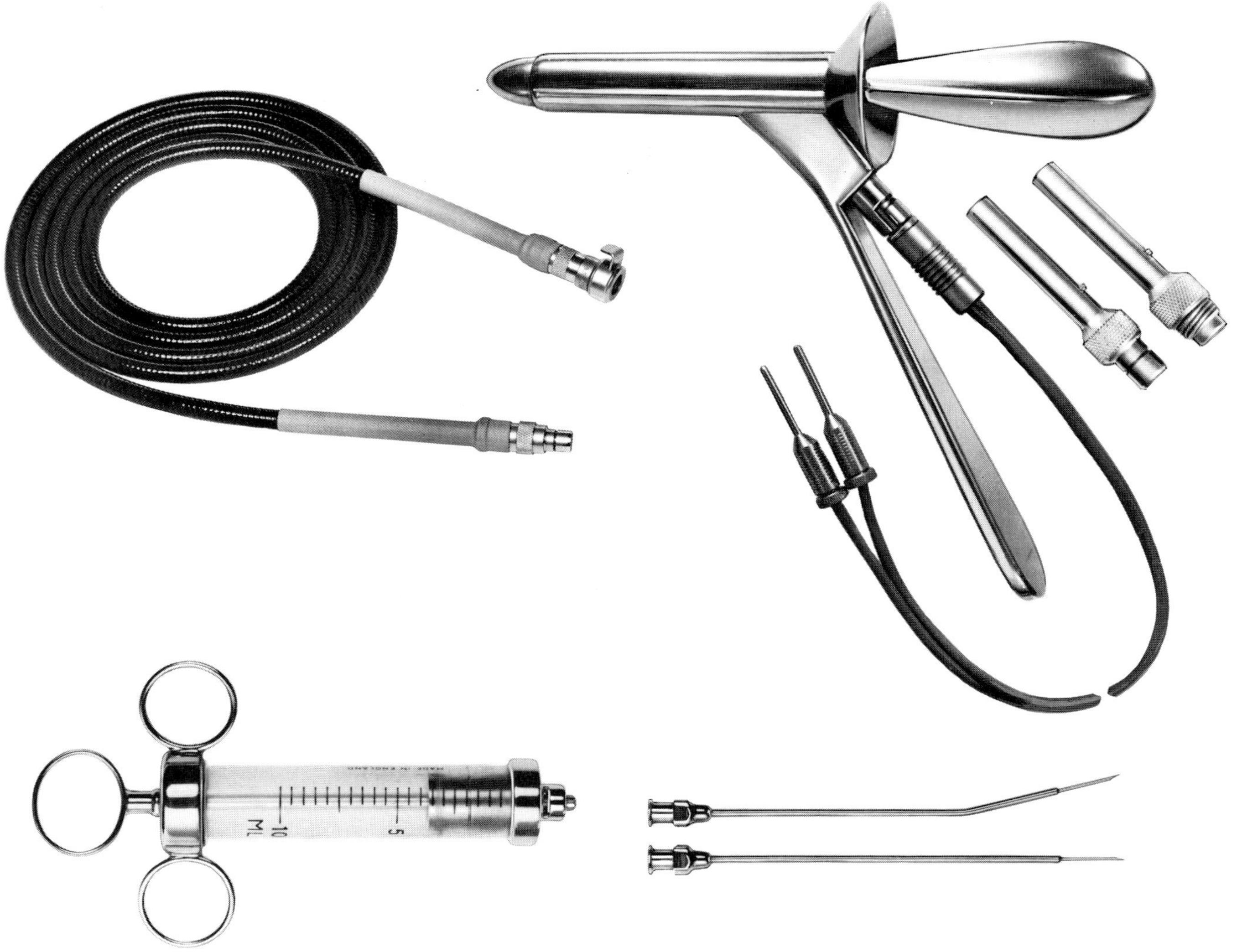

Fig. 2.6 St. Mark's Hospital pattern proctoscope with Gabriel's Haemorrhoid injection syringe and needles. Illumination by tungsten-filament 3.5 V bulb, or fibre-optic cable and light (Seward Medical, London).

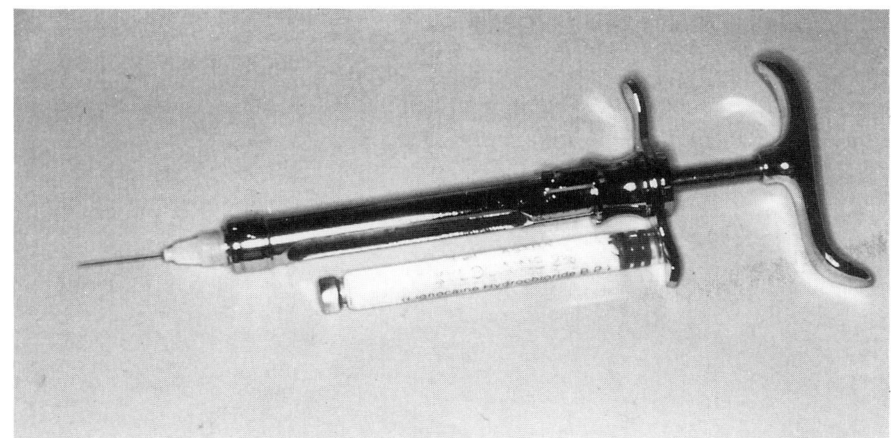

Fig. 2.7 Dental syringe with cartridges of local anaesthetic and 30 g needles; ideal for children and digital nerve blocks (Ash Instruments).

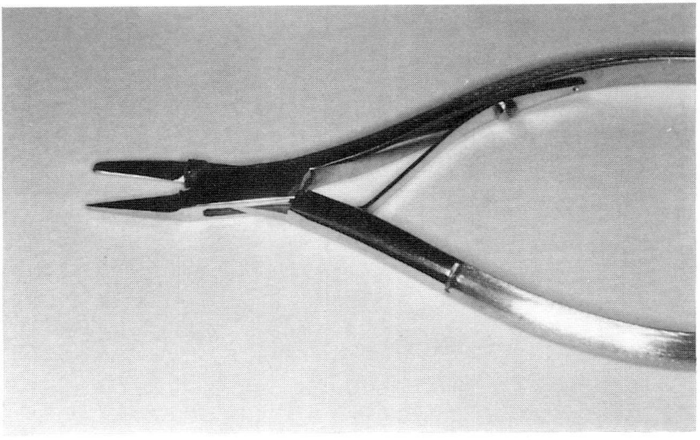

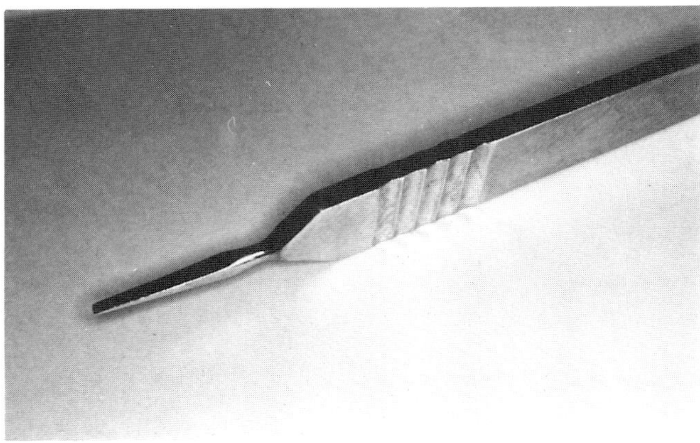

Fig. 2.8 Thwaites nail nipper (English pattern, Nova Instruments).

Fig. 2.9 Nail chisel (Nova Instruments).

2.1 INSTRUMENT AND EQUIPMENT MANUFACTURERS

(See the Appendix)

The list given at the end of this book is far from comprehensive; it includes all the firms which the author has used during the past twenty-five years; however, each practitioner will have his or her own favourite suppliers, and it is certainly worth 'shopping around' for the 'best buy'. All the items of equipment and surgical instruments described in this book can be obtained from firms included in this list.

2.2 SOURCES OF SUPPLY

To build and equip a minor operating theatre using all new materials and instruments could be prohibitively expensive for most general practitioners, particularly as they are unlikely to be able to recoup much of the expenditure either from grants, item-of-service payments or patients' fees.

However, by making careful enquiries and contacting various agencies, a very acceptable treatment room can be equipped for a fraction of what it would cost new. Major items such as operating theatre tables, trolleys, sterilizers and lights may often be obtained from the local Hospital Supplies Officer who knows of obsolete items of equipment no longer required by the hospital. They may often be purchased for a nominal sum, and although classified as 'obsolete' as far as the hospital is concerned, may prove to be exactly what is needed in a small minor operating room.

Often equipment has been purchased for use in hospital, only to be superseded by an improved model after several years; the original is then relegated to the stores, yet is still perfectly serviceable. Similarly, it is worth contacting large surgical equipment manufacturers to see if they have any reconditioned, obsolete, or demonstration models available at a reduced price. Medical representatives from these firms are always most helpful if they can see what is needed, and it is always worth contacting them, usually through the Operating Room Supervisor/Theatre Sister at the nearest hospital.

Charitable organizations will often be prepared to raise money and purchase a piece of equipment, particularly if they can see the benefits which will accrue locally if an improved surgical service is offered.

Finally when all else fails, it is still possible to advertise for equipment and instruments in the various journals and weekly magazines, and be successful.

2.3 ADVANTAGES OF INSTRUMENT PACKS

Where a doctor is performing a regular number of minor operations and particularly if the CSSD (Central Sterile Supplies Department) facilities can be used, there is much to commend compiling a number of 'instrument packs'. For example, Suture pack, Ingrowing toe-nail pack, Meibomian cyst pack, Abdominal paracentesis pack, etc. In this way, just the instruments which are required are sterilized and used in a more efficient way. Individual packs may be sterilized and kept for future use, as well as being available for use both at the surgery or in the patient's home. It is also easier to check the contents of each pack at the end of each operation to ensure no instruments have been lost. Unfortunately the smaller autoclaves are not suitable for instrument packs as they do not have a vacuum cycle, so the practitioner will normally have to rely on a hospital autoclave or, failing this, a hot air oven.

The following instrument packs will be found to be most useful for the general practitioner undertaking minor surgery.

2.3.1 Basic 'suture' pack

1 scalpel handle size 3
1 Kilner needle holder $5\frac{1}{4}''$ (13.3 cm)
1 stitch scissors, pointed, 5" (12.7 cm)
1 toothed dissecting forceps 5" (12.7 cm)
1 straight artery forceps 5" (12.7 cm)
1 scalpel blade size 10
1 sterile braided silk suture metric gauge 2 cutting needle. Ref. Ethicon W 533

2.3.2 Meibomian cyst pack

1 pair chalazion ring forceps
1 scalpel handle size 3
1 pair iris scissors, curved $4\frac{1}{2}''$ (11.4 cm)
1 chalazion curette
1 scalpel blade size 11
1 sterile eye pad and bandage
sterile gauze swabs

2.3.3 Abdominal paracentesis pack

1 scalpel handle size 3
1 scalpel blade size 15
1 trocar and cannula
connecting tubing and screw clip
sterile gauze swabs

2.3.4 Ingrowing toe-nail pack

1 scalpel handle size 3
1 scalpel blade size 15
1 pair artery forceps, straight 5″ (12.7 cm)
1 pair stitch scissors, sharp/sharp 5″ (12.7 cm)
or Thwaites nail nipper (English pattern)
5⅛″ (13 cm) (Nova Instruments)
1 nail chisel (Nova Instruments)
1 Volkmann sharp-spoon curette
2 wooden applicators with cotton wool
sterile gauze swabs

2.3.5 Minor operations pack

1 pair Rampley sponge forceps 9½″ (24.1 cm)
2 Mayo towel clips
3 Dunhill artery forceps 5″ (12.7 cm)
3 Halstead mosquito forceps straight 5″ (12.7 cm)
3 Halstead mosquito forceps curved 5″ (12.7 cm)
2 Allis tissue forceps 6″ (15.2 cm)
1 McDonald's dissector
1 McIndoe dissecting forceps 6″ (15.2 cm)
1 Gillies dissecting forceps 6″ (15.2 cm)
1 McIndoe's scissors, curved 7″ (17.8 cm)
1 Mayo scissors straight 5½″ (14 cm)
2 Gillies skin hooks
2 Kilner, double-ended retractors
1 Volkmann scoop
1 Kilner needle holder
1 scalpel handle size 3
scalpel blades 10 and 15
sterile drapes, gauze swabs,
surgical sutures braided silk
metric gauges 2 and 3 with curved cutting needles. Ref. Ethicon W 533 and W 667

THREE

The minor operating theatre

'There are two kinds of Light, the common and the artificial – the common is not at our disposal – the artificial is at our disposal'

(Hippocrates, 460–377 BC)

The physical dimensions of the treatment room will ultimately decide what equipment can be accommodated, thus the smallest room compatible with reasonable operating conditions would have a floor area of 140 square feet (13 square metres) and in most cases, the larger the room, the better the facilities. It should be emphasized that a separate operating room is not an essential prerequisite; indeed, the majority of minor surgical procedures described in this book may all be performed in the doctor's consulting room using the examination couch as an operating table, and an anglepoise lamp fitted with a reflecting spotlight as the source of illumination. Where pre-sterilized instrument packs are used, the standard of asepsis can be extremely high.

However, there is no doubt that where a purpose-built treatment room is available, a much more satisfactory service can be offered to the patient; not only can all the instrument packs be assembled in readiness, but sterilizers, resuscitation equipment, trolleys, illumination and recovery facilities also prepared.

In general practice this room has the advantage that it can double as a nurse's treatment room, chiropody clinic, examination or recovery room, immunization or family-planning clinic, so the maximum use can always be made of the facilities.

3.1 FIXTURES AND FITTINGS

Fitted cupboards with a good working surface are essential. Wall mounted cupboards can be used if space is at a premium; these are used to store instrument packs, dressings, bandages, suture materials, equipment such as sphygmomanometers electrocauteries etc. as well as resuscitation equipment.

A glass-fronted instrument cupboard, although not essential, makes selection of instruments and drugs very much easier, and this too can be permanently fixed to the wall. One X-ray viewing box is a relatively inexpensive item and if not used for viewing X-ray films, can still be used for viewing colour transparencies. Sufficient hooks for coats should be provided and a separate clothes locker would be even better.

A good quality, stainless steel hand wash-basin is essential, with hot and cold running water, preferably with an elbow operated mixer tap, and an antiseptic/soap dispenser fitted above. Waste disposal is usually by means of bins with plastic liners (Figs 3.1, 3.2 and 3.3).

Disposable paper hand towels and paper sheets are becoming more popular. Several of the large paper manufacturers produce wall-mounted

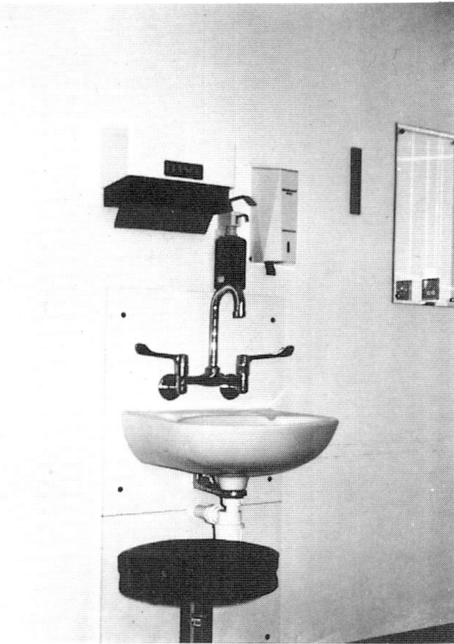

Fig. 3.1 Elbow-operated mixer-taps help to avoid cross-infection.

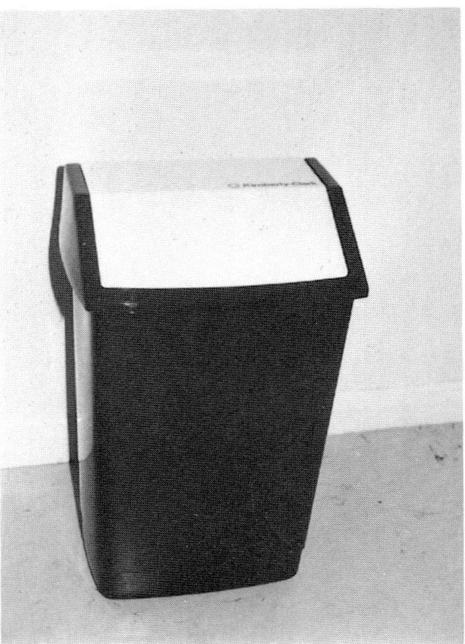

Fig. 3.2 A large waste-bin with disposable bin-liners is very useful (Kimberly-Clark).

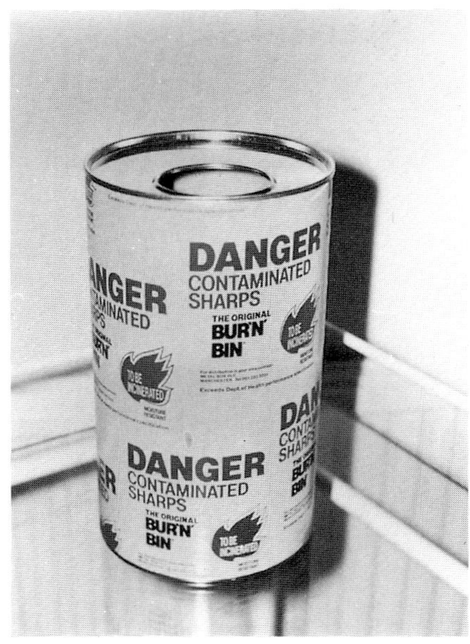

Fig. 3.3 A separate container is necessary for all needles, broken glass, and 'sharps'.

dispensers and holders for the rolls of paper; likewise disposal bags and stands are made by the same firms. The large disposable sheets are excellent for placing on the operating theatre table underneath the patient, for protecting pillows, and for covering trolley shelves (Figs 3.4, 3.5, 3.6 and 3.7). Sufficient electric power sockets should be fitted, and a minimum of eight outlets provided.

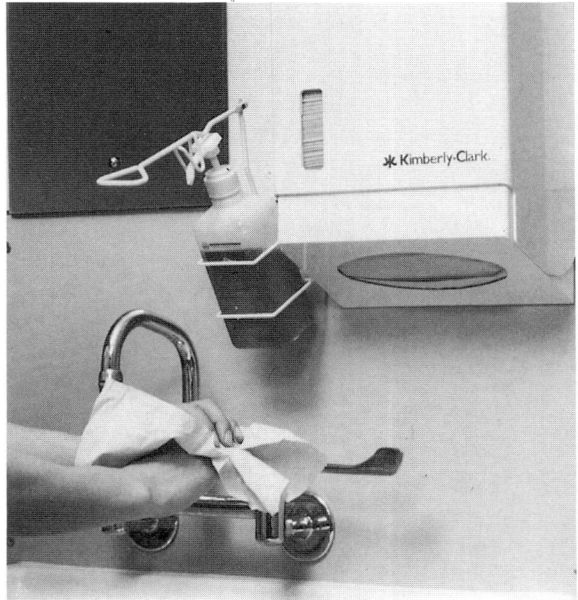

Fig. 3.4 Paper hand-towels: economical and hygenic (Kimberly-Clark).

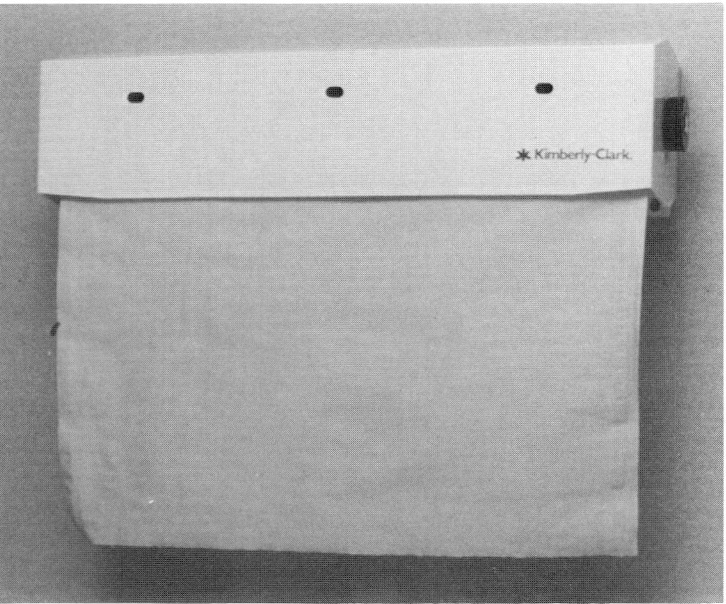

Fig. 3.5 The wider paper towelling is useful for couches and covering the operating theatre table (Kimberly-Clark).

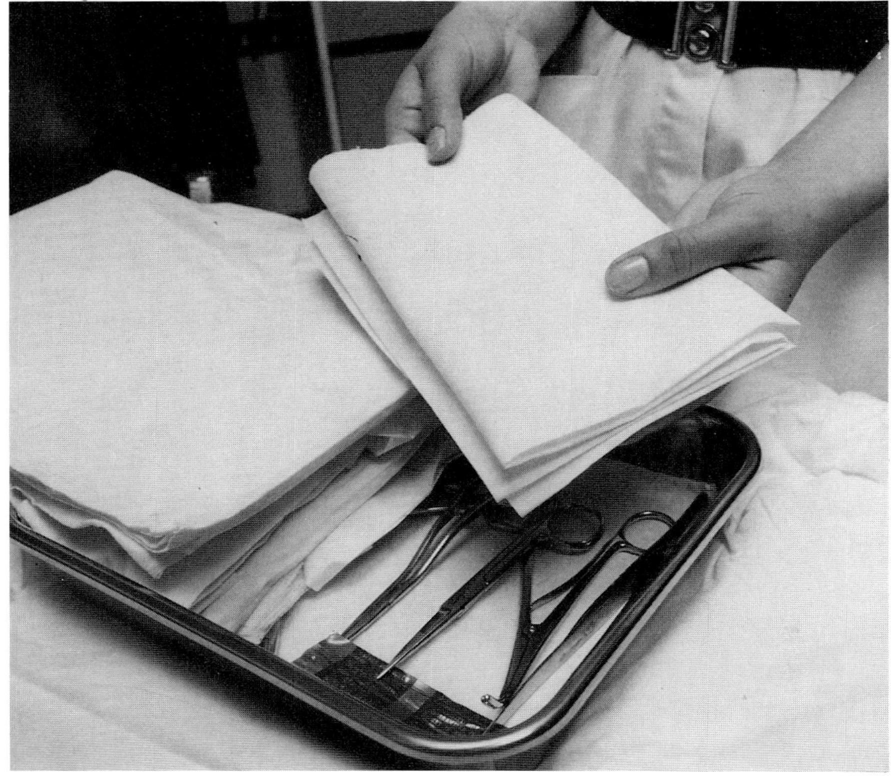

Fig. 3.6 Paper dressing-towels may also be included in CSSD instrument packs (Kimberly-Clark).

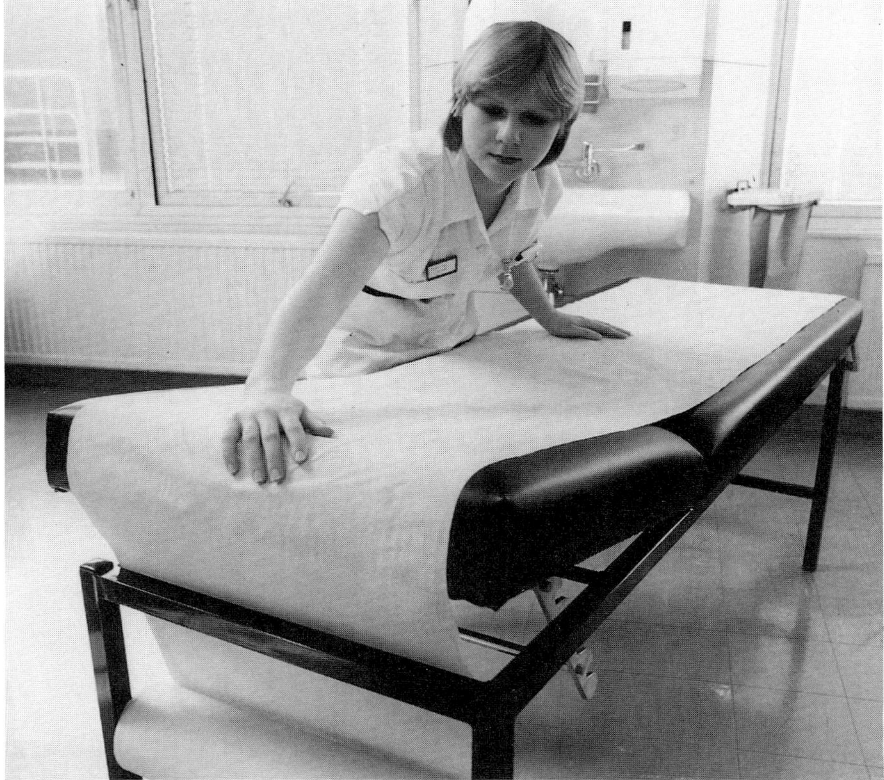

Fig. 3.7 Paper towelling being used to cover examination couch and operating area (Kimberly-Clark).

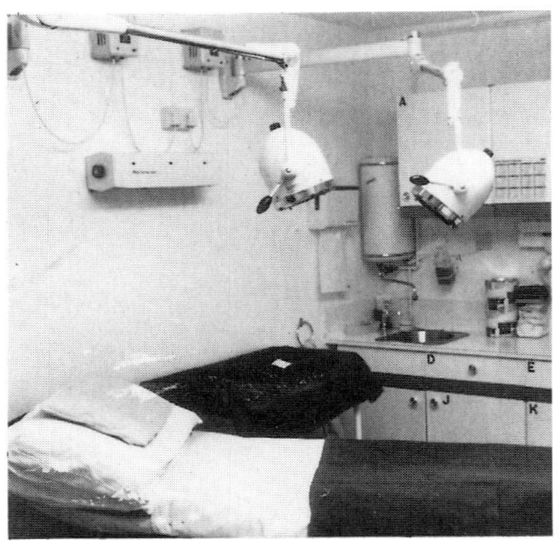

Fig. 3.8 Wall-mounted spotlights are ideal for most minor surgical procedures.

Background illumination may be provided by fluorescent strip lighting which will complement natural light from windows. An extractor fan is not a luxury – there are many procedures such as opening perineal abscesses, sigmoidoscopy, and the use of electrocautery where a rapid change of air is desirable; because of this it is better to choose an extractor fan one or two sizes *larger* than recommended by the manufacturers. Finally, included amongst the fixtures and fittings is a small dangerous drugs cupboard or drawer; this is recommended as some surgical procedures may require a pre-medication injection of such drugs as Diazepam and pethidine (Demerol).

3.2 THE OPERATING THEATRE TABLE

The most important item in any minor operating room is the table (Fig. 3.9) or couch for the patient. New operating theatre tables are expensive for the average practitioner, but by contacting local hospitals and clinics, a second-hand table may be found which will be more than adequate for minor surgery. The ability to raise and lower the patient, or adjust the angle of the neck or limbs is a decided advantage over the fixed examination-couch type tables, and where possible it is worth waiting until a second-hand theatre table becomes available.

Having acquired the table, certain simple accessories such as an arm rest or lithotomy stirrups can be obtained and greatly increase the scope of the operations to be performed. Where space is restricted, a small Mayo-type tray which fixes to the side of the operating theatre table is a small useful addition which can be recommended. One or two instrument trolleys should be purchased: preferably glass topped or stainless steel. Instruments for any operation may then be prepared in advance and the trolley brought to the patient for the operation. Again, new trolleys need not be felt to be essential as many very good second-hand ones can be found in

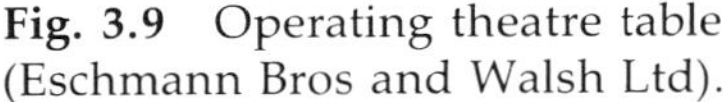

Fig. 3.9 Operating theatre table (Eschmann Bros and Walsh Ltd).

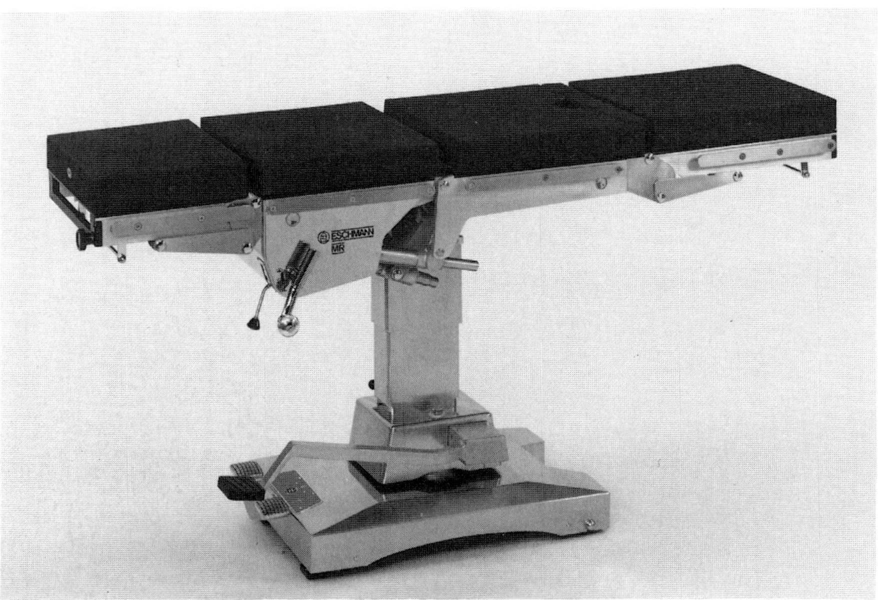

most hospitals – perhaps needing slight repairs such as welding or repainting. One operator's stool, adjustable in height, is needed; most minor operations can be readily performed with the patient lying down and the operator standing, but where any intricate surgery is being done, a comfortable stool for the surgeon makes the task easier.

As many minor operations are performed on the lower limbs, a chiropodist's chair for the patient would be a great help – as they are fairly bulky however, a large treatment room would be necessary.

3.3 ILLUMINATION

As previously mentioned, it is worth spending more on a good quality operating spotlight. For superficial minor surgical procedures, it is not necessary to install the large shadowless main operating theatre lights, but one or two good quality low-voltage spotlights are essential, preferably mounted permanently to the wall or ceiling (Fig. 3.10). Most are now fitted with a plastic heat filter, tinted to give a more natural wavelength of light – many also with adjustable focus. Low voltage (24 V) bulbs are preferred, especially the quartz halogen lamps, but each will need a special step-down transformer or rechargeable battery which needs to be fitted separately (Fig. 3.11).

In recent years, circular fluorescent lights surrounding a central 5″ (12.7 cm) convex lens have been introduced, and these give excellent illumination coupled with magnification, particularly valuable for eye surgery and intricate hand surgery. There are several firms who make such lights, and each will provide lenses of different (or even combined) magnifications depending on the needs of the operator (Figs 3.12 and 3.13). These lights have the added advantages that no heat is generated, the light wavelength nearly approximates to natural daylight, and they are light and manoeuvrable. Their only disadvantage is that they have to be

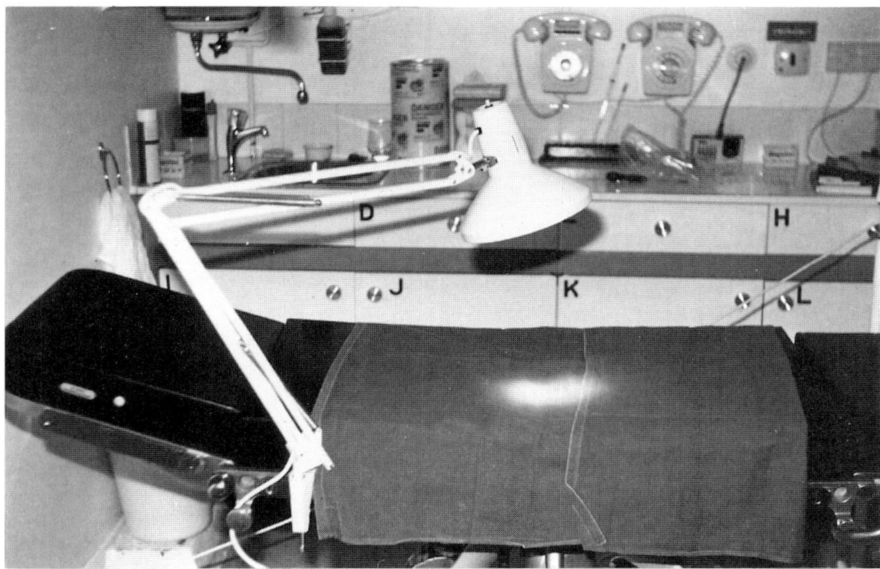

Fig. 3.10 Anglepoise-type spotlights are adequate where space is restricted, and give very good illumination (LEDU Lamps).

Fig. 3.11 A useful spotlight using low-voltage reflector bulb; may be wall or ceiling mounted or on castors (1001 Lamps Ltd).

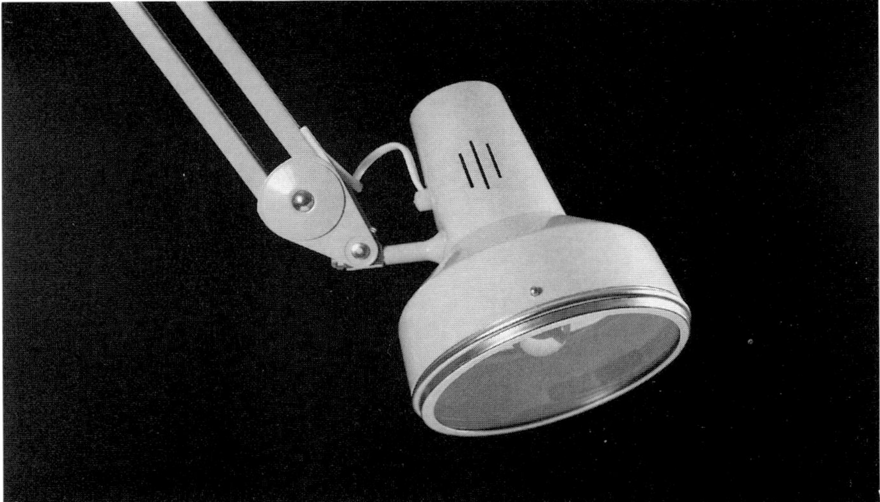

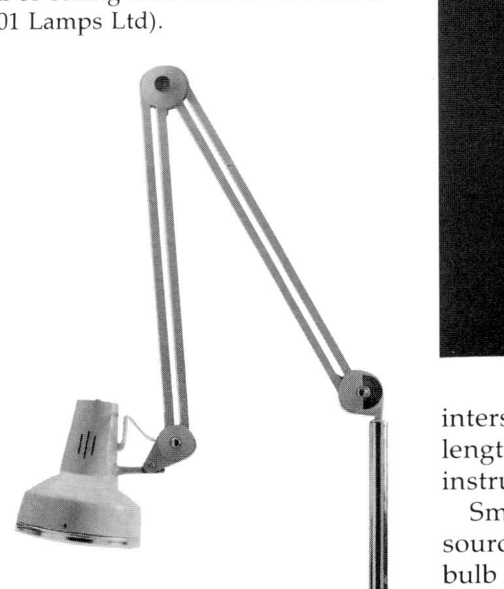

interspersed between the patient and operator; and, where short focal-length lenses are used, there is a risk of the operator's hands and instruments accidentally touching the under-surface of the unit.

Small head-mounted spotlights are favoured by some surgeons, the source of illumination may be a tungsten filament bulb or quartz halogen bulb mounted behind a convex lens, or a fibre-optic transmission system from a light source adjacent to the operator. Although giving good illumination, particularly inside cavities, they have the disadvantage that the operator is connected to batteries, transformer or light source and is not able to move about freely.

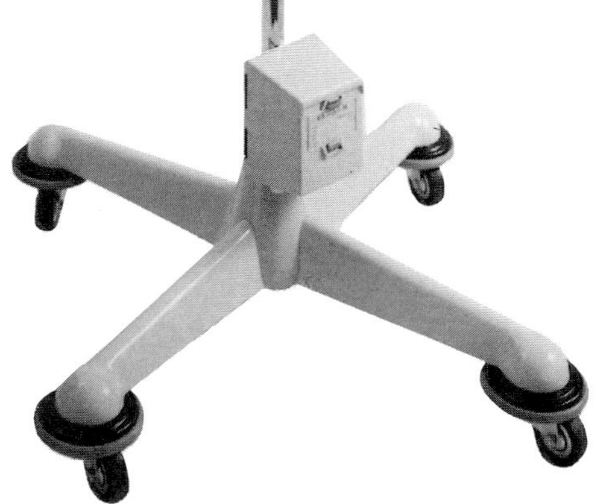

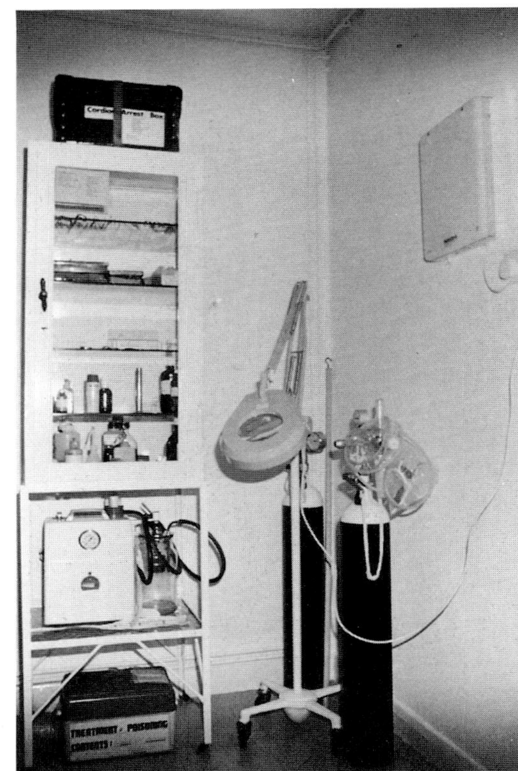

Fig. 3.12 Magnifying light on castors, instrument cupboard and resuscitation equipment.

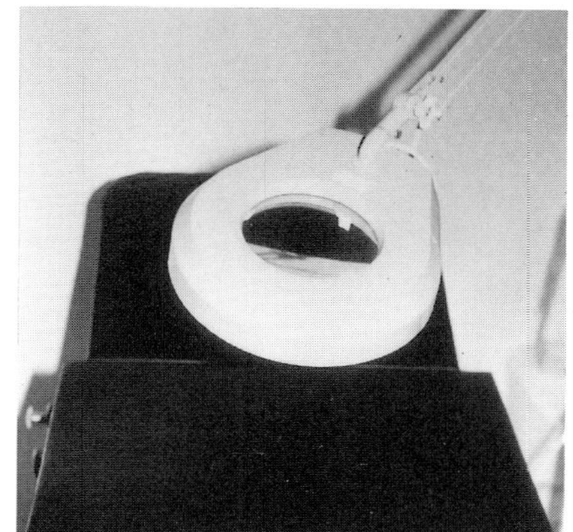

Fig. 3.13 Fluorescent circular magnifying light; extremely valuable for fine work e.g. eyes and removing splinters.

3.4 THE ELECTROCAUTERY

One of the most useful instruments for minor surgical procedures is the electrocautery: it consists essentially of a platinum wire which can be heated to red heat by means of an electric current (Figs 3.14 and 3.15).

Application of the red hot wire to tissues will either cut them or seal any bleeding points by coagulation. It is thus ideal for removing small skin tags

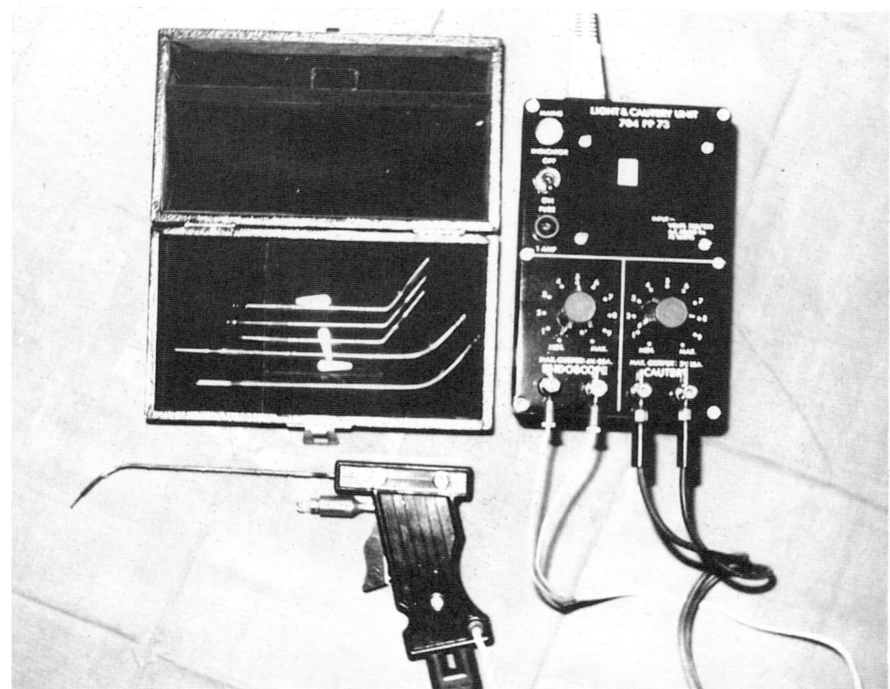

Fig. 3.14 Electrocautery transformer and selection of burners (Rimmer Bros Ltd).

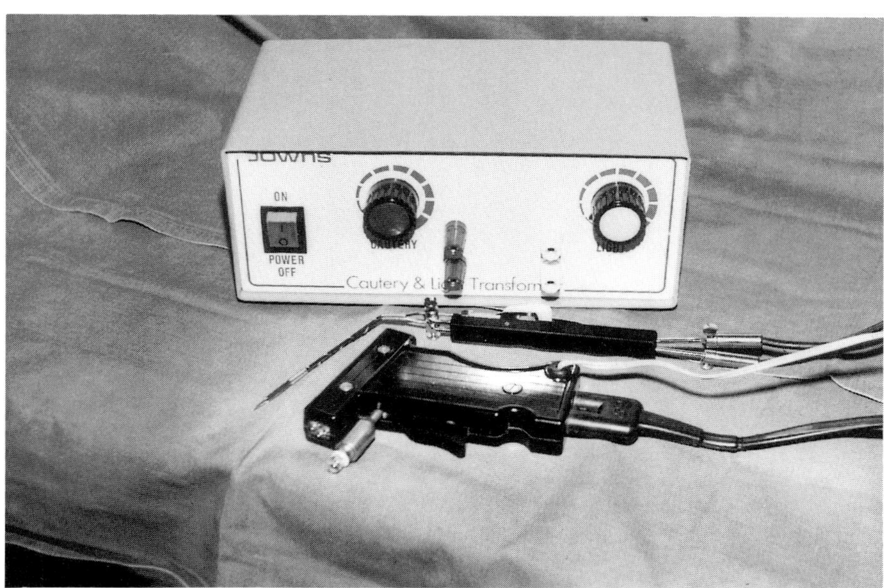

Fig. 3.15 Alternative electrocautery transformer with pistol-grip handle (Down Bros).

and papillomata, and for controlling the bleeding following curetting warts, granulomas, and similar lesions.

The earliest electrocauteries used a standard battery, and rheostat to control the temperature of the tip; subsequently with the change in domestic electricity supplies from direct current (d.c.) to alternating current (a.c.) it was possible to use step-down transformers and rheostats as the source of current, with the great advantage that it avoided 'flat' batteries, provided the patient was within reach of a mains voltage socket.

More recently with the introduction of nickel/cadmium rechargeable batteries with their ability to withstand high current drain without damage, many firms now produce portable rechargeable electrocauteries which combine all the advantages of portability, reliability and cheap maintenance.

A variety of different shaped platinum tips are produced for different applications, but for general use the simple Λ wire is all that is needed; with careful handling it will last for many years, does not corrode, and can be immediately sterilized merely by switching on the current and heating the tip for a few seconds.

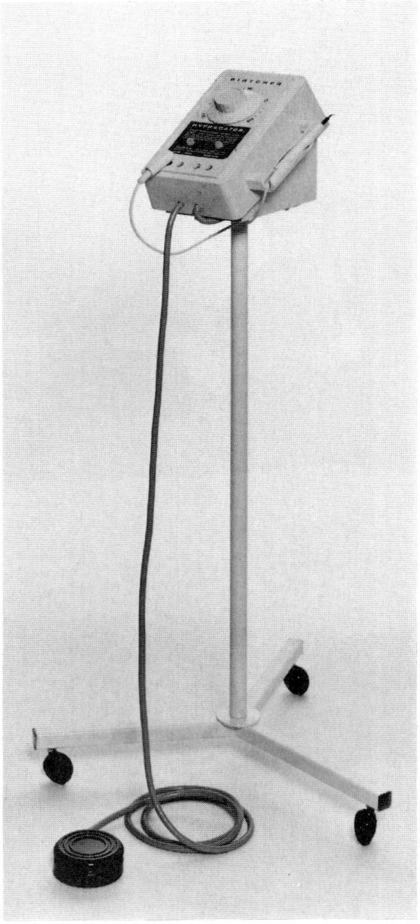

3.5 THE 'HYFRECATOR' OR UNIPOLAR DIATHERMY

Most surgeons will be familiar with the standard bi-polar diathermy apparatus in use in most large operating theatres. In this, a very high-frequency current is passed through the patient's body and generates heat. By making one electrode relatively large and strapping it firmly to one limb, and by making the other electrode a pointed movable tip, sufficient heat is generated at the tip to coagulate or cut tissues. For major surgery such coagulating/cutting is standard practice, but the equipment is expensive, has to pass stringent tests for electrical safety, and is not really necessary or ideal for minor surgery.

One answer has been to produce the unipolar diathermy or 'Hyfrecator' (Fig. 3.16). This is a small, portable, instrument which by means of an adjustable spark gap or solid-state circuitry and transformer, produces a very high voltage and low current, sufficient to cause a spark to pass from the electrode tip to the patient without needing a second large pad electrode to complete the circuit. Three types of electrode are commonly used; the first is a fine wire electrode which may be inserted into the lesion to be destroyed. Passing a current through the tissues generates heat, which in turn coagulates the blood and cells; this 'desiccation' is particularly suitable for vascular haemangiomata. The second type of electrode is larger than the needle electrode, and is held a short distance away from the tissues; when the current is switched on, a stream of hot sparks passes between the patient and the electrode, and this is sufficient to destroy small areas of tissue. This technique is referred to as 'fulguration'. Thirdly, the Hyfrecator can be used for coagulation by using a double electrode which is connected to a lower voltage winding on the high-frequency transformer. By placing this double electrode on the surface to be treated and passing a slightly heavier current between the poles of the electrode, the underlying tissues are coagulated and destroyed.

Fig. 3.16 The Birtcher Hyfrecator Model 733 on stand 708-1 (Birtcher Corporation, USA, Schuco International, London).

The advantage of using the Hyfrecator is the absence of bleeding; it's effect is very similar to that of the electrocautery, and the heat generated automatically sterilizes the area treated; a sterile dry dressing or no dressing at all is, therefore, all that is needed to promote healing. The disadvantage is that histological examination of the treated lesion is not usually possible due to the distortion of the cells from the heat, thus a preliminary biopsy needs to be done where the diagnosis is in doubt.

3.6 RESUSCITATION FACILITIES

Every doctor's surgery should possess some form of simple resuscitation equipment. Because patients suffering from a variety of diseases are constantly passing through the premises, sooner or later one will collapse with a myocardial infarction, major epileptic convulsion, cardiac arrest, simple haemorrhage or just a vasovagal 'faint'. Where any form of treatment is being offered, be it one hypodermic injection or minor surgical procedure, the incidence of reactions will increase, and the practitioner must be prepared for the patient who will faint, or suffer an unexpected allergic reaction to the treatment. Should a patient 'collapse' on the premises the first prerequisite is a room or area sufficiently large to be able to allow the patient to lie on the floor with sufficient space around him or her for equipment, doctors and assistants. The second requirement is the management of the unconscious patient – to maintain an airway and circulation, to prevent the inhalation of secretions or vomit, to establish a diagnosis and render treatment.

Fortunately the majority of 'attacks' will be vasovagal, all of which will be expected to recover rapidly once the patient is lying flat, with or without elevation of the legs to assist venous return to the heart.

A clear resuscitation sheet, based on the first aid manuals [3], supplemented with additional information for cardiac arrest and anaphylactic reactions should be on a wall in the treatment room for all staff to see.

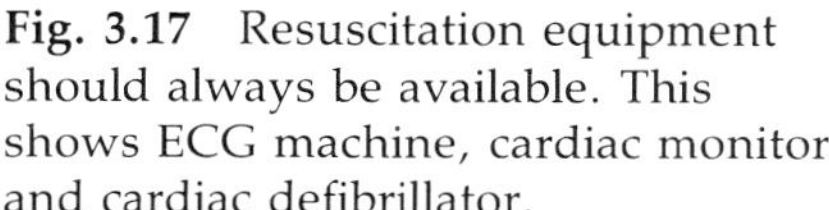

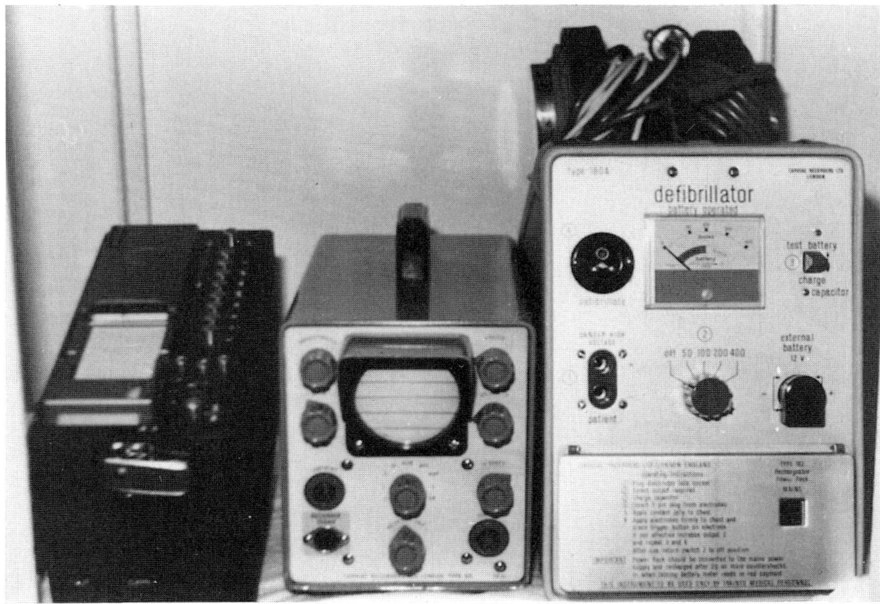

Fig. 3.17 Resuscitation equipment should always be available. This shows ECG machine, cardiac monitor and cardiac defibrillator.

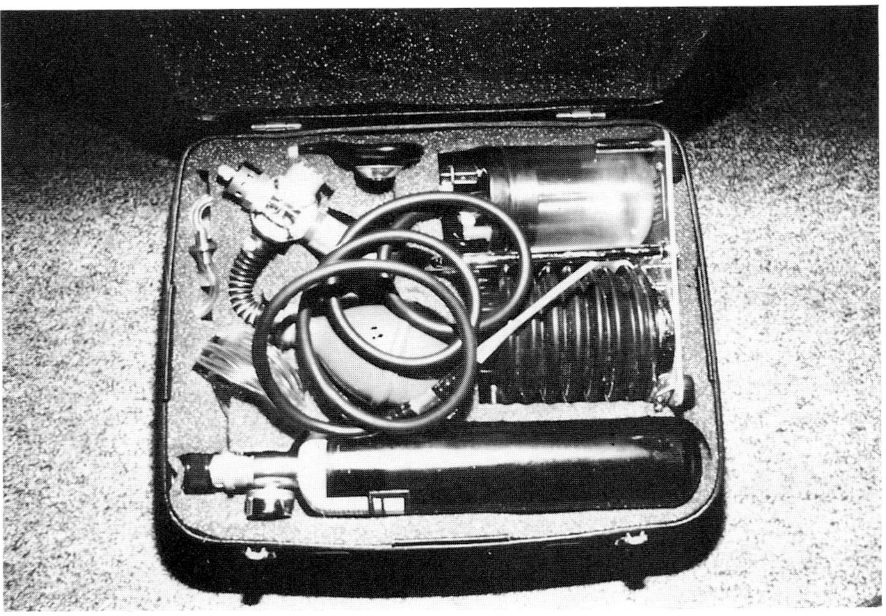

Fig. 3.18 Portable resuscitation kits have the added advantage that they can be taken to the patient's home in addition to use at the surgery.

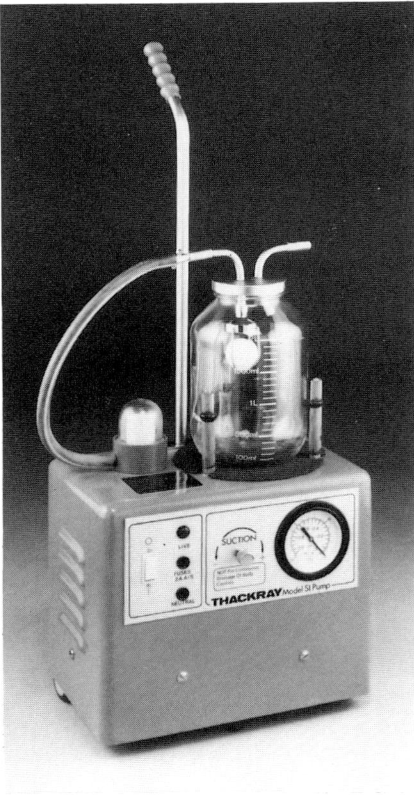

Fig. 3.19 Adequate suction equipment is valuable (Chas F. Thackray).

Resuscitation equipment should comprise syringes and needles, a selection of drugs to be administered including Diazepam, morphine, adrenaline, Lignocaine, Atropine, verapamil, plasma expanders and hydrocortisone, together with intravenous cannulae, intravenous giving sets, bandages and adhesive plasters. Simple disposable airways are valuable, and an Ambu type positive pressure resuscitator is worth having. Where funds permit, and particularly where regular surgery sessions are undertaken, additional resuscitation equipment such as electric suction, ECG machines, oxygen giving sets and cardiac defibrillators are a good idea even though the need for any of them hardly ever arises. In general practice it would be difficult to justify the purchase of such items as cardiac defibrillators, but it is the type of equipment often donated by charitable organizations or groups of patients, and the possession of more sophisticated types of resuscitation equipment greatly adds to the practitioner's (and patient's!) peace of mind (Figs 3.17, 3.18 and 3.19).

3.7 STERILIZERS

Some means of sterilizing or disinfecting instruments and equipment should be included in the minor operating theatre. In recent years there has been a trend towards CSSD (Central Sterile Supplies Department) packs, where the instruments are cleaned, prepared and packed at a central sterilizing department, autoclaved in sealed paper envelopes, and delivered to the treatment room or surgery. Where such an arrangement can be made by the practitioner, this is ideal; every instrument is guaranteed to be sterile, together with all dressings, drapes, towels and gowns which are included in the pack. Where CSSD facilities do not exist, alternative methods can be employed.

Traditionally the method of disinfecting instruments was by boiling in

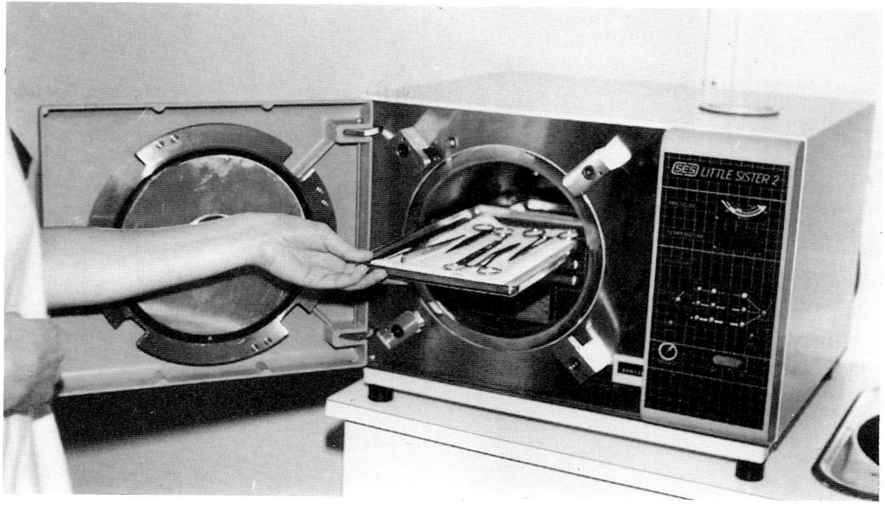

Fig. 3.20 Instruments being loaded into 'Little Sister Mk II' autoclave.

water for 5 min; bacterial spores and viruses may not be destroyed and thus the term sterilization should not strictly be employed. Most hot water disinfectors have a variable heat control indicator light and thermostat together with trays to hold instruments. Alternatively a dry heat oven may be employed, heating the instruments to 160° C (320° F) for 1 hour; this is better than boiling, but has the disadvantage that plastics, paper drapes and dressings tend to be damaged. Where heat cannot be used for certain instruments such as fibre-optic cables, and endoscopes, soaking in a solution of glutaraldehyde is acceptable.

Perhaps the most efficient method of sterilizing instruments in a small treatment room is by using a small portable autoclave (Figs 3.20 and 3.21). These utilize the same principle as the larger hospital equipment, viz. steam under pressure resulting in temperatures of 136° C (277° F) under a pressure of 30 lbf/in^2 (207 kNm^{-2}) for 3.5 min. This destroys all known organisms and can be used for most instruments. However, it has the disadvantage that instruments cannot be packed with dressings and drapes inside a sealed paper envelope as the smaller machines do not have a vacuum cycle to extract all the air.

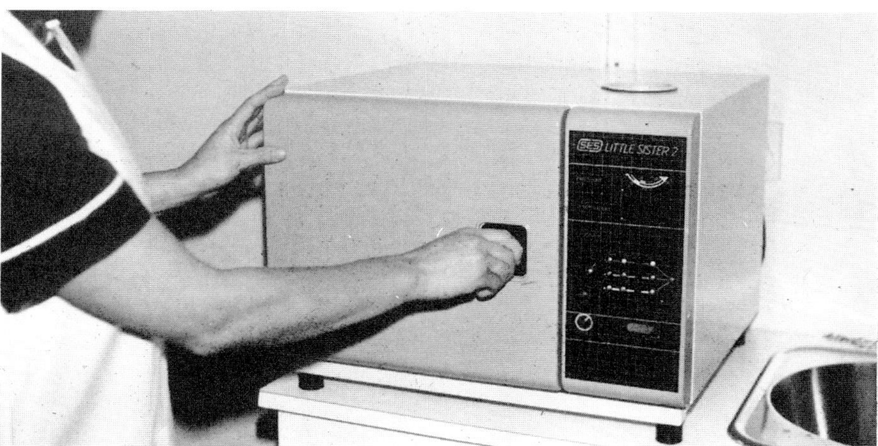

Fig. 3.21 Door being closed prior to autoclaving.

3.8 DISINFECTANT DISPENSERS

Surgical scrub solutions are recommended for routine washing and hand-scrubbing prior to each operation; the two most commonly used agents being Hibiscrub (chlorhexidine gluconate 4% in detergent base) and Betadine surgical scrub (Povidone-iodine 7.5% in detergent base). Each is supplied in a standard container which may be affixed to a wall-mounted dispenser, usually provided free of charge by the manufacturers.

3.9 SYRINGES AND NEEDLES

Standard 1 ml, 2 ml, 5 ml, 10 ml and 20 ml syringes with Luer fitting are needed for local anaesthetics, intravenous drugs, and for sclerotherapy of varicose veins. Three standard size Luer fitting needles are recommended 25 SWG × $\frac{5}{8}$″ (0.5 mm × 16 mm), 23 SWG × 1″ (0.6 mm × 25 mm) and 21 SWG × $1\frac{1}{2}$″ (0.8 mm × 40 mm). In addition a standard dental syringe and 30 SWG × $\frac{3}{4}$″ (0.3 mm × 19 mm) needle will be found to be invaluable for giving local anaesthetics in fingers and toes and particularly for children. Dental cartridges of local anaesthetic can be quickly inserted in the syringe, and as nearly a painless injection as is possible can be made.

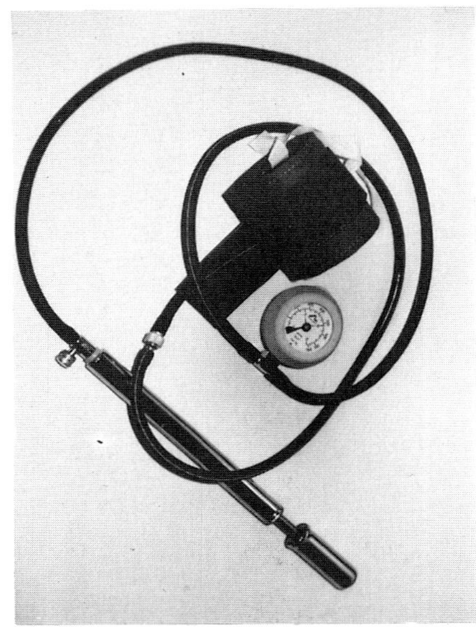

Fig. 3.22 Orthopaedic pneumatic tourniquet; this is better than a blood-pressure sphygmomanometer cuff if intravenous regional anaesthesia is undertaken (OEC Orthopaedic Ltd).

3.10 TOURNIQUETS

Where a bloodless operating field is required such as for ingrowing toe-nails, carpal tunnel decompression, excision of ganglion or release of trigger finger a tourniquet is required. For fingers and toes this need only be a length of rubber tubing and a pair of artery forceps, but for a whole limb, a proper orthopaedic pneumatic tourniquet is used (see Chapter 7 Intravenous regional anaesthesia) (Fig. 3.22).

3.11 WASTE DISPOSAL

Needles, broken glass ampoules and 'sharps' should be first placed in a cardboard receptacle such as a 'burn bin' and subsequently incinerated. Larger items such as soiled dressings, disposable drapes etc., can be placed in plastic bin liners and subsequently left for disposal (Fig. 3.3).

FOUR

Care of instruments and equipment

'The Instruments, and when and how they should be prepared, so that they may not impede the work, and that there may be no difficulty in taking hold of them, with the part of the body which operates.
But if another gives them, he must be ready a little beforehand and do as you direct'.
(Hippocrates, 460–377 BC)

Like all mechanical and electronic equipment, surgical instruments require regular care and maintenance to retain their efficiency and prolong their useful life. Dirty, rusty forceps are not only a potential source of infection, but look unsightly, are difficult to use, and ultimately break prematurely.

Stainless steel is the material of choice for most surgical instruments; it combines a high resistance to corrosion and rust with an attractive finish. Even under ideal conditions the finest stainless steel instruments can become pitted and stained, so great care is needed with washing and cleaning, polishing and lubrication. Rough handling or the use of abrasives can permanently mark stainless steel, so initially all instruments after use should be cleaned with a hard brush under running cool water. Very hot water will cause coagulation of blood and exudate and make subsequent cleaning harder.

If use of an ultrasonic cleaning bath using instrument detergents is available, this will be ideal and restore a high polish to most instruments.

After washing, instruments should be carefully dried to avoid water remaining in any joint and causing corrosion. Lubrication using a water-soluble lubricant is strongly to be recommended and will greatly prolong the useful life of any instrument.

Saline solutions are a major cause of pitting, and instruments should never be soaked in them, nor should a saline solution be allowed to dry on an instrument.

Whenever cleaning or washing instruments, keep all ratchets unlocked and box joints open, and similarly avoid using wire wool or abrasives, iodine, bromine, aluminium chloride or barium chloride. The same advice applies to surgical blades and needles, both of which may rust and corrode more easily than stainless steel instruments.

Plastic instruments or plastic parts of instruments are particularly vulnerable to corrosive agents, heat, rough handling and abrasive cleaners. They should be treated with great respect; generally, washing with warm soapy water with a soft cloth is sufficient. Sterilization may be by either soaking in antiseptic solutions or autoclaving at a lower temperature (115° C under 9 lbf/in^2 (62 kNm^{-2}) for 30 min) than is used for steel instruments. Cleaning and polishing should only be undertaken using recommended cleansers and polishers, as even ordinary domestic polishes can abrade perspex and similar plastics. Most plastics are best stored in a dry state rather than under prolonged soaking in antiseptic solutions.

4.1 ELECTRICAL SAFETY

It cannot be stressed enough that there should be the utmost regard for electrical safety at all times. Many modern instruments and pieces of equipment operate from mains voltage 110 or 240 V a.c. All such instruments have to pass stringent safety tests during and after manufacture and can be assumed to be electrically safe on delivery. However, with use, cables become frayed, earth connections work loose or break, internal components move with vibration or accidental damage or unauthorized alteration to the circuitry or safety fuses occur, resulting in potentially lethal voltages and currents reaching the patient. Obvious simple checks of plugs, fuses, and cables should be made regularly, and routine maintenance be performed by a qualified person at standard intervals as recommended by the manufacturer. Water and electricity do not mix (!) so it is imperative that all mains electrically operated instruments be kept dry. Low-voltage battery equipment is generally safe and may even be designed to work in damp or humid conditions. Earth connections and safety fuses should be regularly checked, making sure that the correct loading fuses are being used. Any frayed cables should be immediately replaced and any loose components such as switches and sockets dealt with. All equipment working from mains voltage should have a circuit breaker in the supply lines.

Cardiac defibrillators deliver a high voltage of several thousand volts, together with a relatively high current, making a lethal combination to the operator if any serious electrical fault should occur; it is thus even more imperative that servicing and maintenance of these instruments be entrusted to a qualified electrical engineer.

Electronic components comprising microchips and integrated circuits are generally very rugged and will withstand rough handling; they also operate at low voltages so are relatively safe, but they respond badly to high temperatures. Overheating should therefore be avoided, and any ventilation apertures left uncovered; given these safeguards, they should give good service.

FIVE

Sterilizing and disinfecting instruments

'In the course of the year 1864 I was much struck with an account of the remarkable effects produced by Carbolic Acid upon the sewage of the town of Carlisle, destroying the entozoa which usually infest cattle fed upon such pastures'

(Lord Joseph Lister, 1827–1912)

Sterilization is the destruction of all living organisms. Contrary to popular belief an item may only be sterile or non-sterile – it cannot be nearly sterile. Disinfection, on the other hand is the reduction of a population of pathogenic micro-organisms without achieving sterility. Not all bacterial spores are destroyed. There are five methods of sterilizing or disinfecting instruments in general practice:

1. Antiseptic solutions
2. Boiling
3. Hot air ovens
4. Autoclave
5. Use of CSSD facilities

It is known that bacterial spores and certain viruses causing hepatitis B, herpes, influenza, polio and mumps are particularly resistant to heat and boiling. One of the most serious infections is hepatitis B or serum hepatitis; it may be transmitted from patient to patient by as little as 0.0001 ml of infected blood. The virus remains active for up to six months in dried blood, consequently instruments which have been poorly cleaned or disinfected may be responsible for infecting other patients, while poor surgical technique may result in the doctor becoming infected from the patient. It has been estimated that there are possibly 200 million carriers of hepatitis in the world, representing up to 20% of the population in African, Pacific and other tropical countries and 0.5% of the population in Northern Europe. Thus, statistically, the doctor has a 1 in 200 chance of treating a Hepatitis B carrier. Similarly in recent years there has been growing concern about other viruses such as herpes which are known to be resistant to boiling. Fortunately the incidence of cross infection would appear to be extremely low, but the doctor should not be lulled into a false sense of security, and should adopt the highest standards of sterilization of all the instruments and of surgical technique. The incidence of cross infection outside hospital is much lower, and this applies particularly to general practice where cross infection rates of less than 1–2% can be expected (see Chapter 13). Without scrupulous attention to detail, cross infection rates will rise and approximate those found in hospital.

From what has just been said, it will be appreciated that sterilization and not disinfection should be the aim in every surgery. In practice this means autoclaving or dry heat ovens for the majority of items.

5.1 ANTISEPTIC SOLUTIONS

Traditionally 70% alcohol was the solution most widely used, subsequently with the addition of 0.5% Chlorhexidine. This is widely used for emergency disinfection of surgical instruments requiring only two minutes immersion. Where instruments are left for longer periods or stored continuously, the addition of one tablet of sodium nitrite BPC 1 gram will prevent rusting. As the tablet dissolves over several days, another is added.

The aldehydes are powerful disinfectors and sterilizers. A solution containing 2% glutaraldehyde will disinfect instruments if they are soaked for ten minutes, and sterilize if left soaking for ten hours. The disadvantages are that the solution needs to be fresh, and it can cause staining if left on the skin.

5.2 BOILING

This is still the most widely used method of disinfecting instruments in the world; it is simple, quick and reasonably effective, but will not destroy certain bacterial spores and certain viruses. Normally, instruments are cleaned, and then boiled for five minutes (100° C or 212° F). It is obviously not suitable for dressings, drapes or paper (Fig. 5.1).

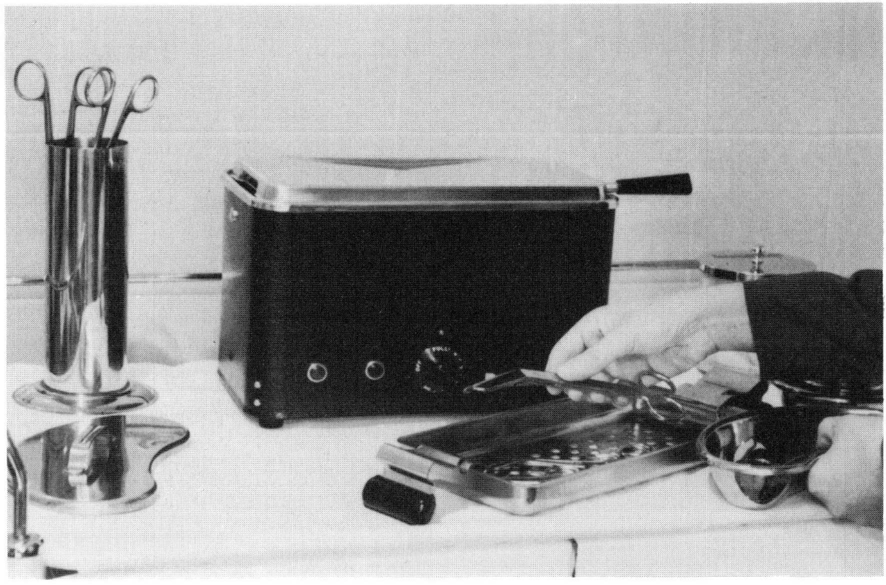

Fig. 5.1 Electric boiling water disinfector with thermostat and removable tray (Surgical Equipment Supplies).

5.3 HOT AIR OVENS

These are thermostatically controlled ovens, with an electric heating element, similar to a domestic electric oven. Instruments to be sterilized are heated to 160° C (320° F) for 1 hour. Sterilization is achieved, but it is not suitable for rubber, plastic or, to a lesser extent, paper items (Fig. 5.2).

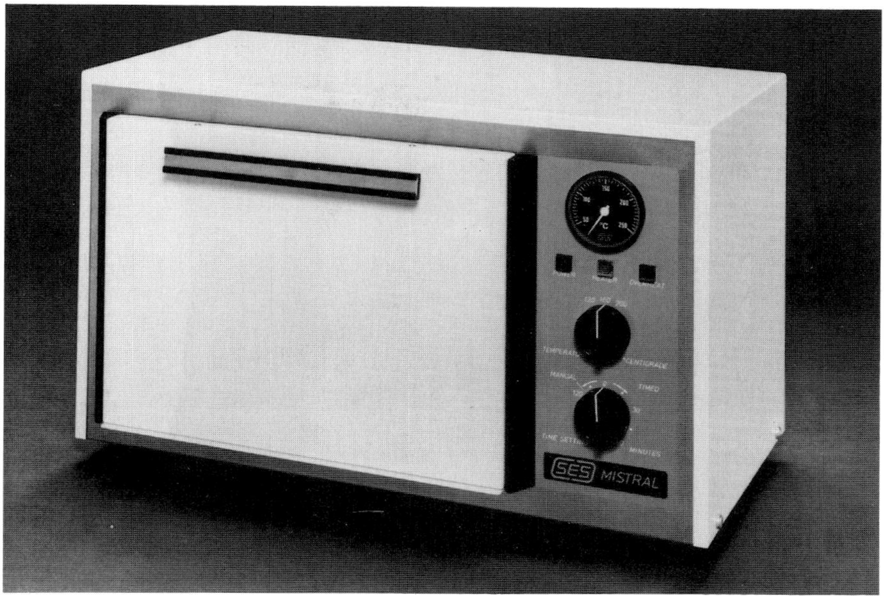

Fig. 5.2 Hot air oven (Surgical Equipment Supplies).

5.4 AUTOCLAVES

Now considered to be the most efficient method of sterilizing instruments, packs and dressings, and suitable for most materials, an autoclave is basically a pressure cooker, and in fact, there is no reason why a domestic pressure cooker should not be used to sterilize instruments. The small autoclaves produced for the doctor's surgery offer a choice of temperatures, pressures and sterilizing times: typically a 'quick' cycle would heat the water to 134° C (273° F) for 3.5 min under a pressure of 30 lbf/in^2 (207 kNm^{-2}) whereas a slower cycle, more suitable for plastics, would

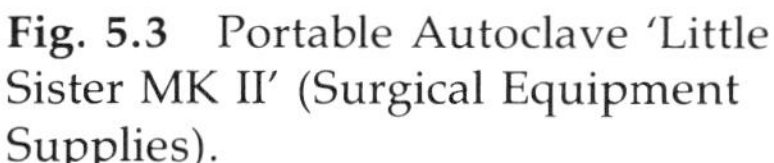

Fig. 5.3 Portable Autoclave 'Little Sister MK II' (Surgical Equipment Supplies).

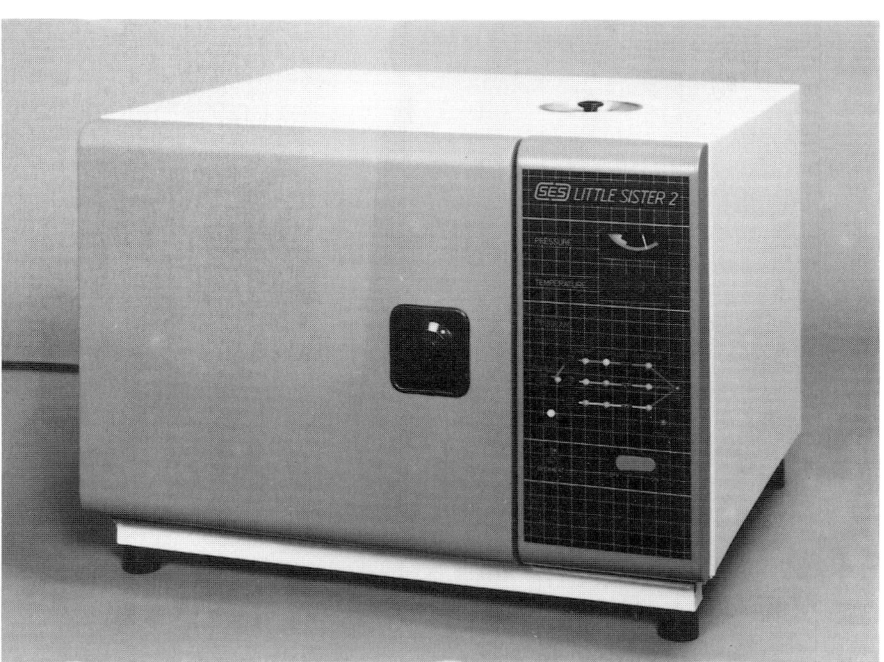

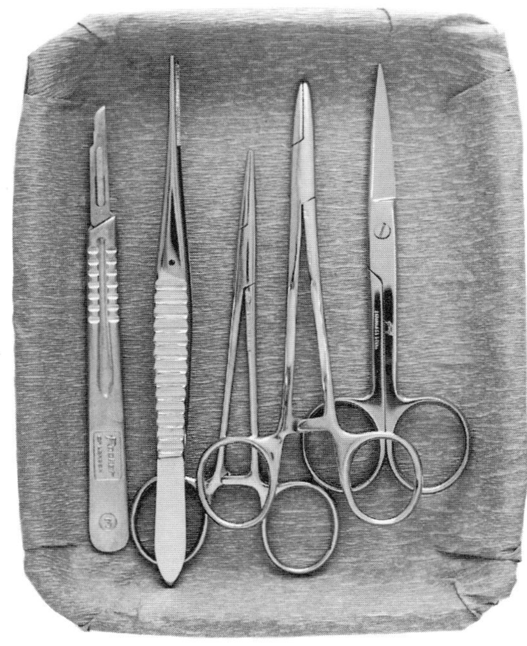

Fig. 5.4 Basic instrument set, ready for autoclaving (Rocket of London Ltd).

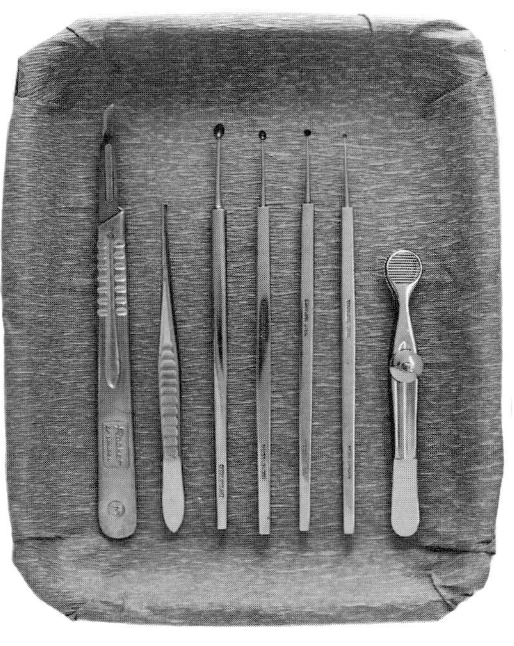

Fig. 5.5 Meibomian cyst pack, ready for autoclaving (Rocket of London Ltd).

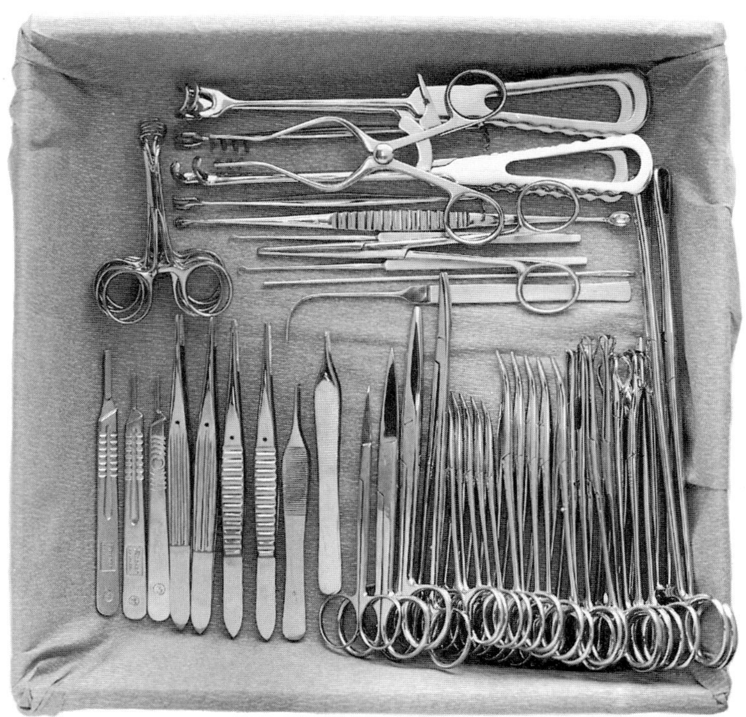

Fig. 5.6 A comprehensive minor operation set of instruments, in tray, ready for autoclaving (Rocket of London Ltd).

heat the water to 115° C (239° F) under a pressure of 10 lbf/in^2 (69 kNm^{-2}). In practice, instruments are placed in the trays, the autoclave turned on, and left for the desired time. At the end of the cycle, the instruments are ready for use. The main disadvantage of the smaller autoclave is that instrument packs cannot be sterilized as there is not a vacuum cycle to extract air and dry the packs. However, most materials including rubber, plastics and metal can be readily sterilized, the only exception being sealed containers (Fig. 5.3).

5.5 USE OF CSSD FACILITIES (Central Sterile Supplies Department)

Most hospitals in Europe and North America now use large autoclaves for all routine instrument sterilization. As well as superheated water under pressure, the large machines have two vacuum cycles, a pre-vacuum pulsing stage which removes air from the load ensuring efficient steam penetration, and a post-vacuum pulse stage which ensures a dry sterile load at the end of the cycle. Thus dressings, drapes, gowns, sheets and instrument packs can be sterilized and dried at the same time. In practice, instruments are pre-packed in plastic or foil trays, together with any selected dressings and drapes, these are then enclosed in a paper envelope which is closed with a heat sensitive autoclave adhesive tape, and the whole enclosed in an outer paper envelope, similarly closed with the autoclave marking tape. This tape changes colour if the desired sterilizing conditions have been reached, and affords a visible proof of sterilization. This type of autoclave offers the best method of sterilization, and it is well worth the practitioner making arrangements, if at all possible, with a hospital Central Sterile Supplies Department. Not only will the GP's instruments and drapes be sterilized, but each will be cleaned and repacked in a sterile envelope ready for future use. Such packs may be stored at the surgery and used either on the premises or taken to the patient's home if needed for such conditions as draining malignant abdominal ascites or a minor operation on a house-bound patient.

SIX

Skin preparation

'I tried the application of carbolic acid to the wound to prevent decomposition of the blood'

(Lord Joseph Lister, 1827–1912, letter dated May 27th 1866 to his father)

For many procedures skin preparation is probably not necessary; the removal of small skin tags with the electrocautery is certainly better done without applying any antiseptic solution to the skin – indeed if the electrocautery or diathermy is used shortly after applying an inflammable antiseptic such as alcohol or ether, serious burns could ensue. In any case, the temperature of the electrocautery wire is sufficiently high to sterilize the tissue during use. Similarly, operations on or near the eye are best performed without any prior disinfection of the skin or conjunctiva, and rarely does one see any infection.

For the majority of other minor operations some form of skin antiseptic is used; many commercially prepared solutions are available, containing either Chlorhexidine 0.5% in isopropyl alcohol (Hibisol ICI,) or Povidone-iodine 10% alcoholic solution (Betadine Alcoholic Solution: Napp). Coloured solutions have the added advantage that the operator can readily see where the antiseptic has been applied. As there are so many preparations available, the final choice depends on the preference of the individual doctor. Each antiseptic solution may either be painted on the skin using an absorbent swab, sprayed over the area from a pressurized applicator, or the affected part if small enough, such as a finger or toe, immersed in the solution.

Removal of hair by shaving is now rarely necessary – the majority of minor surgical procedures can be performed easily without; where sebaceous cysts occur on the head, and there is much hair, cutting away the minimum amount with stitch scissors or iris scissors is all that is necessary.

Although normal surgical practice is to apply skin antiseptics only *before* any operation, occasionally it helps to apply a second application *after* the skin has been closed, before a final sterile dry dressing is applied, to reduce any bacterial colonies secreted through the pores of the skin or which have contaminated the skin, either airborne or from the operator or assistant during the operation.

SEVEN

Anaesthesia

'The powder benumbs the nerves of the tongue depriving it of feeling and taste'
(Albert Niemann, first description of cocaine, 1860)

Modern anaesthetics have revolutionized surgical practice, and it should now be easily possible to perform any minor operation completely painlessly. It is worth taking time to fully anaesthetize the area and to have the confidence that it has been successful; to repeatedly ask a patient 'Can you feel this?' does nothing for their confidence; they will let the operator know if they can feel any pain!

Many different techniques are available, the most widely used being infiltration; some operations such as those on the eye may require two different methods such as surface anaesthesia of the conjunctiva and infiltration of the skin.

7.1 FREEZING

Most doctors have witnessed small abscesses being opened by freezing of the overlying skin with an Ethyl Chloride spray. Those doctors who have had such a procedure done to them will also say how ineffective it is, and how uncomfortable it is as the tissues thaw out. One suspects that most freezing was performed for the benefit of the operator and had a placebo effect at best for the patient! Ethyl Chloride spray freezing was reserved mainly for incision of abscesses; if such abscesses were deeply situated it certainly would not offer much pain relief other than that achieved from the release of pus, and if very superficial probably was unnecessary as the overlying skin was now insensitive to pain. Thus as a method of anaesthesia it tends to have been superseded by other more effective agents (Fig. 7.1).

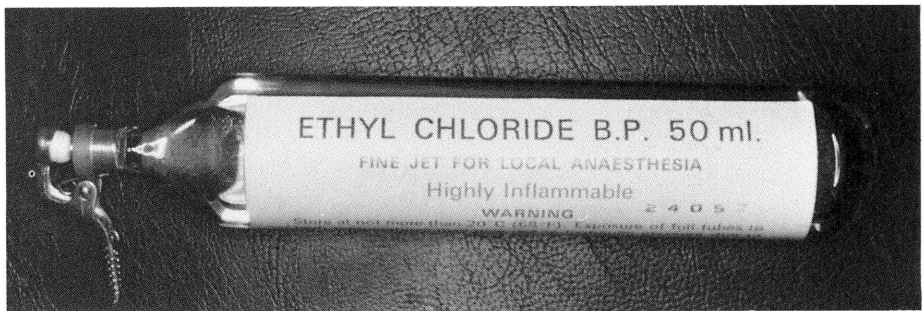

Fig. 7.1 Ethyl chloride spray; suitable for incision of certain abscesses, but not very effective for the majority of procedures requiring anaesthesia.

7.2 TOPICAL OR SURFACE ANAESTHESIA

Mucous membranes fortunately absorb local anaesthetics very rapidly, efficiently, and painlessly. Thus the cornea and conjunctiva can be readily anaesthetized with local anaesthetic drops, of which there are several varieties. Lignocaine (Xylocaine UK; Octocaine USA) is manufactured as a 4% solution eye drops. Individual applications of Oxybuprocaine Hydrochloride 0.4% (Minims Benoxynate SNP 0.4% UK) or Amethocaine Hydrochloride 0.5% (Minims Amethcaine SNP 0.5% UK) are manufactured for once-only application. Onset of anaesthesia is rapid and lasts for up to 1 hour.

Similarly the lining of the nose, buccal mucosa, larynx and pharynx, oesophagus, trachea, tympanic membrane and urethra may all be anaesthetized using topical anaesthetic preparations.

Lignocaine aerosol spray (Xylocaine spray UK, Octocaine spray USA) is particularly useful for the nasal cavity, pharynx and larynx, while Lignocaine sterile gel (Xylocaine gel 2% UK; Octocaine gel 2% USA) is extremely good for anaesthetizing the urethra.

As with all local anaesthetics, the maximum safe dose which can be given to any particular patient should be known and not exceeded; as doses for different anaesthetic agents differ, the doctor is advised to refer to the manufacturer's data sheet. Ask the patient if he or she is on any medication.

7.3 INFILTRATION ANAESTHESIA

Most local anaesthetic agents can be given by injection and this method of infiltration is now widely used for producing anaesthesia, particularly for minor surgery. Certain points need to be borne in mind.

1. The finer the needle, the less the discomfort. A small bleb of local anaesthetic is raised in the skin initially before advancing the needle to deeper tissues.
2. Inject slowly as the needle advances, sudden injections of large volumes, even of local anaesthetic, cause pain.
3. If possible, ensure that the solution to be injected is at body temperature or at room temperature, injection of icy-cold solutions taken from a refrigerator causes discomfort.
4. Wait an adequate time for anaesthesia to develop, so often one sees a rapid injection of local anaesthetic followed immediately by a surgical procedure which can be felt by the patient, only to see full anaesthesia reached after the procedure is completed.
5. Use single-dose snap-open glass ampoules in preference to multi-dose vials; this reduces the risk of cross infection and reactions to the preservative.
6. Use only pre-packed sterilized disposable syringes and needles.
7. Do not open any sterilized pack until the moment of use.
8. Hands should be washed clean with Hibiscrub or similar agent and thoroughly dried – wet hands increase the risk of infection.
9. Do not touch the needle at all, and in particular, do not guide the needle with your finger.
10. Advise the patient that neither of you should talk or cough while the needle is exposed to the air and during the injection; droplet infection can occur otherwise, and for this reason it is still good practice to wear a mask, particularly if aspirating or injecting a joint.

11. Swab the injection site with Betadine alcoholic solution or similar antiseptic before giving the injection.
12. Do not exceed the manufacturer's recommended dose of local anaesthetic.
13. Beware of using local anaesthetics with added adrenalin and **never, never** use these for fingers or toes in case the prolonged vaso-constriction causes ischaemia and gangrene.
14. In a vascular area, occasionally withdraw the plunger of the syringe to check that the needle is not inside a vein. Probably some 'reactions' and 'allergic responses' to local anaesthetics have been due to inadvertent intravenous injection of the anaesthetic with or without added adrenalin.
15. Remember that adrenalin can interreact with certain drugs such as anti-depressants: ask patients if they are taking any medication.
16. Caution should be observed in patients with epilepsy.

7.4 WHICH LOCAL ANAESTHETIC?

Several well known local anaesthetic agents are manufactured, and each gives very adequate anaesthesia. Different surveys have shown slight variations in toxicity between different local anaesthetics, but the three most widely used agents are currently Lignocaine (Xylocaine UK; Octocaine USA) Bupivicaine (Marcain UK; Marcain USA) and Prilocaine (Citanest UK; Xylonest USA). Where small volumes are being used, there is little to choose between the three local anaesthetics; where intravenous injections are used, Prilocaine appears to be the drug of choice at present.

Each of the above anaesthetics is also manufactured with added adrenalin as an option, this has the effect of causing localized vaso-constriction and thus prolonging the action of the anaesthetic drug. However, as previously emphasized, any of the preparations with adrenalin should be treated with great respect and should **never** be used for digital anaesthesia – the constriction of digital arteries could result in gangrene of fingers or toes. This also applies to the tip of the nose, tip of the ear or penis. For this reason, as an added safeguard, all local anaesthetics containing adrenalin should be kept separately from the plain injections, and should be clearly marked.

7.4.1 Maximum dose

As a guide, the maximum safe dose of each of the three local anaesthetics is shown below for an average adult of 70 kg.

Lignocaine	200 mg
Bupivicaine	140 mg
Prilocaine	400 mg

This represents, respectively, 20 ml of 1% Lignocaine (or 40 ml of 0.5% Lignocaine), 28 ml of 0.5% Bupivicaine (or 56 ml of 0.25% Bupivicaine), and 40 ml of 1% Prilocaine (or 80 ml of 0.5% Prilocaine). Dosages should be correspondingly less in the elderly, debilitated and young, and basically it should be remembered that the correct dose is the smallest dose required to produce the desired anaesthesia.

7.5 NERVE BLOCKS

Any nerve in the body can be 'blocked' by infiltrating local anaesthetic around it; this can be put to good use in the sole of the foot by using a posterior tibial nerve block, and the technique can be applied to any other sensory nerve if appropriate. As a method of producing anaesthesia of the sole of the foot it is ideal, as in this area the skin is particularly thick, and injections through the horny layer cause intense pain, and largely defeat any object of painless surgery!

The posterior tibial nerve is a branch of the sciatic nerve; it passes down the back of the calf in company with the posterior tibial vessels to the interval between the heel and the medial malleolus where it ends under the cover of the flexor retinaculum by dividing into the medial and lateral plantar nerves, which between them supply the sole of the foot. The posterior tibial nerve may be blocked as it passes behind the medial malleolus, before it divides.

7.5.1 Technique of posterior tibial nerve block

A point is chosen exactly midway between the medial malleolus and tendo-achilles at the level of the ankle, and the overlying skin painted with Povidone-iodine alcoholic solution (Betadine) or similar antiseptic.

A sterile syringe with 25 SWG needle is used to draw in 5 ml of 1% Lignocaine with added adrenalin 1:200 000. A small wheal of local anaesthetic is raised at the point between the medial malleolus and tendo-achilles, and then the syringe is directed at 45° in a horizontal plane, aiming the needle at the underlying bone. When this is reached, the needle is withdrawn 2 mm and the plunger gently withdrawn to check that the needle is not inside a vein. Then 2–5 ml local anaesthetic solution is injected around the posterior tibial nerve and the needle is withdrawn (Fig. 7.2).

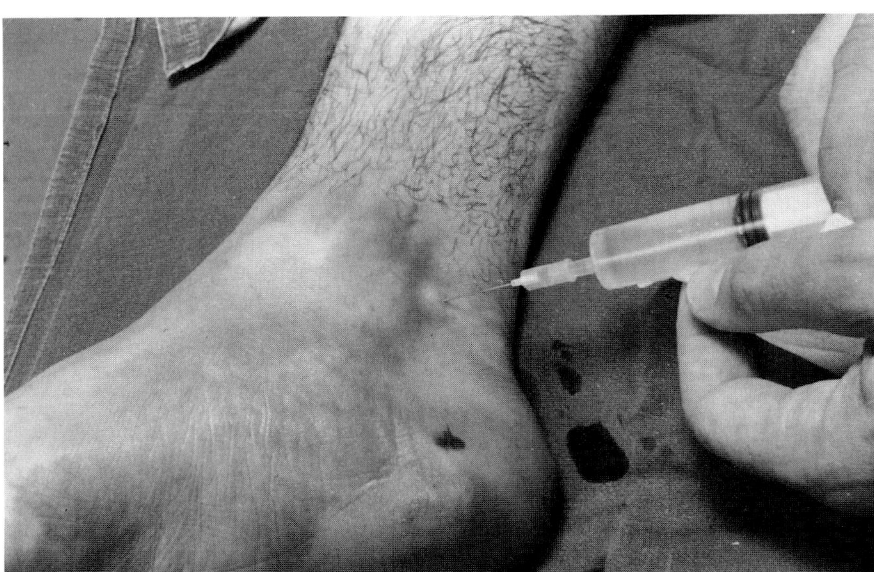

Fig. 7.2 Posterior tibial nerve block. Excellent for producing anaesthesia of the sole of the foot.

Anaesthesia of the sole of the foot gradually develops over the ensuing ten minutes and will last for up to two hours. As the overlying skin at the ankle is so much softer than the horny layers on the sole of the foot, an injection may be given painlessly at this site. The method is particularly useful for suturing lacerations on the sole of the foot or for the treatment of verrucae or other intradermal lesions.

One word of caution – proprioception depends on sensory impulses received from the soles of the feet; therefore it is inadvisable to perform a posterior tibial nerve block on both feet simultaneously otherwise the patient may fall over and be unable to maintain his or her balance.

7.6 EPIDURAL ANAESTHESIA

This method of anaesthesia has achieved great popularity, particularly in the obstetric and general surgery fields. Basically a sterile solution of dilute local anaesthesia is introduced through a lumbar puncture-type needle into the extra-dural space, as opposed to a spinal anaesthetic where the solution is injected into the cerebrospinal fluid. The technique of high epidural anaesthesia is beyond the scope of this book, but caudal epidural anaesthesia is included as a valuable method of pain relief in patients with acute low back pain accompanied by muscle spasm such as is found in prolapsed intervertebral disc lesions.

7.6.1 Technique of caudal epidural anaesthesia

Items required

- 1 50 ml syringe filled with 40 ml 0.9% saline plus 10 ml 0.5% Bupivicaine (Marcain)
- 1 2 ml syringe filled with Methylprednisolone 80 mg (Depo-Medrone)
- 1 2 ml syringe with 1% Lignocaine
- 1 20 SWG spinal needle 3½″ (8.9 cm) long
- 1 sterile dressing pack

The patient is placed prone on the operating theatre table or couch and a cushion placed under the pelvis to tilt the sacrum upwards.

Povidone–iodine (Betadine) alcoholic solution is painted over the overlying skin and 2 ml of 1% Lignocaine is injected through to the sacral hiatus. The spinal needle is now inserted through the hiatus and just below the cornua. Some difficulty may be encountered in determining the exact angle, but it tends to be parallel to the surface of the fifth sacral segment (Fig. 7.3).

After inserting the spinal needle to 5 cm the stylus is withdrawn and no fluid should be seen. If cerebrospinal fluid is seen, the procedure should be abandoned and repeated on another occasion. If blood is seen, the needle should be moved slightly until bleeding ceases.

The saline/Marcain mixture is now very slowly injected, taking five to ten minutes.

After 40 ml has been injected, 2 ml of Methylprednisolone (Depo-Medrone) is injected through the same needle, followed by the remaining 10 ml saline/Marcain solution. The needle is now withdrawn.

After the injection the patient is left lying prone for five to ten minutes

Fig. 7.3 Models to show caudal epidural injection.

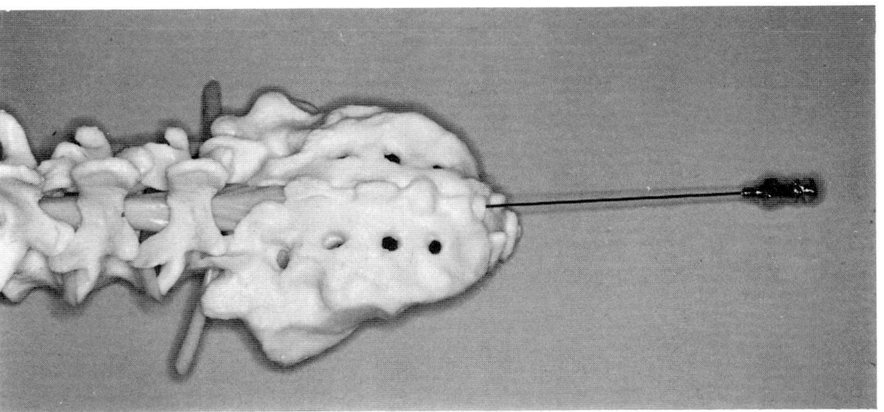

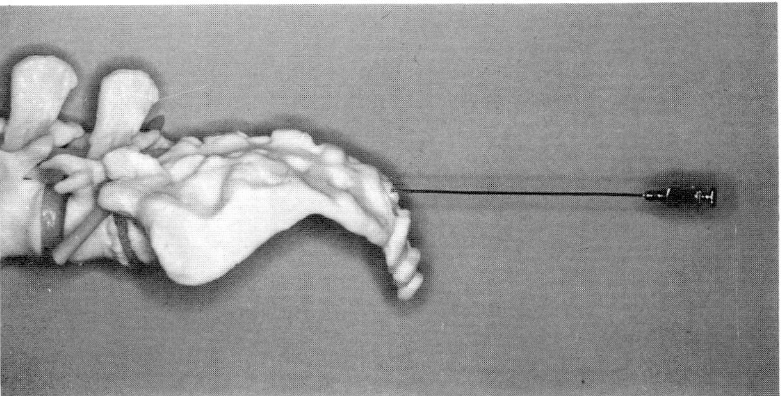

before turning to the supine position. Half an hour later, the patient may return home.

Provided an absolutely meticulous aseptic technique is employed, this is a valuable method of pain relief which can be used in general practice.

7.7 INTRAVENOUS REGIONAL ANAESTHESIA (Bier block)

This is an extremely useful method of producing total anaesthesia, muscle relaxation and a bloodless operating field in an arm or a leg, and enables the general practitioner to increase the scope of minor operations to include carpal tunnel decompression, release of trigger finger, excision of ganglion, exploration for the removal of foreign objects, and even reduction of simple fractures.

The technique was first described by August Bier in 1908 using procain as the anaesthetic [4], but it was not until 1963 that the method achieved popularity using Lignocaine [5]. As a result of numerous side-effects of this drug, in 1965 the editorial of the Journal of the American Medical Association advised against the use of intravenous regional anaesthesia until safer agents were available.

By 1971 Prilocaine had been recommended by Thorn-Alquist [6] and Bupivicaine by Ware [7], who further reported favourably using Bupivicaine in 1979 [8]. In 1983 serious side-effects were reported from various

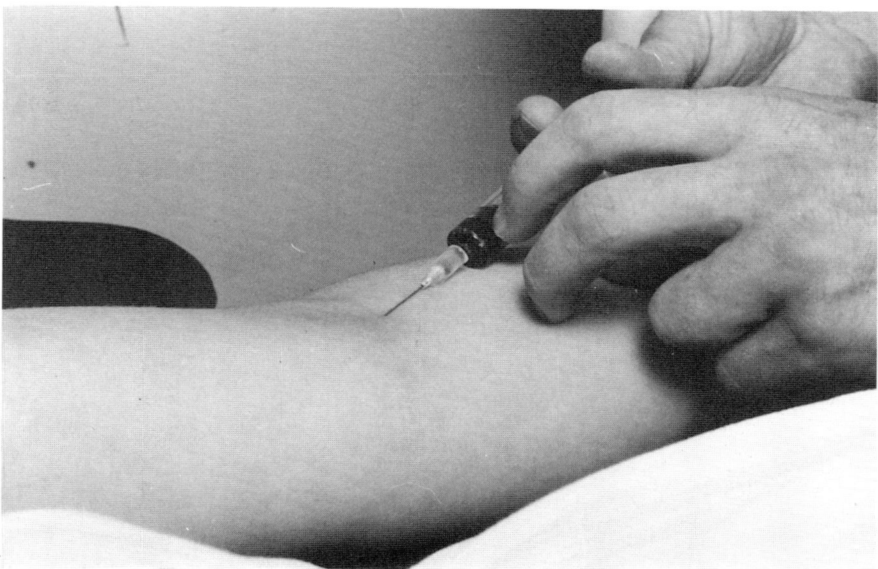

Fig. 7.4 An intravenous 'pre-medication' injection of Diazepam and Pethidine is given.

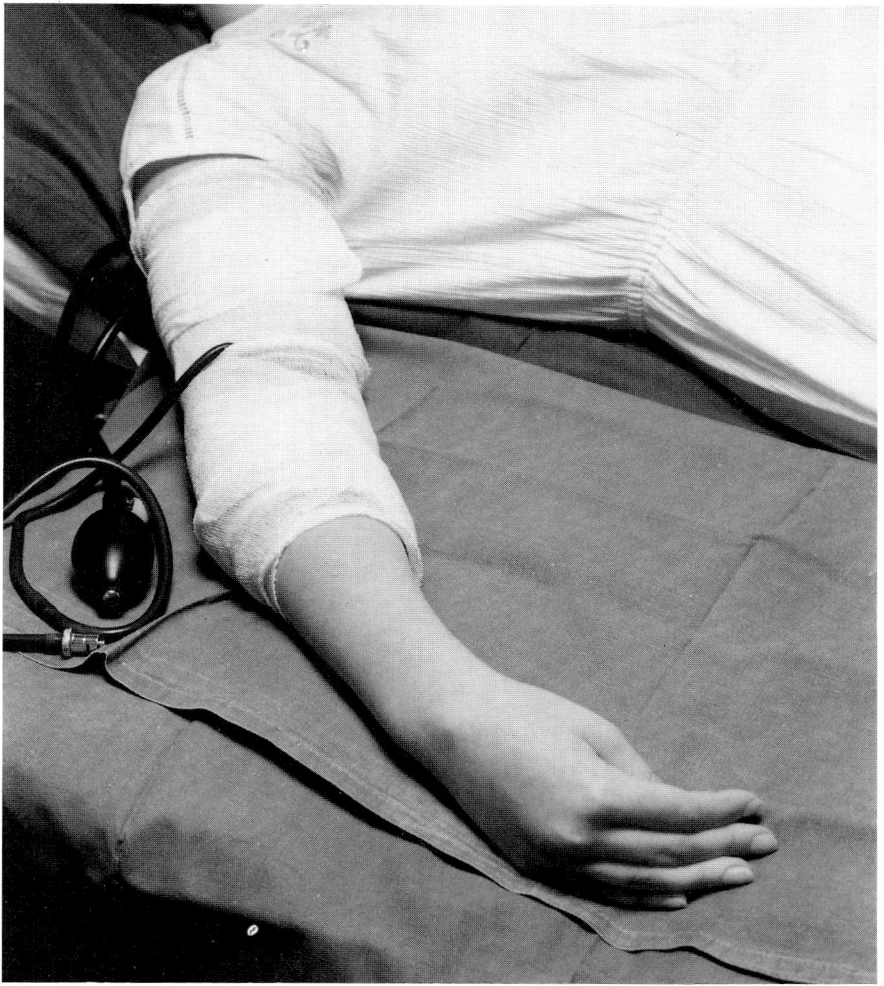

Fig. 7.5 An orthopaedic and sphygmomanometer cuff are applied to the upper arm, and bandaged in place.

centres using Bupivicaine for intravenous regional anaesthesia, and the drug of choice now appears to be Prilocaine (Citanest). A review of the Bier's block technique by Pattison [9] in 1984 concluded that it is a safe, simple, effective, and well tolerated method of regional anaesthesia. He could find no long term complications attributable to the technique. The method consists of exsanguinating the limb and injecting a large volume of dilute anaesthetic intravenously through an indwelling needle; this passes retrogradely via the veins, venules, capillaries, arterioles and arteries, thence to skin, muscle and the whole limb, producing anaesthesia and muscle relaxation. Up to one hour operating time is obtained in a bloodless field with total anaesthesia and muscle relaxation. The following items are required for an intravenous regional block:

1 orthopaedic pneumatic tourniquet
1 standard sphygmomanometer + cuff
1 3″ Esmarch bandage
1 intravenous cannula size 18 SWG (0.09 cm metric)
40 ml 0.5% Prilocaine plain (Citanest)

7.7.1 Technique of Bier block for the arm

1. Cotton wool padding is applied around the upper arm, and an orthopaedic pneumatic tourniquet applied over it.
2. A sphygmomanometer cuff (or second orthopaedic tourniquet) is applied distal to the first tourniquet, covered with a non-stretch bandage, and inflated to just below arterial pressure. This distends the veins at the wrist. This second tourniquet acts as a safe-guard should the first tourniquet fail (Fig. 7.5).
3. The 18 SWG (0.09 cm) intravenous cannula is now inserted in a suitable vein, strapped in position with adhesive tape and the sphygmomanometer deflated (Fig. 7.6). A 1 ml syringe containing Prilocaine is attached to the cannula and strapped in place (Fig. 7.7).
4. The arm is now elevated and the limb exsanguinated using the elastic Esmarch bandage, starting at the fingers, carefully over the indwelling cannula and syringe, tightly over the forearm and extending to, and covering, the second tourniquet (Fig. 7.8).
5. The orthopaedic tourniquet is now inflated to above arterial pressure (in practice 250 mm Hg) and the Esmarch bandage removed. At this stage, the arm is exsanguinated but there is still a cannula fixed inside a vein.
6. 30 ml 0.5% Prilocaine is now slowly injected through the intravenous cannula, and the second cuff inflated to above arterial pressure. (The reason for the interval between inflating the first and second tourniquets is to allow some Prilocaine to infiltrate below the second cuff, producing anaesthesia and reducing discomfort to the patient) (Fig. 7.9).
7. The cannula is left in place as a means of access to the circulation should any complications arise.
8. Anaesthesia develops in approximately 4 min.

7.7.2 Additional safeguards for intravenous regional anaesthesia

Most of the complications and mishaps following the use of intravenous regional blocks have been due to failure of the pneumatic tourniquet, either

Fig. 7.6 After inflating one cuff to 80 mm Hg, an intravenous cannula is inserted in a suitable vein.

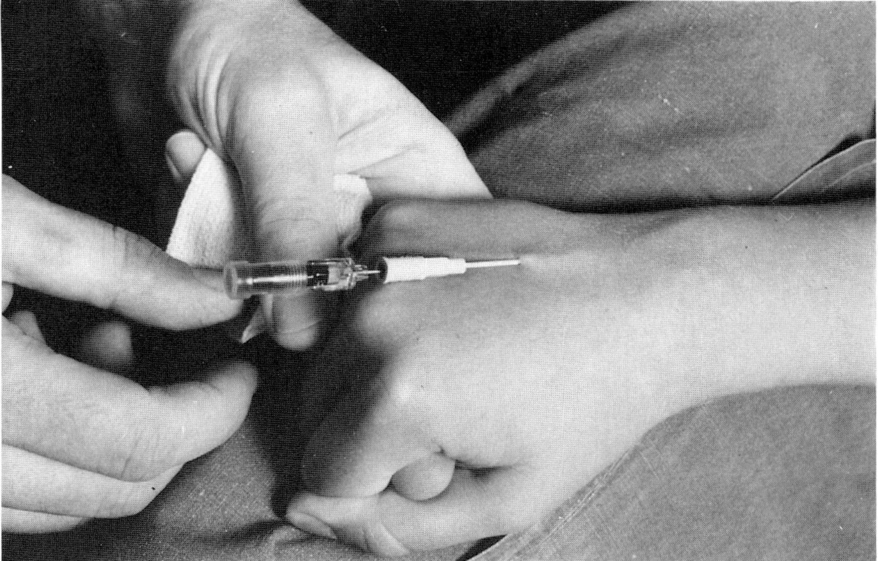

Fig. 7.7 The cuff is now deflated, the stylus withdrawn, leaving the cannula which is connected to a 1 ml syringe and Prilocaine.

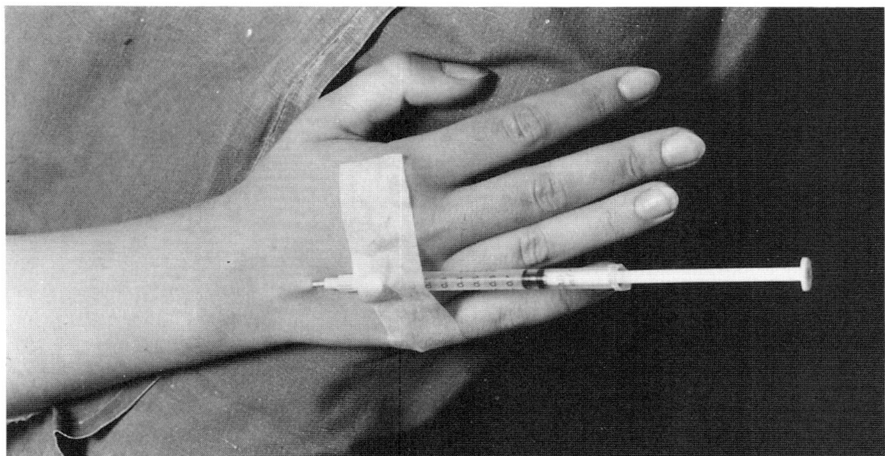

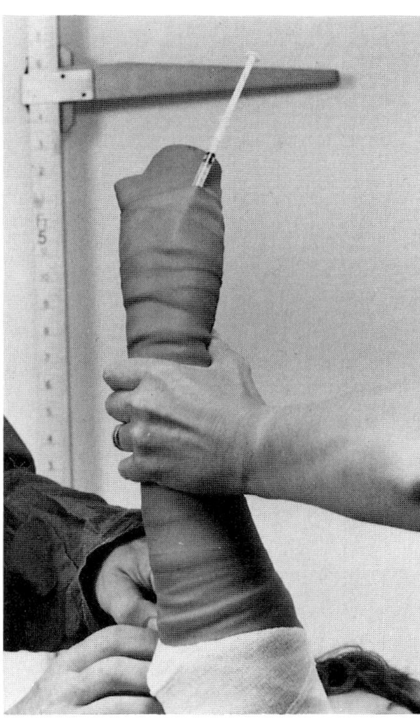

Fig. 7.8 The arm is elevated, and an Esmarch bandage applied. The cuff is inflated to 300 mm Hg and the bandage removed.

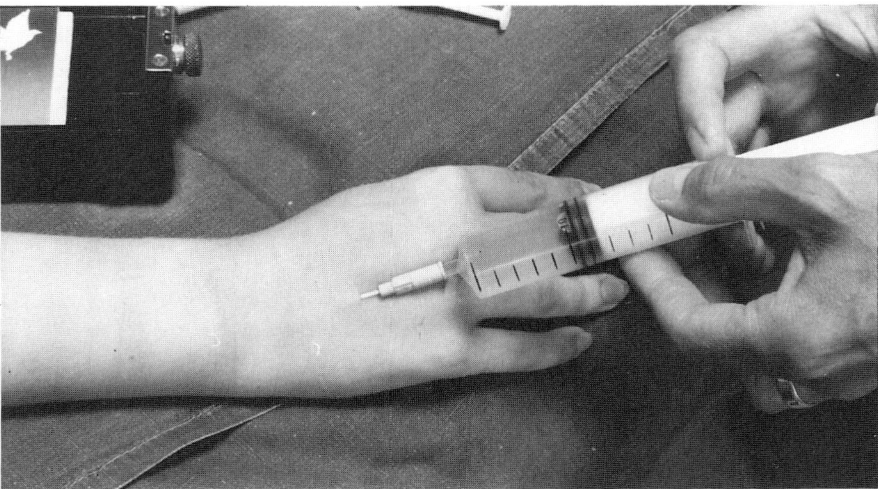

Fig. 7.9 After removing the Esmarch bandage, 30 ml 0.5% Prilocaine is injected through the cannula which is left in place for safety.

from leaking or faulty equipment. This results in a large bolus of local anaesthetic entering the circulation, with possible collapse, convulsions and even death. It is vital that the tourniquet remains inflated above arterial pressure throughout the whole procedure, and in any case should not be deflated in under **fifteen** minutes from injection to allow most of the anaesthetic to percolate through the tissues from the veins. It has also been shown [10] that even with adequate cuffs, some of the intravenous injection finds its way into the general circulation, through an active interosseous circulation. Because accidental failure of the cuff has such potentially serious consequences, an assistant should be present throughout the whole procedure, whose sole responsibility is the supervision of the cuff – checking the pressure continuously, and reporting any signs of reduced pressure. The use of two separate cuffs reduces still further the chances of accidental failure and is to be strongly recommended. If a standard blood-pressure cuff is used for the second 'back-up' tourniquet, it should be bandaged in place with a 4″ non-stretch cotton bandage which will prevent 'ballooning' and loosening of the cuff during inflation. All rubber parts, connections, taps, and pressure gauges should be checked for wear before use and replaced if necessary.

Although most conscious patients can tolerate the discomfort of a fully inflated cuff, nevertheless, it does cause pain to some, particularly after about ten to fifteen minutes. To obviate this, a 'pre-medication' intravenous injection of Pethidine (Demerol) 50 mg with Diazepam 5 mg is valuable and enables the cuff to be tolerated.

Full resuscitation facilities should always be immediately available if this method of anaesthesia is used. Given these safeguards, intravenous regional anaesthesia is a safe, effective and well tolerated procedure which has a definite place in minor surgery.

7.8 AMNALGESIA

In this technique, the awareness of painful stimuli is reduced and although the patient may appear to be fully conversant with what is happening, has no recollection of it afterwards. This is achieved very simply by an intravenous injection of Diazepam with or without an added analgesic such as Pethidine. For the average fit healthy adult, Diazepam 5–20 mg is usually sufficient, with the dosage correspondingly reduced for younger patients and the elderly. This technique is particularly valuable for the patient with malignant ascites who requires paracentesis and who will doze throughout the procedure, and have no recollection of it afterwards.

If given at the surgery, it is wise to allow the patient to rest for one hour afterwards and under no circumstances should they drive a car for the next 12 hours.

7.9 ENTONOX INHALATION

A mixture of equal parts oxygen and nitrous oxide is manufactured as Entonox (British Oxygen; Nitronox, USA), and is widely used for obstetric analgesia. The apparatus can be patient controlled and is safe. Although not generally used for minor surgical procedures, it has a place for

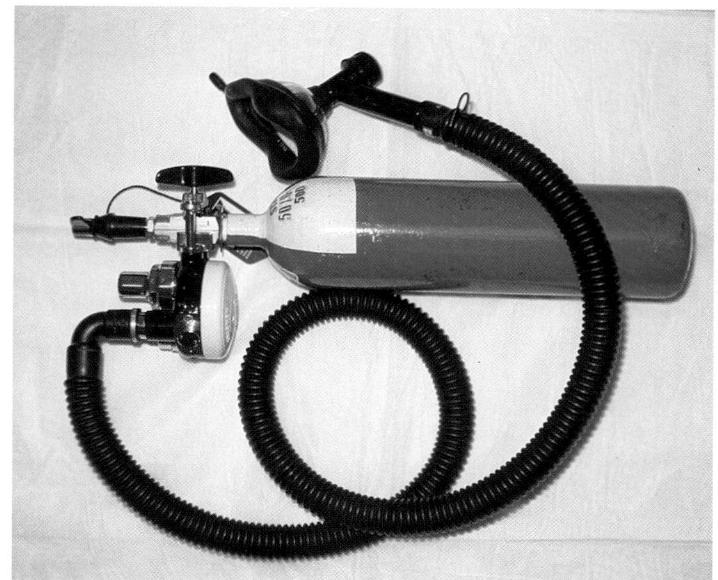

Fig. 7.10 Entonox giving-set.

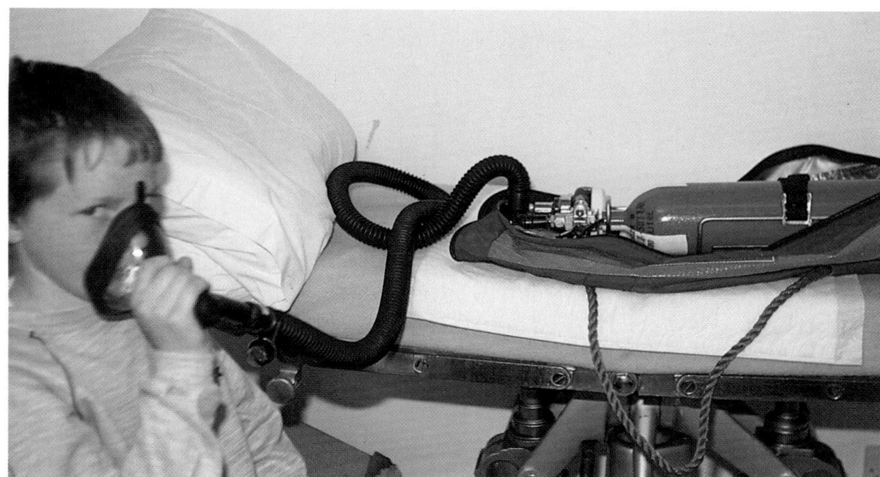

Fig. 7.11 Young patient using Entonox prior to removing a splinter from under finger-nail.

changing painful dressings, incision of small superficial abscesses, and similar procedures.

7.10 GENERAL ANAESTHESIA

Few GPs now give general anaesthetics outside hospital premises. This contrasts with 50 years ago when chloroform, ether, nitrous oxide and pentothal were all widely used in the patient's home and doctor's surgery. Where a practice has facilities to give general anaesthetics, a doctor with a special interest in anaesthetics, and full recovery and resuscitation equipment, there is no reason why some of the minor operations mentioned should not be done under a general anaesthetic, particularly short acting intravenous anaesthetics for such conditions as opening abscesses or the removal of toe-nails. On the whole, however, the doctor will find that all the minor operations described in this book can be very adequately and safely performed under local anaesthesia.

EIGHT

Incisions

'There are three ways of opening an abscess so as to give outlet to the matter: by caustic, by incision, or by the introduction of feton.
The first is more agreeable to timid patients who are afraid of the pain of incision'
(Encyclopaedia Brittanica, 1797)

Patients judge their surgeons by the end result which can be seen, viz., the operation scar. With a little forethought and variation in technique, almost invisible scars can be produced, depending on the knowledge of certain lines on the body, first described by Langer [11] in 1861. Until that time operative incisions were made where they would be most effective to excise the pathological lesion with little regard to the resultant scar. Textbooks of plastic surgery then reproduced pictures of Langer's lines designed to give optimum healing and the neatest scars [12, 13, 14] and it was not until 1950 that some doubt was cast on this atlas of lines for incision by Smith [15] and subsequently in 1951 by Kraissl [16] who compared the traditional Langer lines with wrinkle lines or skin creases. Most wrinkle lines run perpendicular to the action of underlying muscles, and it is common experience that incisions made in these wrinkle lines give the neatest scars with minimum disruption of function. Thus, in planning the elective incision the following points should be borne in mind:

Fig. 8.1 Showing wrinkle lines and optimal sites for incisions on the face.

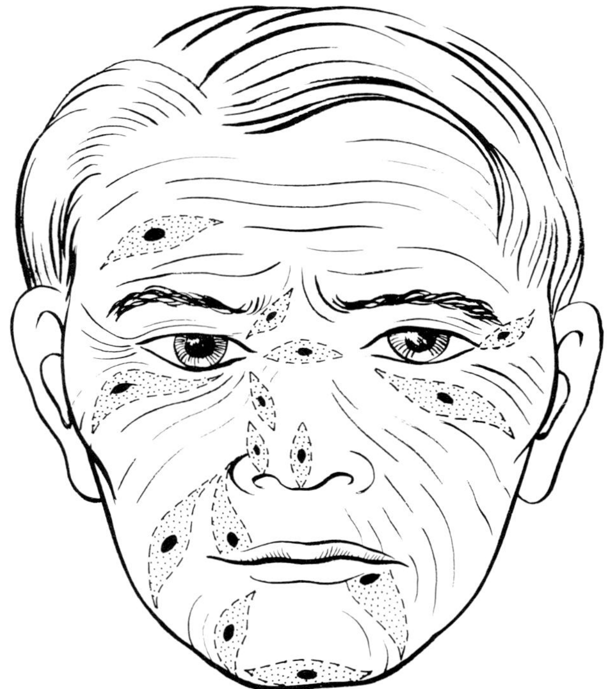

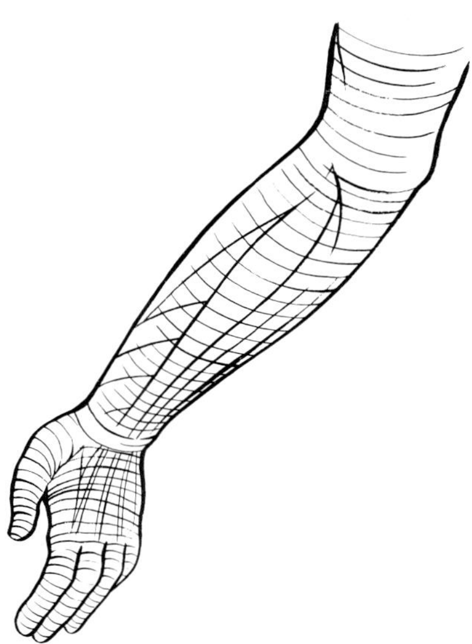

Fig. 8.2 Showing Langer lines for the forearm, and sites for incisions, across underlying muscles.

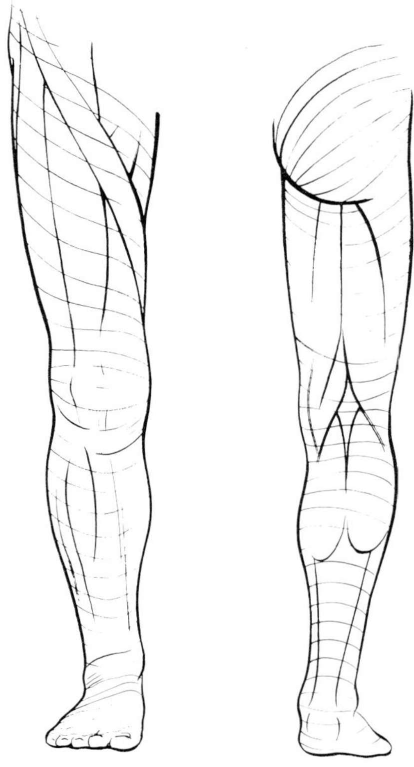

Fig. 8.3 Showing Langer lines for the lower limb, crossing the direction of the underlying muscles.

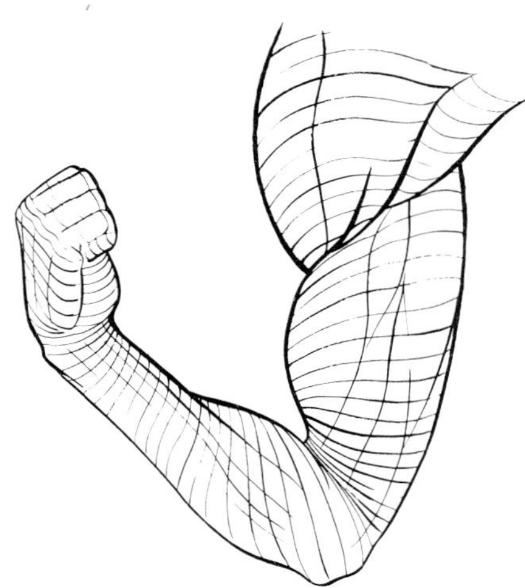

Fig. 8.4 Showing Langer lines for upper limb.

1. Look for natural creases and if possible follow these lines (Figs 8.1, 8.2, 8.3 and 8.4).
2. Where there is an underlying joint the incision should be placed transversely across it to prevent loss of function.
3. To demonstrate some wrinkles, gently compress the relaxed skin in different directions to ascertain the line, or ask the patient to contract the underlying muscles.
4. In many parts of the body, traditional Langer lines are at variance with natural wrinkle lines; in these situations it is better to use the skin creases.

One of the most important aspects in achieving a neat scar is the avoidance of tension; this may mean careful undercutting to approximate the skin edges, and the placing of many fine sutures rather than widely placed interrupted sutures of inappropriately thick suture material. Tension may also be minimized by subcutaneous absorbable sutures, and externally by the use of Steri-strips in addition to sutures.

Infection is a potent cause of unsightly scars – often as a result of an infected subcutaneous haematoma. The latter can be minimized by careful attention to haemostasis at the time of the operation, the obliteration of any dead spaces, and, where appropriate, the insertion of a small drain for 48 hours post-operatively.

8.1 HISTOLOGY

It is important that arrangements be made for all specimens which have been removed to be examined histologically, and where appropriate, cytologically. However sure one is of the diagnosis, sooner or later a surprise occurs such as the dreaded amelanotic malignant melanoma or squamous cell carcinoma. Having every specimen examined also improves the operator's diagnostic acumen, and provides a permanent record of the histological diagnosis, and whether excision was complete or incomplete and whether the lesion was malignant or benign.

Most specimens should be placed in a jar containing a solution of Formalin 10% in normal saline as a preservative; the jar should be carefully labelled with the patient's name, nature of the specimen, the date, and accompanied by a histology request form giving as many details as possible for the pathologist. It is also helpful to indicate whether the specimen is a biopsy or a total excision to avoid confusion in the laboratory.

NINE

Skin closure

'Sutures are best made of soft thread, not too hard twisted that it may sit easier on the tissues, nor are too few nor too many of either of them to be put in'

(Aulus Cornelius Celsus, 25 BC–AD 50)

Following any operation, if skin edges are closely approximated without tension, healing will generally occur in ten days. Traditionally surgeons have used interrupted sutures to hold the skin edges together, but stitches are not always necessary or desirable and many alternative methods have been used in an attempt to give as neat a scar as possible.

The simplest method of skin closure is self-adhesive tape; where tension can be avoided, excellent results are obtained and it is particularly suitable for small superficial lacerations on the face and fingers. Ordinary, non-stretch, self-adhesive plaster tape can be used, but better results are obtained with purpose made sterile strips (Steri-strips 3-M) which can be readily applied and which have good tensile strength (Figs 9.1 and 9.2).

It is important if using sterile strips that good adhesion is obtained; thus the skin must be thoroughly dry, and if in an area where increased perspiration occurs, extra adhesion may be obtained by first painting the skin with tinct. benz. co. or collodion prior to applying the Steri-strips. Additional external support can be given by careful bandaging, and if the original wound is clean, may be left undisturbed for up to ten days. Most lacerations on fingers and toes can be satisfactorily closed using Steri-strips supplemented with tubular cotton stockinette bandage. It is important that the strip does not completely encircle the digit in case oedema occurs and the Steri-strip then acts as a tourniquet with ensuing ischaemia or necrosis. In very young children sutures may be preferable to sterile strip closure in case the child inadvertently pulls off the dressing and strips before healing has occurred.

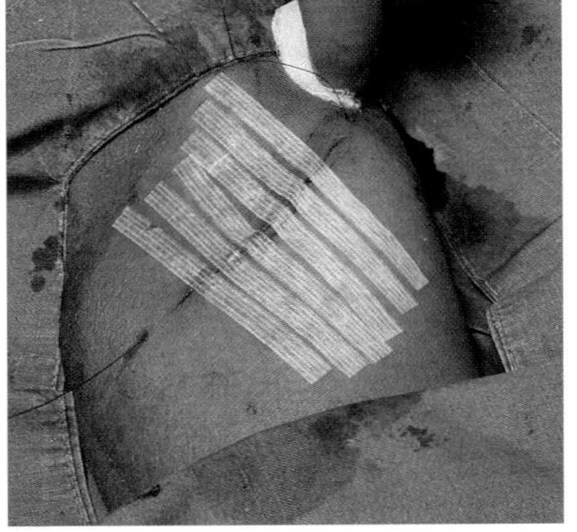

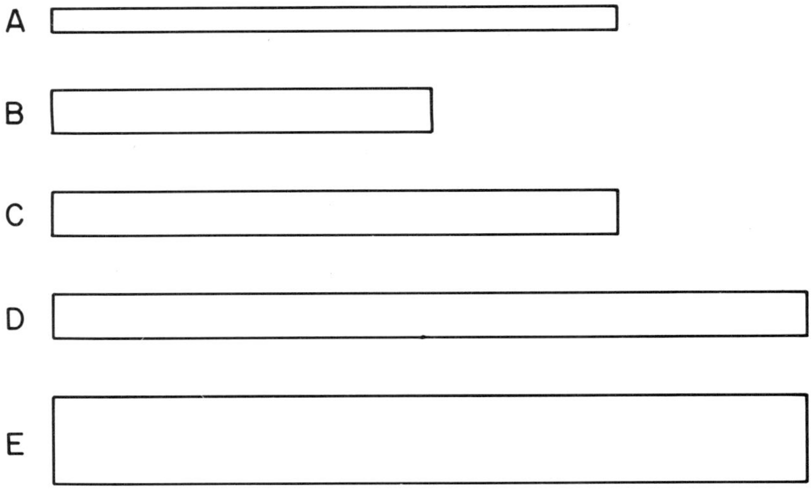

Fig. 9.1 Steri-strips may be used both to close a wound and also to give additional support for sutures (3-M).

A

B

C

D

E

Fig. 9.2 Skin closure strips are ideal for small wounds and for giving additional support during healing.
Size A 3 mm × 75 mm
Size B 6 mm × 50 mm
Size C 6 mm × 75 mm
Size D 6 mm × 100 mm
Size E 12 mm × 100 mm

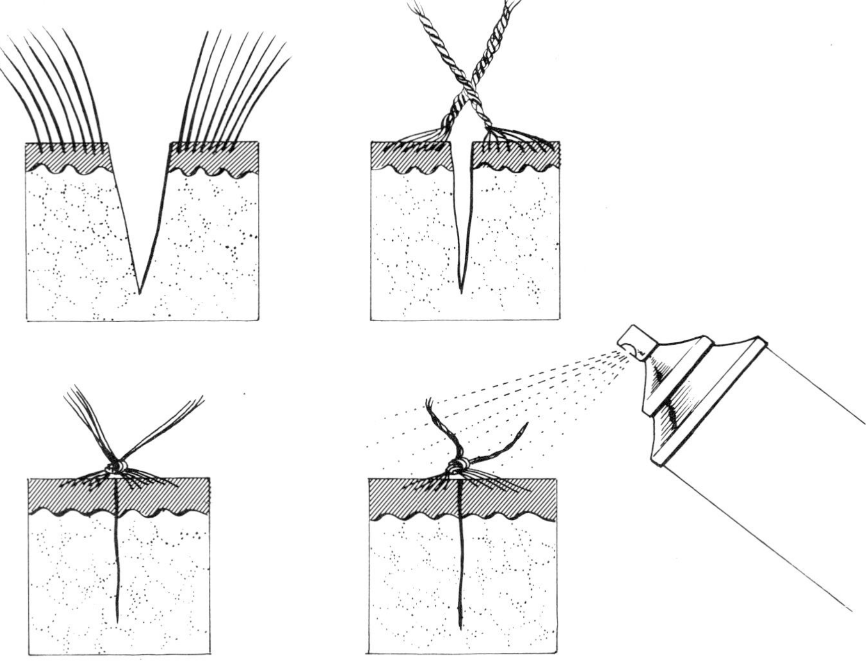

Fig. 9.3 Showing a simple method of closing a small laceration of the scalp, knotting a few strands of hair on either side of the wound.

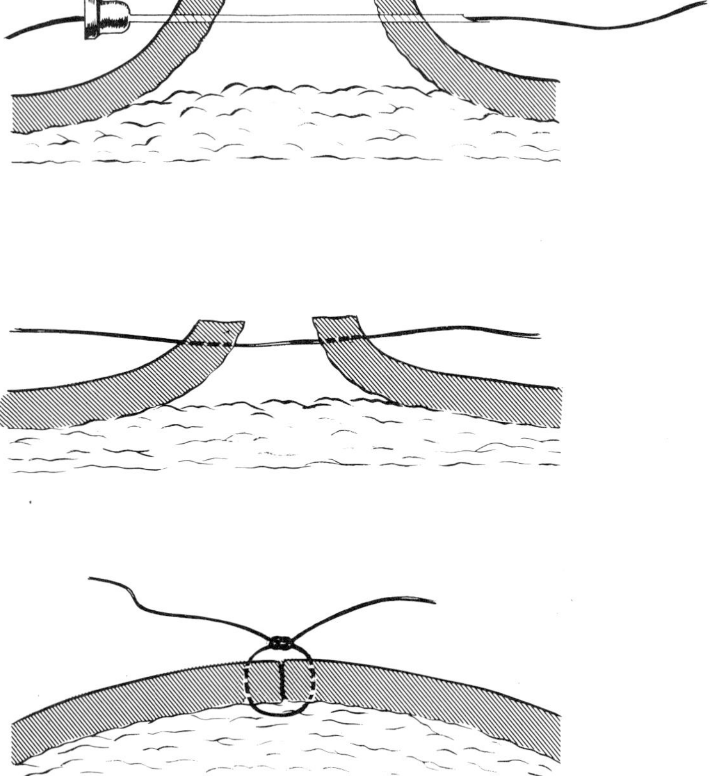

Fig. 9.4 Showing another simple method of suturing a wound using a hypodermic needle and some nylon 'fishing line'.

Faced with a small laceration on the scalp satisfactory skin closure may often be achieved merely by twisting a few strands of hair on either side of the wound and knotting them together over the laceration (Fig. 9.3). Spraying the knot with nobecutane spray, tinct. benz. co. or collodion will prevent the knot slipping, and the knot may then be cut free after ten days when healing has occurred. Another 'first-aid' method of skin closure in the absence of suitable suture materials uses hypodermic needles and nylon fishing line! The needles may be inserted through the skin edges from one side to another, the nylon thread passed through the lumen of the needle which is then withdrawn over the thread, leaving the nylon ready to be tied. Very satisfactory skin closure may be achieved using this simple procedure (Fig. 9.4).

9.1 SUTURES

The doctor looking through a catalogue of surgical sutures will find a bewildering array of materials in all sizes, colours, absorbability, needle sizes etc. Basically the majority of surgical sutures will be either absorbable or non-absorbable. Absorbable sutures as their name implies slowly dissolve as the tissues heal, and therefore do not need to be removed; non-absorbable sutures do not dissolve, and need to be removed. The different sutures are described in the following sections.

9.1.1 Interrupted, plain

This is the commonest method of suturing. The needle is inserted through the skin, across the subcutaneous part of the wound, through the skin on the opposite side, and then knotted, bringing the edges together. As most suture materials have a tendency to slip, a reef knot with one additional throw (Surgeons Knot) is used.

9.1.2 Interrupted, Mattress

Where skin edges may not approximate accurately due to laxity of the tissues or any other reason, good apposition may be achieved by including the skin edges in the suture (Vertical Mattress). Such sutures give a neat scar but are occasionally quite difficult to remove.

9.1.3 Subcuticular sutures

These are becoming increasingly popular and will give an extremely neat scar providing the skin is not under tension (Fig. 9.5). A straight needle is preferable, although cutting curved needles can be used. The needle is inserted through the skin about 1–2 cm away from, but in line with, the incision. It is passed under the skin to emerge in the subcuticular layer on one side of the wound; it is then passed backwards and forwards across the wound, eventually emerging beyond the other end of the incision corresponding to where the suture commenced. By applying traction to both ends of the suture, the skin edges are approximated neatly, and the part of the suture remaining visible is fixed to the skin either with tape, dressings or a single 'button'. Removal is effected by cutting one end flush with the skin, and firmly pulling the other.

9.1.4 Continuous and blanket stitch

These tend to be used for longer scars, and are generally seldom used for minor surgical incisions. As their name implies, a continuous stitch extends from one end of the wound to the other; it is quick to insert, difficult to achieve even tension and even spacing of the stitch, not easy to remove, has an increased risk of infection during removal, and does not allow the removal of individual sutures should fluid collect under the scar and require drainage.

9.2 SUTURE MATERIALS

Every doctor has a personal selection of preferred suture materials; listed in the following sections are the various types available.

9.2.1 Plain catgut

This is made from purified ribbons of animal intestines, which are spun into a strand, electronically gauged, and then polished. It is absorbed by body enzymes; originally it was very popular, but has tended to be superseded by synthetic absorbable sutures in recent years.

9.2.2 Chromic catgut

This is made from ribbons of animal intestines, spun into a strand, exactly as plain catgut, but treated so that the strength of the suture is maintained for a considerably longer time than plain catgut. Still used in obstetrics, and for approximating subcutaneous tissues, but being superseded by synthetic materials.

9.2.3 Braided silk (Mersilk)

The raw silk is treated and de-gummed prior to braiding, resulting in a compact braid which ties easily; it is extremely popular and widely used for skin closure.

9.2.4 Monofilament polyamide 6 and 66 (Ethilon)

These are synthetic, monofilament sutures, whose smooth surface does not appear to support bacterial growth. They can be difficult to knot, but are useful for subcuticular sutures.

9.2.5 Monofilament polypropylene (Prolene)

The advantage of polypropylene is that it is supple, ties securely and handles well. As with other monofilament synthetic sutures, knots need to be square ties with additional throws, and in addition, damage from forceps and needle-holders should be avoided to prevent fracture of the material. It is extremely smooth and suitable for subcuticular stitches.

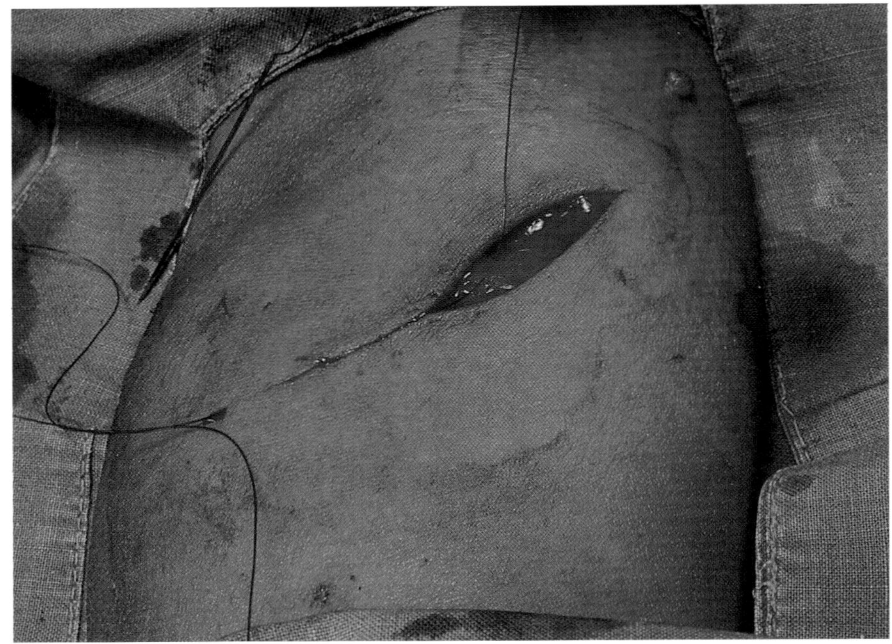

Fig. 9.5 A sub-cuticular stitch gives a neat scar and takes less time to insert than interrupted sutures.

9.2.6 Polyglycolic acid synthetic absorbable sutures (Dexon)

These sutures, introduced in recent years, are extremely popular, they appear to cause virtually no tissue reaction as they dissolve, compared with considerable histological tissue reaction with catgut. Their rate of absorption is considerably slower than even chromic catgut, and may take several weeks. It is an ideal suture material for all subcutaneous, subcuticular, and skin closures.

All suture materials are now graded by metric gauge, which indicates the actual diameter of the suture in tenths of a millimetre, and this gauging system has now been adopted by both European and United States Pharmacopeia, replacing the former system of O gauges.

A selection of the most widely used suture materials is now included in the Drug Tariff and doctors in the UK can now prescribe these for use on their National Health Service patients. For minor surgical procedure, the following 'short-list' will provide a basic treatment set.

1. Sterile braided silk metric gauge 2 (formerly 3/0) Black, 45 cm long, with 25 mm curved super cutting needle, reference Ethicon W533. Ideal for most skin closures.
2. Sterile polyamide 6 suture monofilament B.F. metric gauge 0.7 (formerly 6/0) Black, 35 cm long with 16 mm curved cutting needle, reference Ethicon W506. Ideal for the face, fingers and children.
3. Dexon polyglycolic acid synthetic absorbable sutures on atraumatic $\frac{3}{8}$ circle 24 mm reverse cutting needle, metric gauge 2 (formerly 3/0) 76 cm long, reference Davis and Geck 7618–41. Ideal for all general closure and subcuticular stitches.

9.3 SKIN CLOSURE CLIPS

These are generally not used for minor surgical procedures, although some surgeons favour their use; the disadvantages are that they require a special

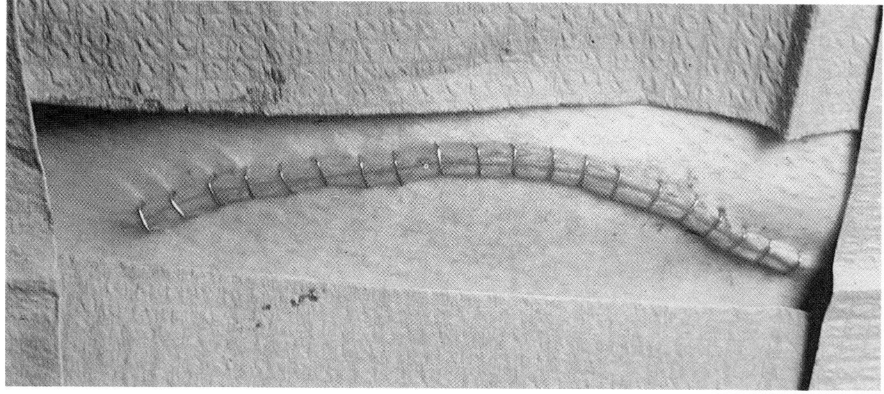

Fig. 9.6 Wound closure using the proximate skin stapler.

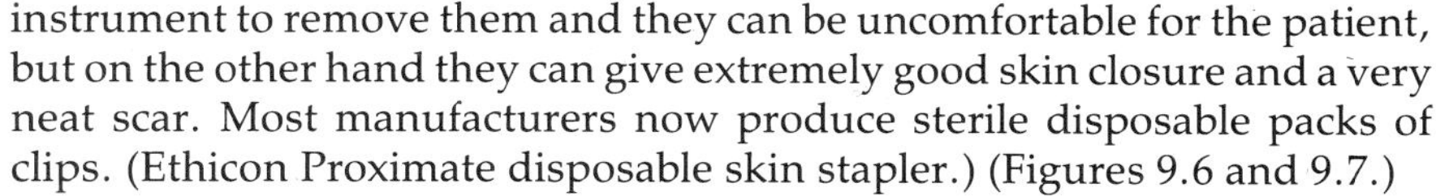

instrument to remove them and they can be uncomfortable for the patient, but on the other hand they can give extremely good skin closure and a very neat scar. Most manufacturers now produce sterile disposable packs of clips. (Ethicon Proximate disposable skin stapler.) (Figures 9.6 and 9.7.)

9.4 DRAINS

Although widely used for operations on the neck, breast, thorax and pelvis, drains are generally not necessary when performing minor surgical procedures. Where good haemostasis has been achieved, and any dead space closed, haematoma formation is unlikely. If drainage is thought necessary, a small piece of rubber or plastic tubing may be inserted under the sutures and removed after 48 hours.

Fig. 9.7 Illustrating use of proximate stapler.

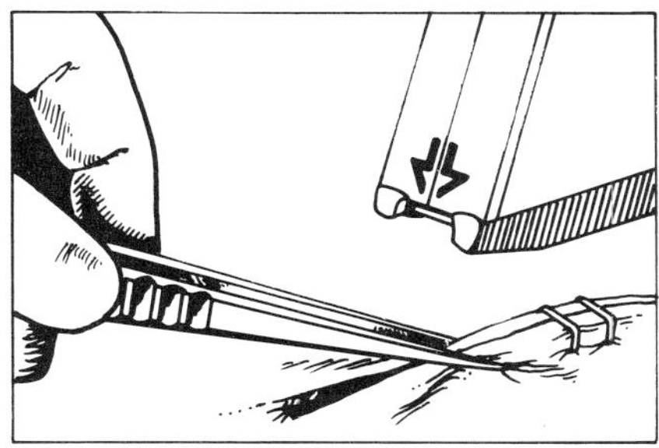

1. Evert and approximate skin edges as desired. Several techniques are suggested:
(a) With one tissue forcep, bring skin edges together until edges evert.

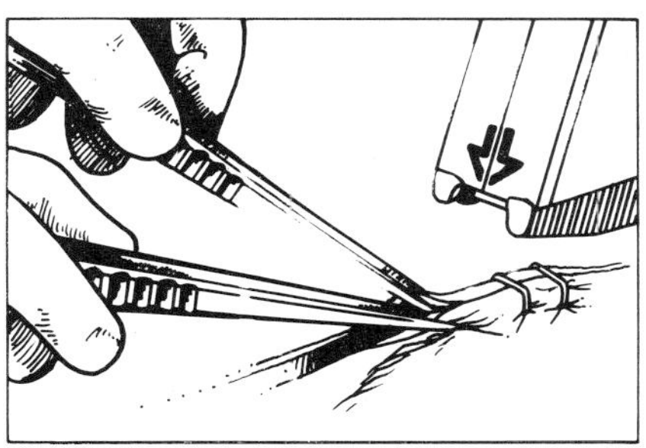

(b) With two tissue forceps, pick up each wound edge individually and approximate the edges.
(c) Apply tension to either end of the incision, such that the tissue edges begin to approximate themselves. One forcep can be used to insure that the edges are everted.

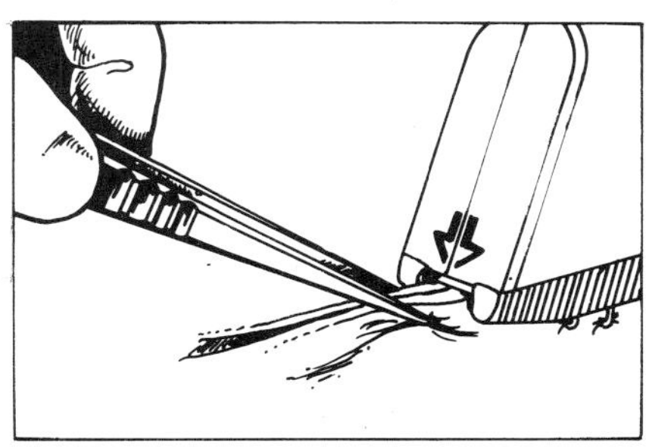

2. Position the instrument very lightly over the everted skin edges, aligning the instrument arrow with the incision. Pressing down on the instrument too heavily may make staple removal difficult.

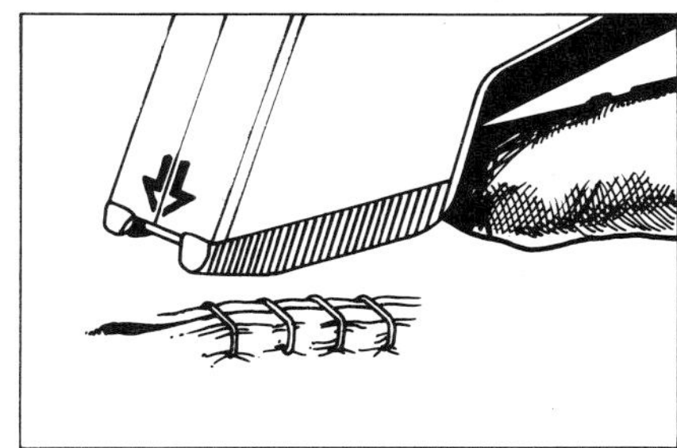

3. With one firm action squeeze the trigger until the trigger motion is halted. Release the trigger and back the instrument off the staple, the anvil easily slides out from under the staple.

TEN

Dressings and removal of sutures

'Now, after thou hast stitched it, thou shouldst bind it with fresh meat the first day. Thou shouldst treat it afterwards with grease and honey every day until he recovers'
(Edwin Smith, Surgical Papyrus, 3000–2500 BC)

It has been suggested that dressings on surgical wounds are unnecessary, that they merely prevent the doctor and patient observing what is happening underneath, and this is certainly true on many occasions. Every doctor will have observed how well incisions heal on the scalp and face, where no dressings are used.

10.1 REASONS FOR USING DRESSINGS

Where dressings are used, they probably help in four ways:

1. absorption of any secretions,
2. protection from contamination,
3. additional support during the healing phase,
4. limitation of excessive movements during healing.

10.1.1 Absorption of secretions

Any wound which is discharging or oozing will be helped by the application of an absorbent sterile, dry dressing, which must be changed frequently.

10.1.2 Protection from contamination

If a surgical operation has been performed under sterile conditions, and primary skin closure is expected, a sterile dry dressing firmly applied at the end of the operation should be left *undisturbed* until the sutures are removed. Peeping under the dressing 'to see how it is healing' is to be condemned: this only increases the chances of cross-infection. Only if there is a definite indication such as unexpected pain, swelling, fever or signs of infection should the original dressing be disturbed – in every other case leave well alone!

10.1.3 Additional support

Sutures alone may not give adequate support to a healing wound, and in this case a dressing firmly bandaged in place will give additional external support, reduce tension on the stitches, and promote healing.

10.1.4 Limitation of movement

Wounds on the limbs may be subjected to excessive forces during healing, for example transverse wounds near the knee joint may tend to pull apart during walking and kneeling; by applying a thick layer of bandage, limitation of movements of the joint will be achieved, and promote healing. Similarly on the hand or fingers where sterile strips may have been used in preference to sutures, but by themselves are not strong enough to withstand full movements, supportive bandaging will supplement the Steri-strips and avoid the need for suturing.

10.2 TYPES OF DRESSING

10.2.1 Non-adherent dressings

Where there is considerable discharge either from an ulcer, burns, blisters or sinuses, ordinary dry dressings may become adherent and difficult to remove. In such cases non-adherent dressings may be used, such as Melolin X-A, Johnsons N.A. dressing, vaseline impregnated gauze or similar preparations.

10.2.2 Antibacterial dressings

These consist of tulle gras dressings impregnated with antibacterial substances. They are of limited use and carry the risk of causing skin sensitization. In certain situations such as ingrowing toe-nail operations where there is known to be heavy infection, the routine use of such dressings appears to accelerate healing.

10.2.3 Acrylic resin aerosol dressings (Nobecutane)

These consist of acrylic resin dissolved in a mixture of acetate esters in aerosol containers. By spraying on the skin from a distance of 20 cm a protective film is produced. This is useful on sites where conventional dressings would be difficult to keep in place e.g. the scalp; in other sites it may be used instead of a dry gauze dressing particularly after sutures have been removed.

10.2.4 Cotton conforming bandages (Kling, Crinx and Kurlex)

These lightweight bandages are so designed that they will bandage irregular surfaces and maintain even tension. They are cheap, efficient, and widely used.

10.2.5 Elastic bandages

Where firm external elastic support is required, for example on the legs to control varicose veins, elastic web bandages are ideal. Wounds and ulcers on the lower leg tend to heal more slowly, the more so when oedema is present. The early application of firm elastic bandages reduces oedema and accelerates healing. They are frequently used in the treatment of varicose veins and varicose ulceration.

10.2.6 Elastic net stockinette (Netalast)

This elastic tubular dressing is designed to hold dressings in place in sites such as the axilla, breast, perineum, buttock and scalp; it is manufactured in different widths, and with ingenuity all parts of the body can be covered. It has the advantage of being extremely comfortable but does not give much compression.

10.2.7 Elasticated tubular stockinette (Tubigrip)

For additional elastic support, elasticated tubular stockinette is used; particularly for wounds on arms and legs. As with the elastic net stockinette it is manufactured in various sizes to suit most parts of the body. It is used to give compression for sclerotherapy for varicose veins.

10.2.8 Cotton surgical tubular stockinette (Tubegauz)

This is a non-elastic, cotton stockinette, which is ideal for bandaging fingers and toes. It is manufactured in various widths, and is applied with a special tubular applicator using a twisting action to increase compression if required.

ELEVEN

Suture removal

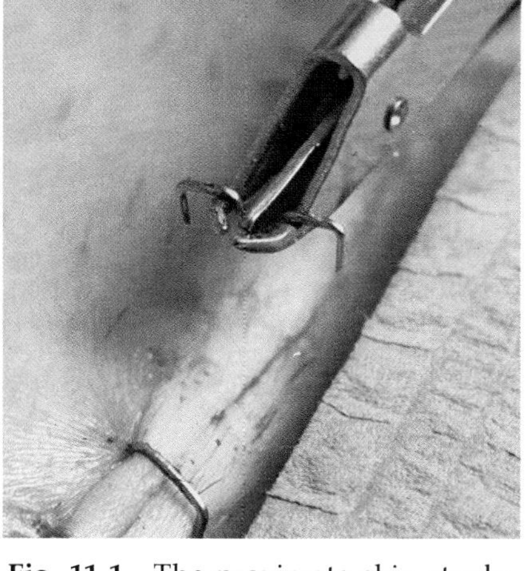

Fig. 11.1 The proximate skin staple remover in use.

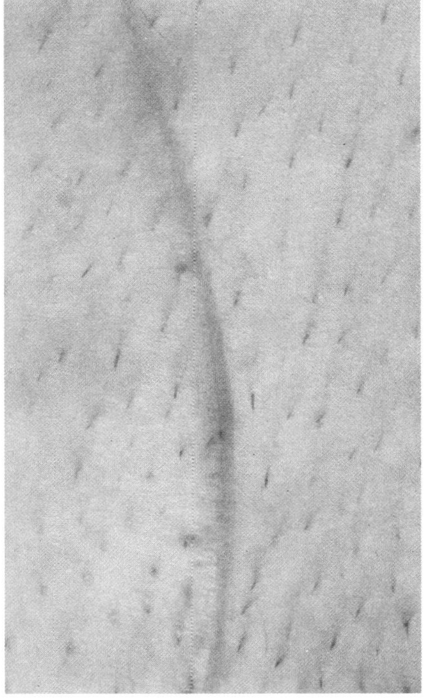

Fig. 11.2 Typical scar following skin stapling.

'If thou examinest a man having a wound in his lip, piercing through to the inside of his mouth, thou shouldst examine his wound as far as the column of the nose: thou shouldst draw together that wound with stitching'

(Edwin Smith, Surgical Papyrus, 3000–2500 BC)

The shorter the time sutures are *in situ*, the neater the scar. However, if they are removed too soon, there is a risk of the wound gaping; consequently a compromise has to be reached, and the optimum time will vary in different sites on the body. Thus the majority of sutures are removed on the tenth post-operative day, but on the face it is preferable to remove them very much earlier, and on the foot it might be advisable to leave them a day or two longer. It is also possible to remove alternate sutures one or two days before the remainder, and this improves the appearance of the final scar. Where it is desirable to remove sutures early, but the practitioner feels the wound may not be firmly adherent, additional external support may be given using sterile self-adhesive strips.

11.1 TECHNIQUE OF SUTURE AND CLIP REMOVAL

Unfortunately, a wound which has healed well may be contaminated by poor suture removal technique resulting in stitch abscesses and an infected scar. Where possible, the sterile dressings applied at the time of the operation should be left undisturbed until the sutures are to be removed. A sterile dressing pack should be used, and a no-touch technique employed using sterile instruments. The doctor or nurse should either wear a mask or not talk during the actual procedure to reduce droplet cross-infection.

Fine sutures are best removed using a pair of iris scissors and dissecting forceps, most other sutures may be removed using either standard pointed stitch scissors or pre-packed disposable stitch cutters and forceps. To minimize any risks of contamination, the knot should be picked up with forceps and one side of the suture cut flush with the skin; it may then be removed by carefully pulling on the knot.

11.1.1 Subcuticular stitch removal

One end of the subcuticular stitch is cut flush with the skin, while the other end is grasped with artery forceps and traction applied. Additional support may be given by the application of sterile self-adhesive strips, which can be applied either at the time of the original operation or at the time of suture removal.

TWELVE

Statistical analysis

'You know, my children, that Surgical Operations are divided into two classes: those that benefit the patient, and those that more often kill . . . abstain from undertaking dangerous and difficult treatments'

(Albucasis, AD 1013–1106)

By keeping simple records of every operation performed, valuable statistical analysis is possible, which in turn may be of help in planning future requirements for the practice. A register of operations may be compiled using a hard-back book in which is entered the date, patient's name, address, age and sex, together with the type of operation. This list may be numbered chronologically or include a code for additional data retrieval or computer storage. At the end of each year, a breakdown of the year's operations is made, from which can be compiled a summary and analysis.

12.1 RECORD KEEPING

The importance of keeping accurate comprehensive and legible records of every operation cannot be emphasized enough. Details should be written down immediately the operation is finished, and not committed to memory; such details as which digit, whether left or right, which joint, whether infected or not, size, situation and extent of the lesion, history, signs and symptoms, findings at operation, method of anaesthesia, dose of anaesthetic used, skin preparation, method of excision, whether histology was requested, haemostasis, closure, type and number of sutures used, type of dressings used, estimated date of suture removal and subsequent management – all these should be entered on the patient's notes and signed and dated. At this stage the doctor should personally check that any specimen which is being sent for histology is correctly labelled and corresponds to the histology request form.

12.2 ORGANIZING A MINOR OPERATING LIST

It is much better to set aside a time each week for a minor operating list rather than doing each as it arises. Not only can the patient make preparations, the surgery staff and nurses can prepare instruments, equipment and forms in advance, clean the room and generally anticipate what will be needed. It is also a more efficient use of everyone's time, the only disadvantage of arranging a list is the risk of cross-infection, particularly if an unsuspected abscess or heavily infected lesion is treated at the beginning of the list before the remaining 'clean' cases. With scrupulous attention to aseptic technique, and the use of CSSD packs, cross-infection should not occur; nevertheless it is good practice to put 'clean' operations such as carpal tunnel decompression or excision of ganglion, where

FRIDAY, JANUARY 1st

2.00 John Smith
10, London Road.

Excision Sebaceous Cyst
on Scalp.

2.30 Karen North (Aged 11)
247, Westbury Close

Ingrowing Toe-Nail

3.00 Ingrid McKewary
3, The Meadows

Injection Varicose Veins
Left Leg.

3.20 Winifred Lott
194, London Road

Left Meibomian Cyst

Fig. 12.1 An appointment book can also be used for the 'operating list' each week.

infection could be disastrous, first on the list, and arrange 'dirty' cases such as infected ingrowing toe-nails and abscesses at the end.

Having decided to reserve a set time regularly for minor operations, an appointment book should be made, giving time and date, details of the patient's name and address, nature of operation and estimated time allowed. Initially, the doctor should keep this appointment book personally, and personally see every patient. With experience, an accurate estimate of the time each operation takes will be learned and at this stage the appointment book may be taken over by a receptionist or secretary, with clear instructions from the doctor about arrangements for transport and subsequent follow-up. Telephone numbers of patients should be recorded in case it is necessary to change the order of the list and contact the patient at short notice.

A typewritten list of the operations should be prepared with copies for the treatment room, nurses, receptionists, filing clerks, and doctor. By so doing, appropriate patient notes may be prepared, histology forms and containers labelled, and necessary instruments and dressings prepared.

12.3 INFORMING THE PATIENT

The doctor should personally discuss with the patient every detail of the operation: what is involved, the type of anaesthetic, the site and size of any scar, the removal of any sutures, how long the procedure will take, whether transport will be required to take the patient home or whether they will be able to drive or walk home, alone or accompanied. It is important to give an estimate of how long the patient may need to be away from school or work, and any risks of the operations carefully explained. It is also important to advise patients whether the operation will be 100% curative (e.g. excision of simple naevus or cyst) or whether recurrence may be expected and what proportion can be expected to recur (e.g. varicose vein sclerotherapy, excision of ganglia, ingrowing toe-nails). It is well known that much of the information given to patients is not remembered, consequently it is helpful to have pre-printed leaflets to give to the patients to take away with simplified details of their operation, appointment times and any necessary arrangements. These leaflets may also act as an *aide-mémoire* for the doctor and staff (Fig. 12.2).

12.4 COMPLICATIONS

With careful selection, good operating technique and the provision of sterile instruments and dressings, complications from minor surgical procedures are rare. The commonest complication is sepsis – this may be unavoidable if the lesion is already infected (e.g. ingrowing toe-nails, infected sebaceous cysts, and abscesses) or may occur as a result of cross-infection during the operation or post-operative period.

Tissues should be handled as little as possible, a no-touch technique developed by doctor and assistant, breathing and coughing over the wound avoided, sterile drapes utilized to keep the operating field as free from contamination as possible and careful application of skin antiseptics should be made, making sure not to miss any areas. The widespread use of

INGROWING TOE-NAILS POST-OPERATIVE INSTRUCTIONS

1. A small strip of nail, including the nail bed has been removed, and the base treated with pure phenol to prevent this narrow strip from re-growing again.
2. When you arrive home, please rest on a settee with the feet elevated on a cushion for the remainder of the day: this reduces the discomfort and the tendency to bleeding.
3. Any simple analgesic tablet such as aspirin, Disprin, or Panadol may be taken for any post-operative discomfort.
4. Please make an appointment to see Nurse on ________________ at _____ and a second appointment to see Nurse one week later on________________ at _____.

INJECTION TREATMENT FOR VARICOSE VEINS

Injection treatment for varicose veins consists of injecting an irritant fluid into the vein and applying a firm dressing over the injection site. The object of the treatment is to create an inflammation inside the distended vein, and then by compressing the inflamed surfaces together, hope that they will adhere to each other, thus obliterating the lumen of the vein.

The following simple instructions should be followed:

1. The bandages should be left on (day and night) for 3 weeks. Some discomfort should be expected during the first few days. The outer layers should be removed and reapplied if they work loose, but do not disturb the cotton wool rolls over the injection sites.
2. Walk at least 3 miles every day.
3. If you wish to have a bath, the bandaged leg may be kept dry by putting it inside a large watertight polythene bag with an elastic band round the upper end.
4. After 3 weeks, please would you make an appointment to see me when the dressings will be removed.

J. Stuart Brown

Fig. 12.2 Pre-printed information leaflets which may be given to the patients after their operation.

powerful antibiotics as a 'cover' is unnecessary and should be condemned as bad practice; however, the judicious use of antibiotics in a few carefully selected patients is justified and may result in healing by first intention. These may be given orally, by injection, or directly into the lesion (e.g. Fucidin Caviject inserted in abscess cavities prior to closure).

12.4.1 Haemorrhage

This is rarely a problem; most is venous and can be controlled by firm pressure, and the use of diathermy or electrocautery. Small arteries can be clipped with curved mosquito artery forceps and tied if necessary, but most can be controlled by skin sutures alone.

12.4.2 Damage to nerves, tendons and arteries

Again, all these complications are extremely rare; knowledge of the underlying anatomy is essential, the awareness of variations from normal and the use of bloodless operating fields for such operations as carpal tunnel decompression are mandatory. Should damage occur to any nerve, tendon or artery, this fact should be carefully recorded, accurate measure-

CARPAL TUNNEL OPERATION - POST-OPERATIVE INSTRUCTIONS

1. The median nerve passes through a narrow tunnel at the wrist, and your symptoms of pain and pins and needles have been due to pressure on this nerve.
2. The operation consists of splitting the thick tissue which lies in front of the nerve, thus releasing the nerve and removing the pressure.
3. It may take several months before the symptoms disappear, depending on how long the nerve has been trapped: in some instances the pain and pins and needles disappear immediately, but the majority improve gradually.
3. Keep the arm in the sling for two days, and do not disturb the bandages for ten days.
4. There is only one single nylon suture holding the wound together: please make an appointment to see Nurse to have this stitch removed on ______________ at ________.

POST-OPERATIVE INSTRUCTIONS (GANGLION)

A ganglion is a cyst filled with clear jelly: some disappear spontaneously, the majority require operation. Even with careful dissection, a proportion of ganglia recur, in which case they may need a 2nd or 3rd operation.

1. Keep the arm in a sling for 2 days. This reduces swelling and pain.
2. Should there be any discomfort, take aspirin, Disprin, Panadol, paracetamol or similar analgesic in adequate doses every four hours (even through the night if necessary).
3. Leave the bandages undisturbed until the stitches are due to be removed, usually about 10 days.
4. An appointment has been made for you to see our nursing sister to have the stitches removed on ______________________.

ments taken, and a decision taken whether to attempt repair or refer to a specialist colleague. Provided the blood supply to the affected part is adequate, closure and referral at a later date is recommended unless immediate help is available. It is wise that the patient be informed and any action to be taken discussed with him or her.

12.4.3 Medico-legal aspects

Many doctors hesitate to undertake minor surgical procedures, feeling they are at risk from possible litigation should complications arise. Provided the doctor can show that he or she has acquired the necessary skill to perform an individual operation, and has followed accepted guide-lines in the technique and management, there need be no fear and the GP will be supported fully by his or her medical defence organization. Because most doctors are acutely aware of possible risks with minor surgery, they tend to take extra precautions, and overall, the risks of problems occurring in this field are probably less than in many other branches of medicine. Extra safeguards are necessary if the doctor considers performing vasectomies; not only should counselling be comprehensive, but also printed information sheets should be given to the patient, each resected vas, labelled left

	Year 1	Year 2	Year 3	Year 4	Year 5	Year 6	Year 7
Suture of lacerations	26	30	26	31	27	21	27
Sebaceous cysts	11	29	25	26	26	19	27
Meibomian cysts	5	12	6	12	6	13	9
Aspiration of cysts	1	2	0	0	3	3	3
Excision of ganglion (IVRB)	16	9	4	16	7	12	6
Excision synovioma (IVRB)	2	2	4	1	2	2	3
Aspiration bursae	1	1	1	0	0	5	5
Excision dermoid cyst	0	1	2	2	0	0	0
Aspiration hydrocele + phenol	4	1	0	6	2	1	0
Abdominal paracentesis	1	0	4	0	0	2	2
Epididymal cyst + phenol	0	1	0	0	0	0	0
Bartholin's abscess	0	0	0	2	1	3	2
Incision abscess	1	1	3	3	6	6	7
Injection carpal tunnel	5	3	9	12	19	17	7
Decompression carpal tunnel (IVRB)	8	6	6	14	16	10	10
Injection trigger finger	1	3	3	2	3	4	4
Release trigger finger (IVRB)	1	4	4	2	1	1	1
Injection piles	15	11	11	13	21	18	18
Thrombosed external piles	0	9	10	8	9	7	6
Sclerotherapy varicose veins	19	24	34	28	22	22	13
Ligation varicose veins	0	0	2	2	8	1	2
Ingrowing toe-nails	8	17	43	38	31	17	23
Removal nails	15	9	1	5	4	1	4
Curette & diathermy warts	20	24	17	30	41	35	35
Excision papilloma	4	13	8	18	14	11	21
Excision naevus	8	9	9	17	21	16	17
Kerato-acanthoma	0	1	2	0	2	2	1
Excision fibroma	0	4	3	8	5	1	4
Gland biopsy	0	0	1	0	1	0	1
Needle biopsy (breast lump)	0	0	1	3	0	3	1
Sigmoidoscopy	0	0	0	40	37	45	43
Skin biopsy	0	1	2	0	1	0	4
Excision tattoos	2	2	2	3	0	0	0
Excision lipoma	1	4	2	4	7	2	3
Intra-articular injections	2	1	0	0	12	11	15
Injection tennis elbow	12	10	13	10	16	22	24
Injection supraspinatus tendon	3	6	4	4	2	4	4
Nerve block	0	1	1	0	1	2	2
Lumbar puncture	2	2	1	2	0	0	0
Intrathecal nerve block (phenol)	0	0	1	1	0	0	0
IUCD insertion	45	42	30	16	18	22	12
Minor gynaecological	2	2	0	5	1	12	12
Curette & diathermy rodent ulcer	0	0	0	0	10	2	2
Hyfrecate haemangioma	0	0	0	0	15	10	2
Removal pace-maker postmortem	0	0	0	0	1	0	0
Arthrodesis claw toes	0	0	0	0	2	1	0
Miscellaneous	0	0	6	12	6	15	26
Nitrous oxide cryoprobe	0	0	0	0	0	33	29
Total for the year	241	297	301	396	427	434	437

Fig. 12.3 Analysis of minor operations performed over seven years by the author.

and right, should be sent for histological confirmation, follow-up sperm counts arranged and copies filed, the guaranteed reliability explained and the patient's written permission obtained. Most problems of litigation still arise from poor communications with the patient, and the disregard of accepted principles of treatment and should be avoidable.

THIRTEEN

Suturing lacerations

'If thou examinest a man having a wound in his ear, cutting through the flesh, the injury being in the lower part of the ear, and confined to the flesh, thou shouldst draw it together for him with stitching behind the hollow of his ear.'

(Edwin Smith, Surgical Papyrus, 3000–2500 BC)

One of the first skills to be acquired by medical students in their clinical training is the suturing of wounds; in the emergency department they meet a variety of injuries and lacerations, and on the maternity wards they learn how to repair perineal tears and episiotomies. House-surgeons assist at many surgical procedures and are often responsible for suturing the wound at the end of the operation. Thus all doctors by the time they qualify are able to suture the majority of wounds likely to be encountered in any minor surgical operation. If it is considered necessary to suture a wound, the following general principles should be borne in mind:

1. Healing will occur more readily if the skin edges are accurately and carefully opposed to each other.
2. There should be minimum or no tension on the skin edges if at all possible. This may be achieved by careful undercutting of the skin prior to suturing.
3. The skin edges should be slightly everted; this is done by applying slight traction to the skin edge and including slightly more of the dermal layer than skin in the stitch.
4. Many fine sutures, equally placed close together are preferable to larger sutures spaced further apart.
5. Any 'dead space' should be closed either with subcutaneous absorbable sutures, or by including this layer in the skin stitches.
6. All stitches should only remain in place as long as they are needed to give support. Thus stitches on the face may be removed as early as 48 hours–5 days, whereas those on the abdominal wall and foot should remain for 10 days or more.
7. All wounds should be as clean as possible.
8. There should be the minimum of handling and tissue trauma from forceps.
9. Additional support may be given by the use of sterile adhesive strips which can remain in place after the stitches have been removed.

13.1 INSTRUMENTS REQUIRED

The following 'basic set' is recommended for routine suturing and many simple surgical procedures (Fig. 13.1):

1 Kilner needle holder $5\frac{1}{4}''$ (13.3 cm)
1 scalpel handle size 3
scalpel blades 10 and 15

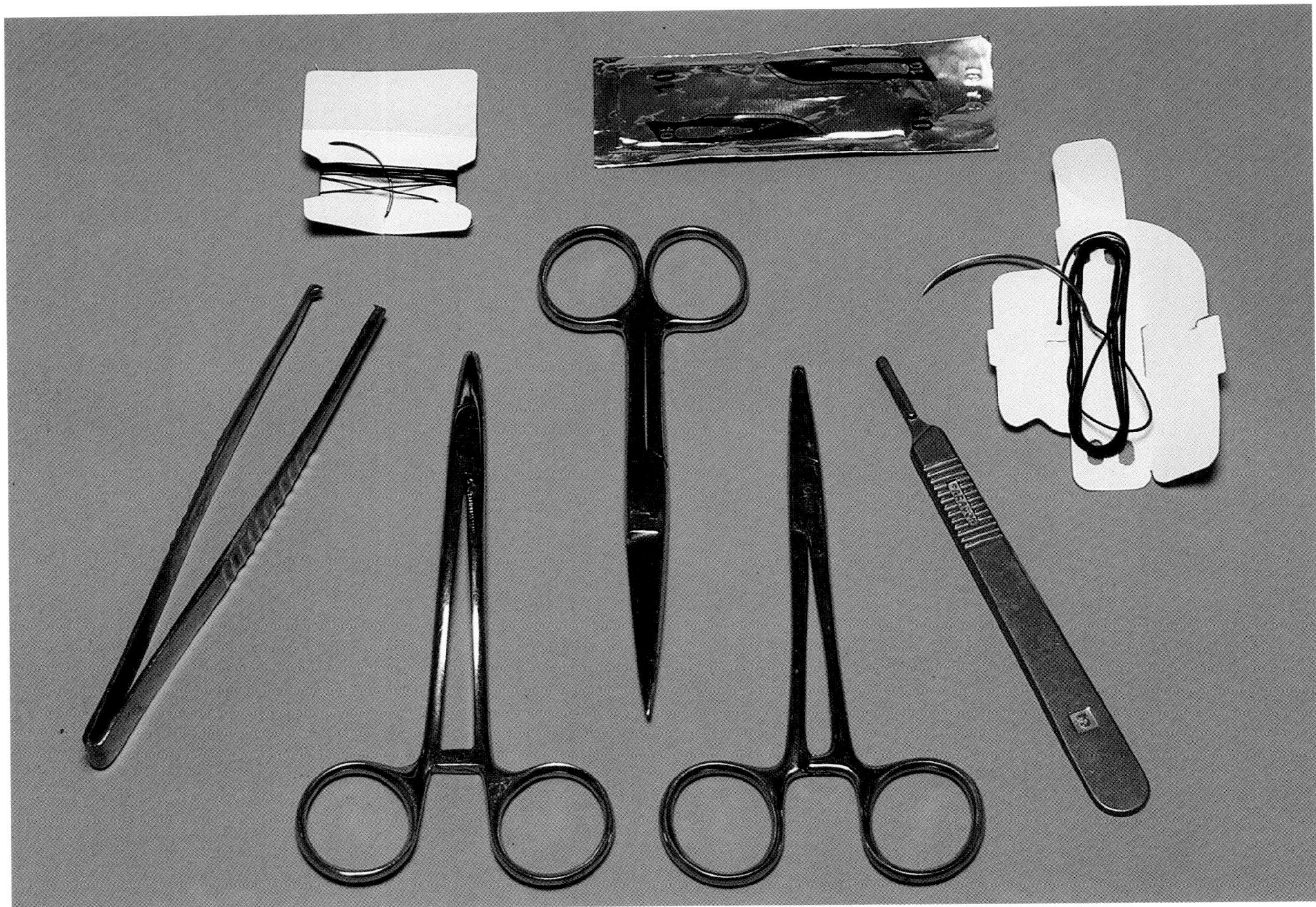

Fig. 13.1 Basic instrument set suitable for most suturing.

1 pair standard stitch scissors (sharp/sharp) 5″ (12.7 cm)
1 pair toothed dissecting forceps 5″ (12.7 cm)

Suture material – individual preference but Ethicon sterile braided silk ref. W667 metric gauge 3 (2/0) on curved reverse cutting needle is very popular and versatile. W533 and W501 are finer gauges if preferred.

Syringes and needles and local anaesthesia: The 2 ml syringe is sufficient for small lacerations, 10 ml or even 20 ml for larger. The finest gauge needles should be selected, and a dental syringe with a screw-on 30 SWG (0.3 mm) needle is ideal for children.

13.2 TECHNIQUE FOR SUTURING LACERATIONS

The patient should be lying comfortably on a couch or operating theatre table, this is preferable to the patient sitting or standing as the most unexpected patients faint during a simple suturing procedure; it is also more comfortable for both the patient and doctor. Good illumination is essential, and the wound should first be carefully inspected to determine the extent and nature of the injury, and to ascertain whether any other

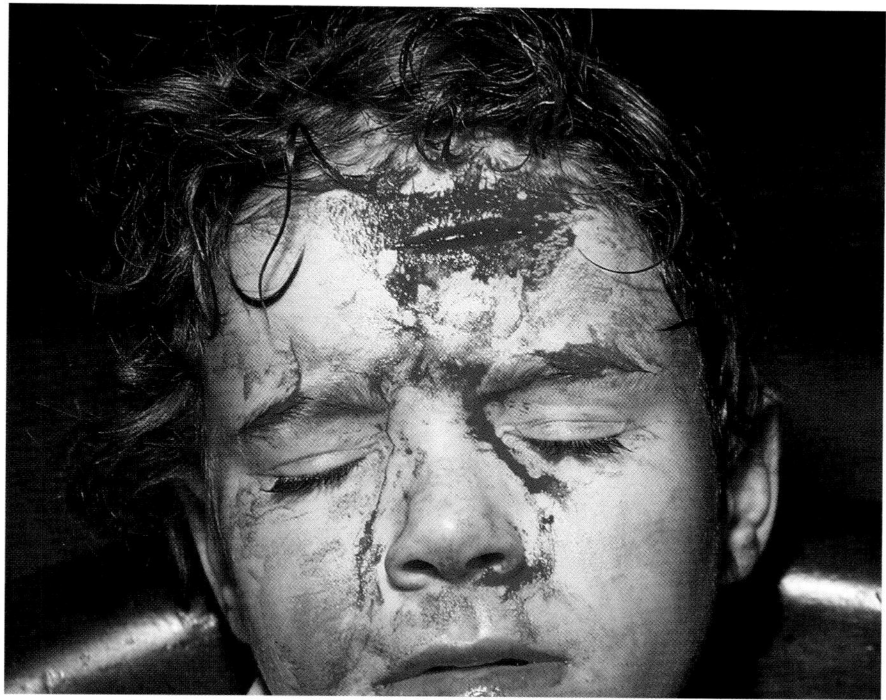

Fig. 13.2 A common injury.

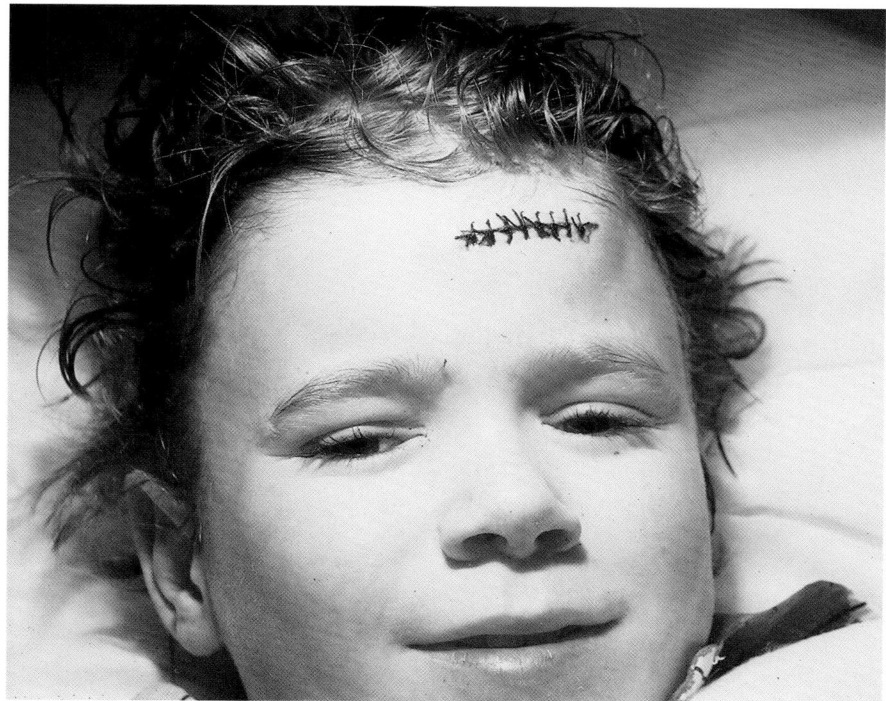

Fig. 13.3 'No hard feelings!'

injury to underlying structures has occurred. Having excluded other injuries, the area should be anaesthetized. This is most conveniently done by infiltration as described in Chapter 7 using first a dental syringe and 30 SWG (0.3 mm) needle, changing to a longer needle and larger syringe if necessary, always remembering the maximum dose of anaesthetic which may be given to this particular patient (take care with the very young and very old).

After allowing a few minutes for anaesthesia to develop, the area may be again inspected, carefully palpated, cleaned thoroughly, and any hairs clipped away from the immediate operative field.

At this stage the doctor will need to decide whether deep tissues will require suturing as well as skin, and if so, catgut or dexon sutures should be inserted. As a general guide, the less deep sutures that are inserted the better, compatible with achieving haemostasis and closing any 'dead' spaces.

Any bleeding points may be dealt with by electrocautery, ligature, clipping, or just firm pressure for a few minutes. Next an attempt should be made to bring the edges of the wound together to see if undue tension will be created. If this is likely, the skin should be widely undercut to help approximate the edges. Any ragged edges should be carefully trimmed, and dead tissue excised.

Using the toothed dissecting forceps to hold the skin edges, interrupted sutures are inserted, tying the knots on the same side, and avoiding any tension, taking into account the fact that tissues may swell during the first two days following injury (Fig. 13.4).

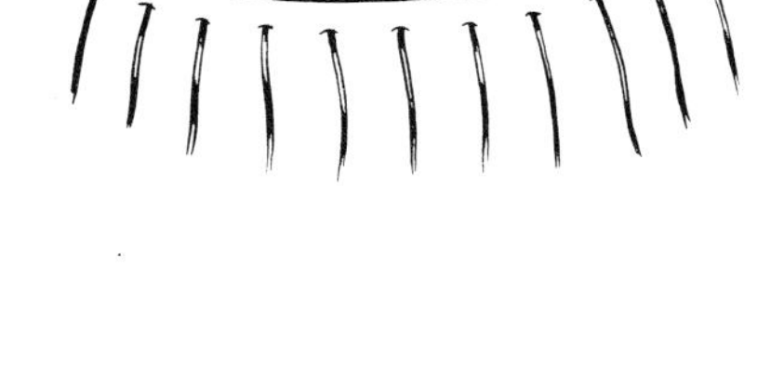

Fig. 13.4 Skin closure with interrupted sutures.

If an assistant is available, 2 Gillies skin hooks can be used, one at either end of the wound, applying traction, which aligns the wound nicely, and makes insertion of sutures easier. A dry dressing may now be applied, with or without a covering of Nobecutane spray on the skin.

Deep, dirty, penetrating wounds should be cleaned as thoroughly as possible, and the patient given prophylactic antibiotics and a reinforcing tetanus immunization if not up-to-date. Dirty contaminated grazes can be scrubbed using Chlorhexidine in detergent (Hibiscrub) after first anaesthetizing the area with infiltration anaesthetic.

13.3 CHOICE OF SKIN CLOSURE

Mention has already been made about alternative closures to sutures, these should always be borne in mind when faced with a laceration. It may be more appropriate to use a subcuticular stitch, sterile self-adhesive strips, or clips or just a firm dressing.

FOURTEEN

Injections and aspirations

'In the cure of ascitic hydropsy proceed thus: after having placed the patient on his back, draw the skin upward. Then take a knife and pierce as far as siphac (peritoneum). Have to hand a cannula and place it in the puncture and draw away as much of the watery matter as the patient may endure. But bear ever in mind that it were better to take too little than empty wholly for the loss of strength that cometh thereby'.

(Mundinus, Abdominal Paracentesis, AD 1275–1326)

Instruments required

sterile syringes and needles
trocar and cannula for abdominal ascites
intravenous cannula size 18 SWG (0.9 mm) for hydrocele
local anaesthetics
steroid injections.

14.1 TENNIS ELBOW (Lateral epicondylitis)

This is one of the easier lesions to inject, but the results are often disappointing inasmuch that many recur after an apparently successful injection.

It is also worth noting that the natural history of lateral epicondylitis or tennis elbow is almost complete resolution in two or three years even without any treatment; therefore the doctor is dealing with a self limiting condition and the effect of any injection is, hopefully, to accelerate healing. In the first instance it is important to establish a correct diagnosis as cervical nerve root entrapment can cause similar pain, particularly C6 lesions referred to the lateral epicondyle. The patient usually complains of pain in the elbow, worse on attempting to pick up wide objects, and can usually localize the point of maximum tenderness. Gripping causes pain, but flexion and extension of the elbow is usually painless. On examination, there is marked tenderness on palpating the extensor insertion into the external (lateral) epicondyle, and pain on resisted dorsiflexion of the wrist. As would be expected the right elbow is affected much more than the left.

14.1.1 Technique

With the patient sitting comfortably facing the doctor and the elbow flexed to a right angle, the point of maximum tenderness is identified (Fig. 14.1).

The overlying skin is painted with Povidone-iodine in alcohol (Betadine alcoholic solution) or similar antiseptic. A mixture of steroid and local anaesthetic is now drawn into a sterile 2 ml syringe using a no-touch technique. Two preparations are commonly used:

1. Methylprednisolone and Lignocaine marketed as Depo-Medrone 40 mg with Lidocaine 10 mg pre-mixed in a 1 or 2 ml vial.

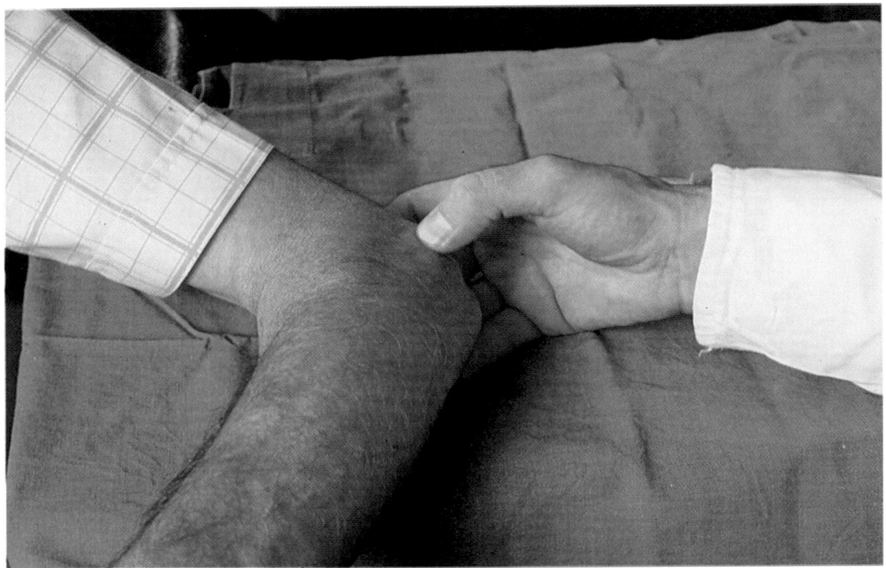

Fig. 14.1 Injection of tennis elbow (lateral epicondylitis) palpating the most tender spot.

2. Triamcinolone Hexacetonide marketed as Lederspan 20 mg in 1 ml vials. This is not pre-mixed with Lignocaine and, if required, must be mixed in the syringe with 1 ml of 2% Lignocaine, giving a final dilution of 1% or 10 mg.

Having drawn the solution into the syringe, the needle is carefully removed and replaced with a new sterile 25 SWG × $\frac{5}{8}''$ (0.5 mm × 16 mm) needle, fixing it very firmly; this reduces still further any risks of cross infection. The patient and doctor should not talk or cough over the exposed needle, and for the same reason it is a good idea to routinely wear a mask.

Without touching the site of the injection or touching the needle, the point of maximum tenderness is located, and the injection made directly into it. Considerable pressure is needed, hence the reason for fixing the

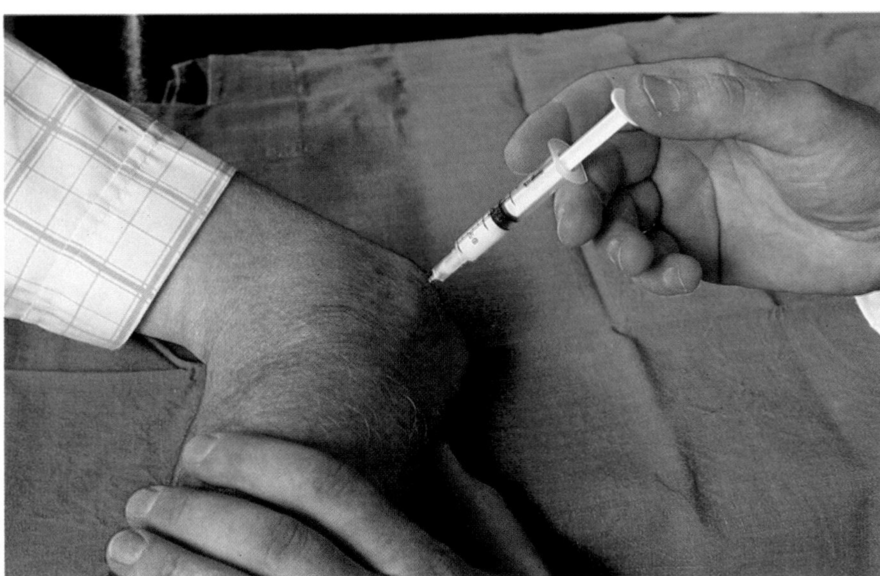

Fig. 14.2 Injection of steroid and local anaesthetic being given into the most tender spot for tennis elbow.

needle firmly to the syringe; the object is to distribute the injection around the bone interface where most of the pain nerve endings are found. The remainder of the injection is placed in the tissues adjacent to the epicondyle (Fig. 14.2).

Having given the injection, the patient is asked to 'work it in' during the next few hours by repeatedly extending the elbow joint pronating the wrist and at the same time palmar flexing the joint. It is also worth warning the patient that the injection site may be extremely painful during the first 24 hours, and thereafter relief may be expected. With meticulous technique there should be no danger of infection, but one of the commonest side-effects to be seen is atrophy of tissues beneath the injection site resulting in a small depression in the skin; this is seen in other situations where subcutaneous steroid injections are given, and is not confined to tennis elbows.

Aftercare is equally important, it is not a good idea to strenuously exercise the hand and fingers – 'to see if it has worked' – on the contrary, the lesion must be rested for several days to allow sound healing.

Despite this, recurrences are common, and the question of a second injection arises. This is unlikely to be as successful as the first, and most doctors therefore limit the number of injections to two or three, preferring to let the condition cure itself spontaneously thereafter.

14.1.2 Alternative treatments

Relief may also be obtained from analgesics, physiotherapy in the form of friction and ultrasonics, and the application of a firm, non-stretch bandage or splint around the body of the forearm muscles just distal to the painful insertion.

14.2 GOLFER'S ELBOW (Medial epicondylitis)

This has the same signs and symptoms as a tennis elbow except that the tenderness is over the medial epicondyle and is reproduced by resisted palmar flexion of the wrist. Treatment is exactly the same as that for tennis elbow, but the volume of injection may be slightly less. The most tender spot is located by extending the elbow and externally rotating the wrist; the overlying area painted with Povidone-iodine in spirit (Betadine alcoholic solution) and the injection made from the anterior surface. It must be remembered that the ulnar nerve lies in a groove just behind the medial epicondyle and any injection should be accurately placed to avoid damage to this nerve. Likewise, it is important to look for any operation scars around the elbow joint in case the patient has had a transposition of the ulnar nerve from behind the epicondyle to in front, for previous nerve entrapment.

14.3 THE PAINFUL SHOULDER

This is a common complaint, and accurate diagnosis of the exact cause is often difficult. Many are due to referred pain from the cervical spine, others from inflamed bursae, tendons or capsule, and it is in this latter group that steroid injections offer much relief.

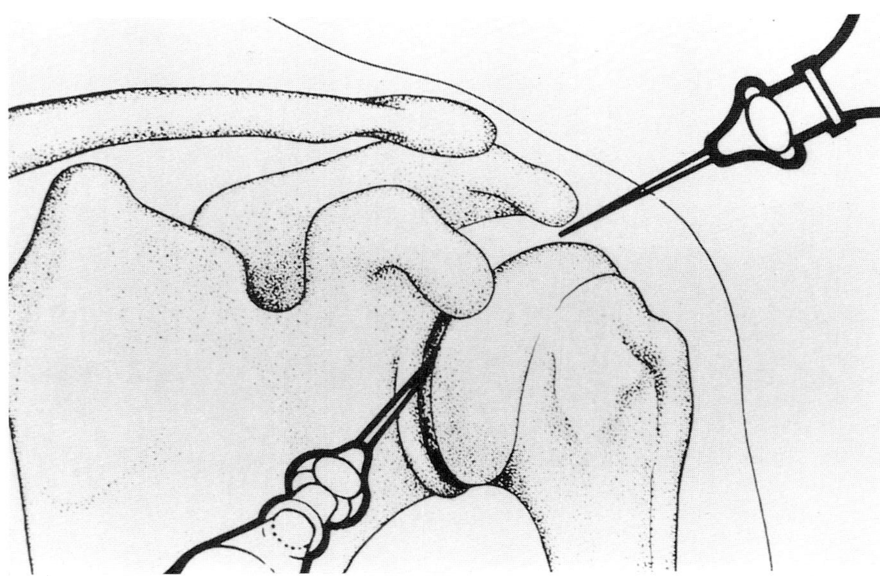

Fig. 14.3 Injection sites for the painful shoulder.

The six common lesions are supraspinatus tendinitis, subacromial bursitis, infraspinatus tendinitis, subscapularis tendinitis, 'capsulitis' and arthritis. Fortunately each can be treated by a common approach, namely the posterior aspect of the shoulder.

14.3.1 Technique

With the patient sitting with his or her back to the doctor, the spine of the scapula is palpated and followed laterally until it becomes the acromial process; using the index finger, the coracoid process is located anteriorly; the line joining these two points gives the direction of injection. The overlying skin is painted with Povidone-iodine in spirit (Betadine alcoholic solution) and 2 ml Methylprednisolone 40 mg with Lignocaine 10 mg (Depo-Medrone with Lidocaine) drawn into a 2 ml syringe. The needle is discarded and replaced with a new 21 SWG × $1\frac{1}{2}$″ (0.8 mm × 40 mm) needle. The needle is inserted about 1″ (2.5 cm) so that it runs below the acromial process towards the coracoid process. There should be no resistance to injection as the needle is in the upper recess of the shoulder joint (Fig. 14.3).

As with tennis and golfer's elbows, the patient should rest the joint for one or two days, then gently exercise; likewise he or she should be warned that the pain may be exacerbated during the first 24 hours before relief is obtained. Injection may often by combined with physiotherapy to achieve maximum benefit.

14.4 INTRA-ARTICULAR INJECTIONS

Any joint in the body may become inflamed, develop an effusion or arthritis, and the majority may be entered with a sterile needle either to withdraw fluid or inject steroids or both. The knee is a suitable joint for both aspiration and injection and will be used as an example.

Certain points need to be borne in mind:

1. An absolute sterile technique is mandatory as a septic arthritis is a disaster.
2. A knowledge of the anatomy of the joint is essential, together with the best method of approach.
3. It should always be remembered that steroid injections rarely cure the underlying pathology – merely suppress the active inflammation.
4. Repeated injections in any one joint are inadvisable unless all other measures have failed.

14.4.1 Technique of aspiration and injection of the knee

Generally an effusion will be present; the best approach to the knee is laterally at the junction of the upper pole of the patella and the patellar tendon.

Povidone-iodine in spirit (Betadine alcoholic solution) is liberally applied, and three separate syringes prepared: the first is a 2 ml syringe loaded with 2% Lignocaine and 25 SWG × $\frac{5}{8}''$ (0.5 mm × 16 mm) needle with which to infiltrate local anaesthetic; the second is a 20 ml sterile syringe with 21 SWG × $1\frac{1}{2}''$ (0.8 mm × 40 mm) needle for aspirating the effusion, and the third is a 2 ml syringe loaded with Triamcinolone Hexacetonide 20 mg/ml 2 ml (Lederspan), the needle on this third syringe is disconnected.

After painting with skin antiseptic, the skin and subcutaneous tissues down to the joint are infiltrated with Lignocaine (Fig. 14.4). Using the same track and the 20 ml syringe, any effusion is aspirated, put in a container for laboratory examination, and the colour noted; it may be clear, cloudy or blood-stained. If clear, this suggests osteoarthritis and if bloodstained, a recent haemarthrosis; in both it is safe to inject steroids. This may be done simply by disconnecting the 20 ml syringe from the needle, and connecting the loaded 2 ml syringe. Gentle aspiration to confirm the needle is still inside the joint is followed by injection of steroid. The needle is then withdrawn, and a sterile dressing applied together with a firm compression bandage. If the aspirate is cloudy, it is not safe to inject steroids before

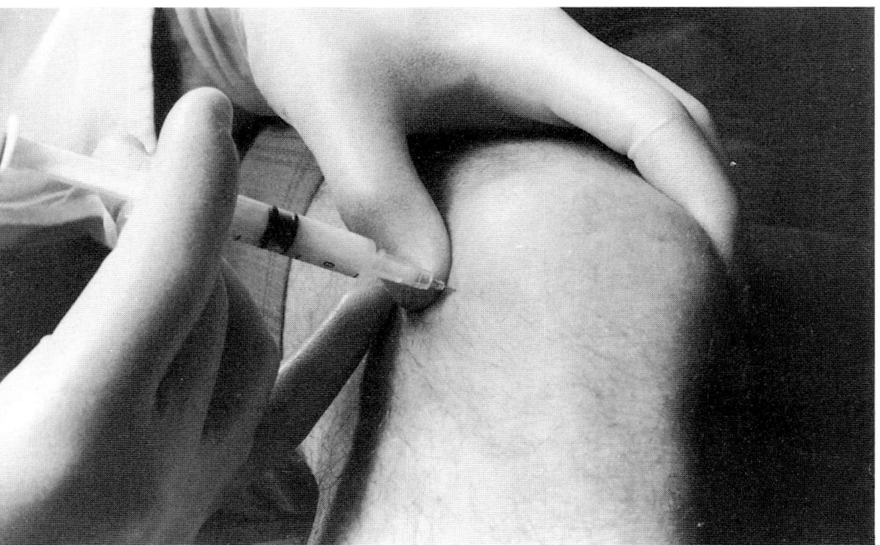

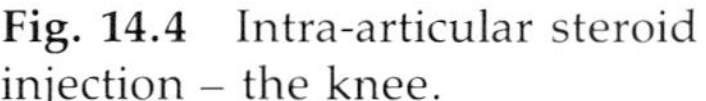

Fig. 14.4 Intra-articular steroid injection – the knee.

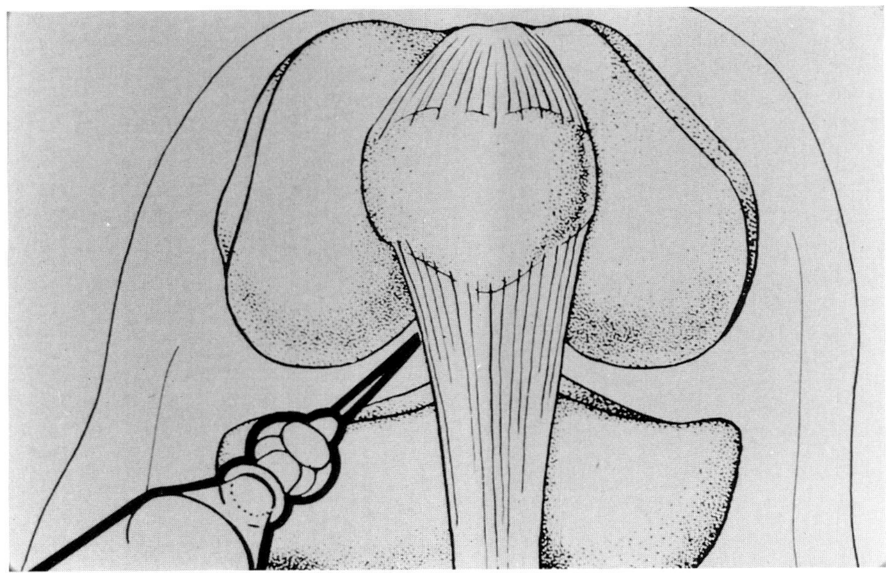

Fig. 14.5 Injection of the knee joint; relationship of needle to underlying structures.

excluding a septic arthritis; the fluid should be examined by Gram's stain and culture, and by polarized light for birefringent crystals found in gout.

It is a good idea to routinely send any fluid aspirated for culture; not only can the unsuspected infection be diagnosed, but, if subsequently any infection occurs, it is helpful to know that it was there at the time of the injection and not introduced by the operator.

14.5 INJECTION OF THE CARPAL TUNNEL

Symptoms from compression of the median nerve in the carpal tunnel are very common and consist of numbness or pain over the middle three fingers, worse at night when the patient typically hangs the arm out of bed or shakes the hand in an attempt to alleviate the discomfort; pain may also be experienced radiating proximally to the elbow, and eventually wasting occurs in the thenar muscles (see Chapter 39). The injection of steroids into the carpal tunnel often relieves all the symptoms permanently, and even if the symptoms recur following injection at least the doctor will know that the diagnosis was correct and that surgical decompression will be successful.

14.5.1 Technique

The injection site is on the palmar surface of the hand, just lateral to the mid-line in the line of the skin crease dividing the forearm and hand. The median nerve lies just beneath the tendon of the palmaris longus muscle (Fig. 14.6).

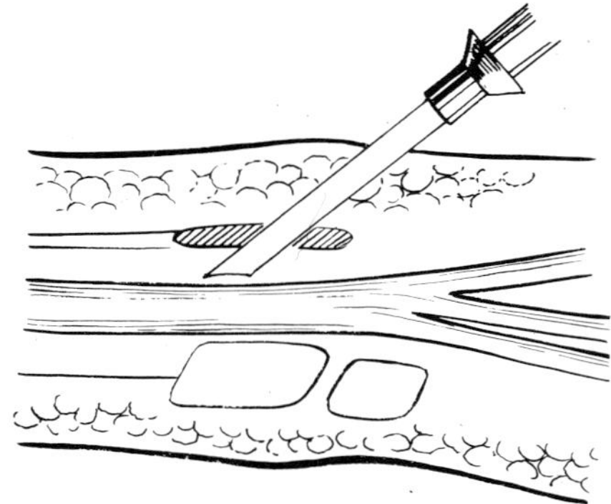

Fig. 14.6 Injection of the carpal tunnel showing angle of needle and bevel in relation to the median nerve.

With the patient sitting by the side of the doctor, his or her hand is placed palm upwards on a sterile sheet from a sterile dressing pack. The overlying area is liberally painted with Povidone-iodine in spirit (Betadine alcoholic solution). Neither patient nor doctor should speak or cough over the injection site.

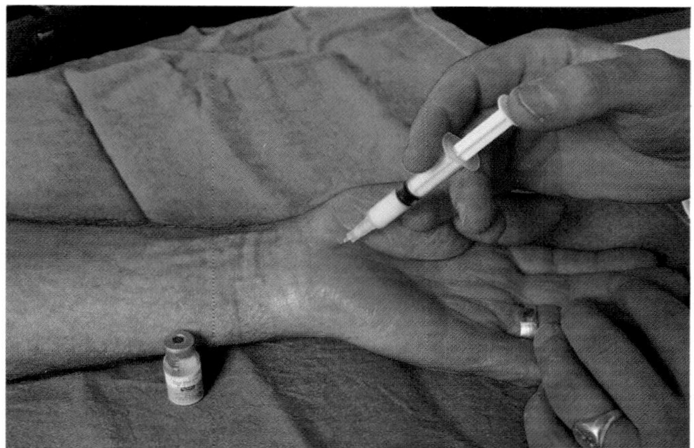

Fig. 14.7 Injection of the carpal tunnel, facing the patient; entry point of the needle is in the thick palmar skin.

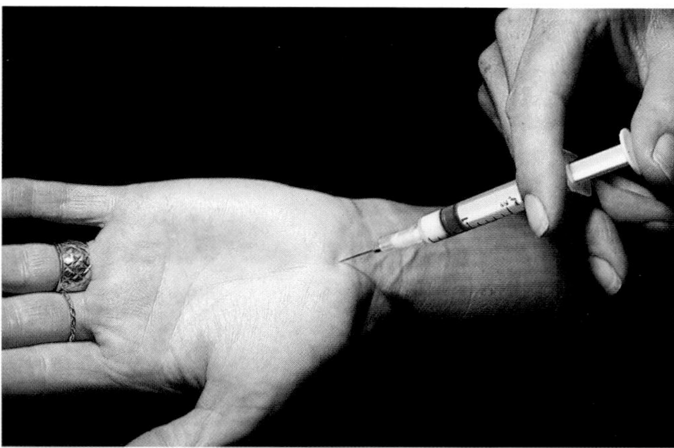

Fig. 14.8 Injection of the carpal tunnel, facing away from the patient; entry point of the needle is in the thinner skin of the wrist.

A 2 ml sterile syringe is used to draw in 1 ml of Methylprednisolone acetate (Depo-Medrone), the needle is then discarded and replaced with a new, sterile 25 SWG × $\frac{5}{8}''$ (0.5 mm × 16 mm) needle. Lignocaine is not added on this occasion as local anaesthetics injected around the median nerve would produce unacceptable anaesthesia of the fingers and in most cases the injection of steroid alone is not painful.

The needle is inserted through the skin, pointing slightly medially and towards the palm, with the bevel pointing downwards and parallel with the underlying nerve. Gentle pressure is applied to the syringe plunger during insertion; as the needle passes through the transverse ligament resistance is encountered, but, immediately the carpal tunnel is entered, loss of resistance is experienced, very similar to that experienced when performing an epidural injection (Figs 14.7 and 14.8).

At this stage the patient may describe mild electric shock feelings in any of the fingers supplied by the median nerve. Then 0.5 ml of the steroid solution is gently injected, stopping if the patient complains of severe pain. The needle is withdrawn and the patient asked to exercise the fingers for a few minutes to distribute the injection fluid along the tunnel. Symptoms are aggravated for 24 hours, but then usually improve after 2–3 days, and this should be explained to the patient before he or she leaves.

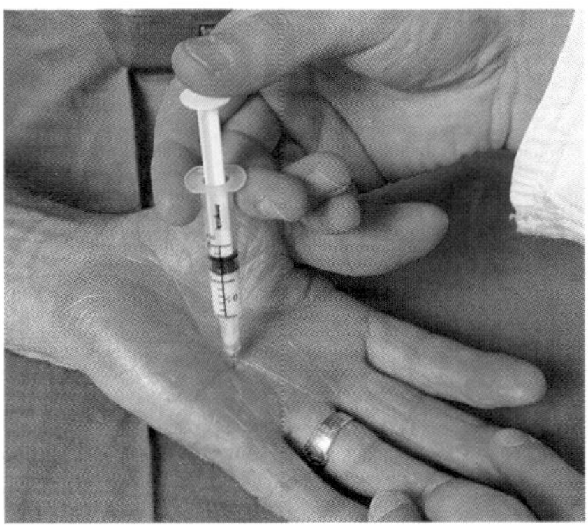

Fig. 14.9 Injection site for trigger finger.

14.6 INJECTION OF TRIGGER FINGER

Trigger finger is due to a tenosynovitis of the flexor tendons of the fingers with a nodular expansion of the tendon which catches in the tendon sheath. The patient complains of locking of one finger or thumb in flexion, which then gives a click when forcibly extended. Treatment by injection is often very successful; the injection is made into the tendon sheath and not the tendon itself.

14.6.1 Technique

The fourth finger is commonly affected and is injected as follows: the patient sits facing the doctor with the hand, palm upwards, resting on a sterile sheet on the desk. Povidone-iodine in spirit (Betadine alcoholic solution) is applied, and 1 ml of Methylprednisolone acetate (Depo-Medrone) drawn into a 1 or 2 ml syringe. The needle is discarded and a new, sterile, 25 SWG × $\frac{5}{8}$" (0.5 mm × 16 mm) needle attached. The injection is made over the site of the triggering, which is commonly in line with the flexor tendon where it crosses the distal palmar crease. As with carpal tunnel injection, the needle should be inserted at an angle with the bevel pointing downwards, parallel to the underlying tendon, applying gentle pressure to the syringe plunger as the needle is advanced. By palpating the tendon sheath with the fingers of the opposite hand, the doctor can usually feel when the injection fluid has entered the tendon sheath. An injection of 0.5 ml of solution is made, the needle is withdrawn, and the patient asked to exercise all the fingers for a minute to evenly distribute the steroid. Improvement usually occurs after 48 hours and may be permanent. Where triggering recurs, surgical division of the sheath is recommended (see Chapter 40) (Fig. 14.9).

14.7 ASPIRATION OF CYSTS AND BURSAE

Simple cysts may occur anywhere in the body, they may contain watery fluid which can be easily aspirated with a needle, or thick semi-solid material which is quite impossible to aspirate through any needle. The two most commonly encountered cysts occur in the breast and thyroid; aspiration in these situations affords immense relief to patient and doctor alike and is often curative. As with all injection techniques, scrupulous asepsis must be observed, the minimum of trauma inflicted by the selection of the finest needle consistent with aspiration, and all fluid aspirated should be sent for cytological examination. Where any possibility of infection exists, the fluid should, in addition be sent for bacterial culture.

14.7.1 Aspiration of breast cysts

The typical breast cyst is smooth, round, very mobile, non-painful, and not adherent to skin or deep structures. Diagnosis may be helped by the use of ultrasonography and mammography, but ultimately the only way to establish an accurate diagnosis is by aspiration. It follows that there will be occasions when a 'typical' breast cyst is found on aspiration to be solid, in this situation, the needle should not be immediately withdrawn, but used for needle biopsy.

To carry out the aspiration it is more comfortable for the patient to be lying down; the skin overlying the cyst is liberally painted with Povidone-iodine in spirit (Betadine alcoholic solution) and the injection site anaesthetized using Lignocaine and a fine 25 SWG × $\frac{5}{8}$" (0.5 mm × 16 mm) needle. A 20 ml sterile syringe with 19 SWG × $1\frac{1}{2}$" (1.1 mm × 38 mm) needle is used for aspiration. The cyst should first be fixed with finger and thumb of the left hand, and the aspirating needle pointed towards the centre of the cyst. By applying gentle traction to the syringe plunger as the needle is advanced, the practitioner will know when the cyst has been entered. Typically the fluid aspirated is a dark green colour; as much as possible should be removed, hopefully emptying the cyst, and sent for cytology. Even if a negative cytology is obtained, the patient should be seen again in four weeks to check that the cyst has not reformed.

14.7.2 Thyroid cysts

Although not as common as breast cysts, thyroid cysts are just as easy to aspirate. It is advisable to confirm the diagnosis by ultrasonography or scan, and the technique, precautions, cytological examination and follow-up are identical to those followed for breast cysts.

14.7.3 Aspiration of semimembranosus bursae (Bakers cysts)

This is a distention of the semimembranosus–gastrocnemius bursa; it communicates with the knee joint via a one-way valve, allowing fluid to travel from the joint to the bursa, but not from the bursa to the joint. Disease of the knee joint which results in an effusion may produce fluid faster than it can be absorbed by the bursa, and a cyst will then form. It follows, therefore, that in many cases, correct management of the distended semimembranosus bursa consists in treating the knee joint.

Where the bursa is grossly distended and causing pain, aspiration and injection may alleviate the symptoms (Fig. 14.10). The patient should be lying prone, with a small pillow under the knee to slightly hyper-extend the joint and distend the bursa. Povidone-iodine in spirit (Betadine alcoholic solution) is applied over the popliteal fossa, and the skin overlying the cyst anaesthetized using Lignocaine and a fine needle. Using a 20 ml syringe and 21 SWG × $1\frac{1}{2}''$ (0.8 mm × 40 mm) needle, the bursa may be completely aspirated and the contents sent for examination. Leaving the needle in the cyst, the 20 ml syringe is exchanged for a 2 ml syringe loaded with Methylprednisolone acetate 40 mg/ml (Depo-Medrone) 2 ml which may then be injected. Recurrence is common for the reasons mentioned.

An alternative treatment to steroid injection is aspiration followed by the injection of 2.5% aqueous phenol. This is a method which gives excellent results in hydrocele and epididymal cysts and is applicable to semimembranosus bursae.

The initial aspiration is performed exactly as described, but instead of using Methylprednisolone, a sterile 2.5% aqueous phenol solution is injected. The volume injected is proportional to the amount of fluid aspirated according to the following formula:

Volume aspirated	Volume injected
0– 20 ml	2.5 ml
20– 50 ml	5 ml
50–100 ml	10 ml

The treatment needs to be repeated on two or more occasions before reduction in the size of the bursa is noticed. As with steroid injections, recurrence is common and attention usually needs to be directed at the underlying disease causing effusion in the knee joint.

14.7.4 Aspiration and injection of hydrocele

A primary hydrocele is an excessive collection of serous fluid in the tunica vaginalis within the scrotum; it occurs at any age, but most commonly in

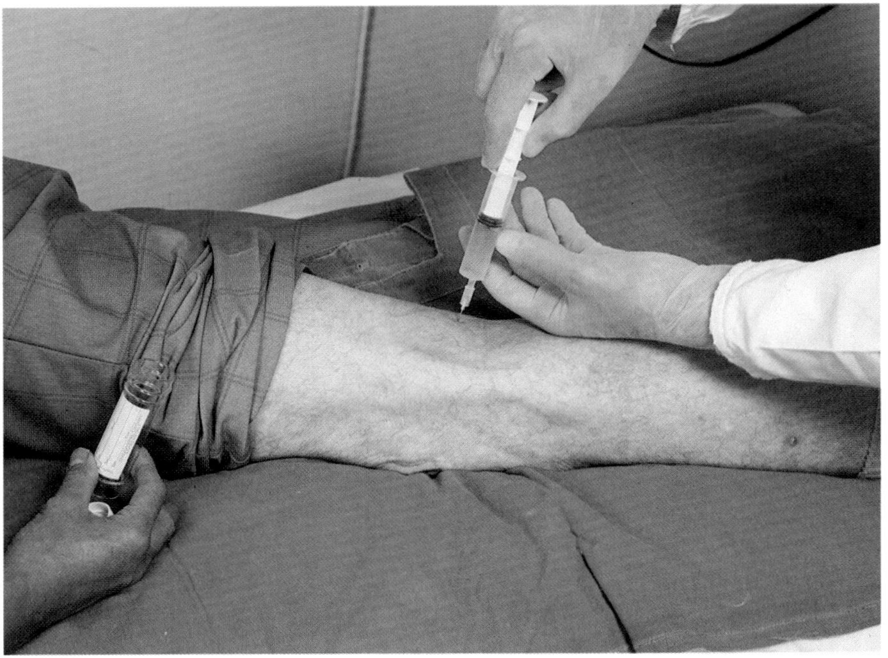

Fig. 14.10 Aspiration of semimembranosus bursa.

adult life. The diagnosis is usually straightforward, particularly if the swelling transilluminates, but it must be remembered that a hernia in an infant also transilluminates.

Aspiration alone rarely cures a hydrocele, but aspiration and the injection of dilute aqueous phenol on two or three separate occasions can offer up to 90% cure [17]; failing this, surgical treatment of the tunica vaginalis is recommended.

A secondary hydrocele occurs as a result of infection or inflammation within the scrotum, thus it is always important to first examine the testis,

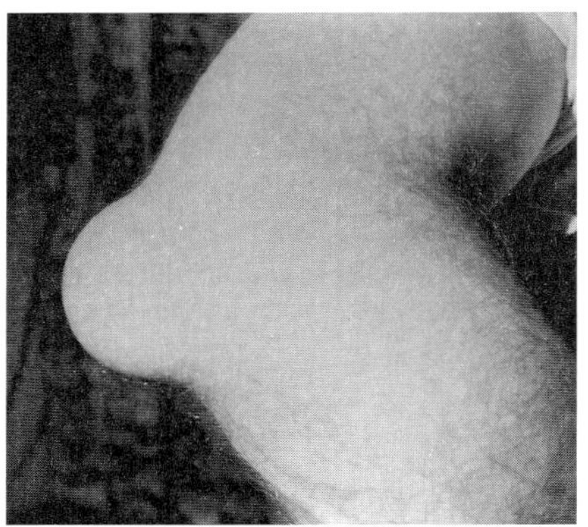

Fig. 14.11 Olecranon bursitis.

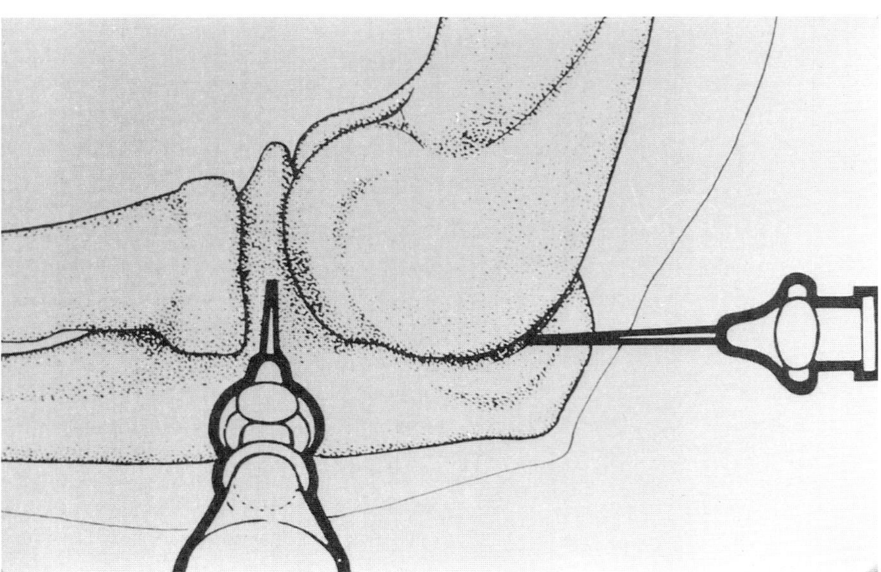

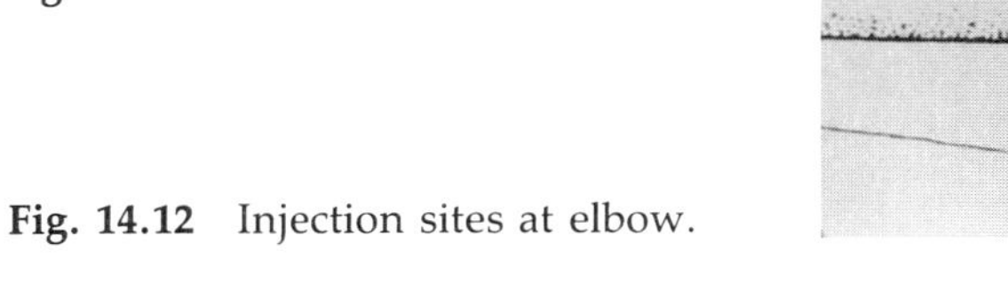

Fig. 14.12 Injection sites at elbow.

epididymis and cord to exclude any disease in these organs. The treatment of a secondary hydrocele is the treatment of its cause.

Instruments required

> 2 ml syringe with 25 SWG × $\frac{5}{8}$" (0.5 mm × 16 mm) needle
> 2 ml 1% Lignocaine
> 18 SWG (0.9 mm) intravenous cannula e.g. Abbocath – T 18
> 10 ml ampoules of 2.5% aqueous sterile phenol
> 20 ml syringes for aspiration and injection

An injection of 2.5% aqueous phenol is not a standard preparation, therefore it needs to be prepared specially; however it has a good shelf life and a small number may be kept in store ready for use.

The technique for aspiration and injection of hydrocele is as follows. The patient should lie on the couch or operating table; good illumination is important, a sterile sheet should be placed under the scrotum and between the legs. Povidone-iodine in spirit (Betadine alcoholic solution) is applied to the scrotum – this may cause a slight stinging sensation – and a point is chosen for aspiration. This point should be on the lower side, away from the testicle and avoiding any blood vessels on the surface of the scrotum. Local anaesthetic is carefully injected through the scrotal wall and underlying tissues, down to the hydrocele sac. This may be confirmed by gently withdrawing the syringe plunger and noting straw coloured fluid entering the syringe. In a relatively small hydrocele it helps to hold the neck of the hydrocele, this makes it tense and prevents it extending into the inguinal canal, it also ensures that the operator has not missed an inguinal-scrotal hernia.

The local anaesthetic needle is now withdrawn, and the 18 SWG (0.9 mm) intravenous cannula inserted through the same needle track. By removing the central cannula needle, a soft, pliable catheter is now situated within the hydrocele sac: this is far less traumatic than the old steel trocar and cannula, and gives equally good results. The serous fluid may either be allowed to run out freely into a container, or aspirated by connecting a 20 ml syringe to the cannula, with or without a three-way tap. As the hydrocele empties the sac is gently compressed with the left hand to remove most of the fluid, and the volume noted. If any doubt exists about the underlying pathology, the fluid should be sent for culture and cytology.

Keeping the cannula in place, a calculated volume of 2.5% sterile aqueous phenol is now injected according to the following formula:

Volume aspirated	Volume injected 2.5% phenol
Up to 50 ml	5 ml
Up to 200 ml	10 ml
Up to 400 ml	15 ml
Over 400 ml	20 ml

The cannula is now withdrawn and a simple collodion dressing applied.

After six weeks the procedure is repeated; most of the hydrocele will have recurred and it is important to have warned the patient that this is likely.

At the second aspiration, if it is noticed that the fluid appears darker or even blood stained, success can be anticipated.

The patient is seen a third time six weeks later, and on this occasion the volume of fluid should be considerably less, or may not have recollected at all. For the elderly patient who would be a poor general anaesthetic and surgical risk, this is undoubtedly the treatment of choice, offering over 90% chance of complete cure.

14.7.5 Epididymal cysts

These are not as common as a primary hydrocele, nevertheless they can be aspirated and injected with 2.5% aqueous phenol exactly as described for hydrocele. Success is even higher offering nearly 100% cure, provided the cyst is not multiloculated, in which case surgical excision is probably the treatment of choice.

14.8 ABDOMINAL ASCITES

By far the commonest cause of ascites seen by the general practitioner is intra-abdominal malignancy. By this stage of their illness, such patients are ill, weak, nauseated and breathless. It is therefore, very much kinder to 'bring the mountain to Mohammed' by taking the instruments and equipment to the patient's bedside, rather than transporting an already terminally ill patient to the surgery or hospital, particularly as the procedure will weaken the patient still further. Additionally, by draining the ascites in the patient's own bedroom, an intravenous 'premedication' injection of pethidine (Demerol) 50 mg and Diazepam 5–10 mg may be given so that the patient actually sleeps throughout the procedure and has no recollection of it afterwards; consequently will have no apprehension should it need to be repeated at another date subsequently.

With modern diuretics, abdominal paracentesis is not performed as frequently as formerly, nevertheless there are significant numbers of patients who obtain good relief of their symptoms by judicious aspiration. It is not necessary, nor desirable, to draw off all the ascites – such a manoeuvre would be likely to precipitate a severe hypotensive reaction and would rapidly deplete the patient of large quantities of protein; the aim should be to remove enough fluid to make the abdomen feel soft, and to alleviate dyspnoea, vomiting and discomfort. If doubt exists about the exact cause of the ascites, a diagnostic aspiration is easily performed, and the fluid sent for analysis, culture and cytology. If this reveals malignant cells, the diagnosis may be easier, and the need for an exploratory laparotomy avoided.

In addition to aspiration, cytotoxic drugs may be injected into the peritoneal cavity through the same cannula.

Instruments required for abdominal paracentesis

1 5 ml syringe with 23 SWG × 1″ (0.6 mm × 25 mm) needle with pethidine (Demerol) 50 mg and Diazepam 5–10 mg pre-mixed (this may appear cloudy but usually clears)

1 5 ml syringe with 25 SWG × $\frac{5}{8}$″ (0.5 mm × 16 mm) needle loaded with Lignocaine 1% and adrenalin 1:200 000

1 needle 21 SWG × 1½″ (0.8 mm × 40 mm)
sterile dressing pack
abdominal paracentesis pack (comprising trocar and cannula, connecting tubing, connector, adjustable screw clamp)
self-adhesive tape 1″ (25 mm)
Povidone-iodine in spirit (Betadine alcoholic solution)
1 standard sterile urine collecting bag with drainage tap
sterile universal containers if required for culture, examination of cytology.
1 many-tailed bandage (optional)
4 large safety pins.

14.8.1 Technique for abdominal paracentesis

The patient will already be in bed and preferably with three or four pillows so that he or she is semi-recumbent. A premedication intravenous injection of pethidine (Demerol) and Diazepam may be offered; some patients will appreciate being asleep for the aspiration, others will prefer to remain awake. Certainly with careful attention to detail while infiltrating with local anaesthetic, the procedure is totally without discomfort.

Depending on the underlying intra-abdominal pathology, a site is chosen away from any masses, usually in the lower abdomen towards the flank; the diagnosis of ascites is verified by gentle percussion, and the patient turned very gently towards the chosen side. Repeat percussion should confirm the presence of shifting dullness. A waterproof dressing sheet (Inco-sheets are ideal) is placed under the patient to protect the lower sheet, and the area chosen liberally painted with Povidone-iodine in spirit (Betadine alcoholic solution). Using the 25 SWG × ⅝″ (0.5 mm × 16 mm) needle on the 5 ml syringe with Lignocaine and adrenalin, a small 'bleb' of local anaesthetic is raised in the skin. Very gradually, the needle is advanced through the skin and underlying tissues, injecting all the time. If the 25 SWG needle is not long enough to reach the peritoneal cavity, it is exchanged for a 23 SWG × 1″ (0.6 mm × 25 mm) or 21 SWG × 1½″ (0.8 mm × 40 mm) needle, and the injection continued (Fig. 14.13). The peritoneum is particularly sensitive, and great care should be used to infiltrate and advance the needle very slowly, allowing adequate time for anaesthesia to develop before advancing the needle. As this is the only part of the procedure which can be uncomfortable if poor technique is used, it is worth spending time to ensure that it is completely painless. This will also increase the patient's confidence and help to allay any anxiety. If the first paracentesis has been painless, the patient will not mind any subsequent aspirations.

Having completely anaesthetized the track from skin to peritoneum, the abdominal trocar and cannula is inserted exactly through the same track. A little pressure is usually necessary, accompanied by a rotating action. Once the peritoneal cavity is entered, the trocar is withdrawn 1 cm and the blunt cannula pushed in to its hub. The trocar is now withdrawn, ascitic fluid spurts from the cannula, which should be rapidly connected via the thin rubber tubing and connector directly to a sterile urine drainage bag with drainage tap; this in turn can be attached to the patient's mattress with two large safety pins. The volume of ascites can be easily measured by reading the quantity on the marks on the urine drainage bag. When full, the bag can

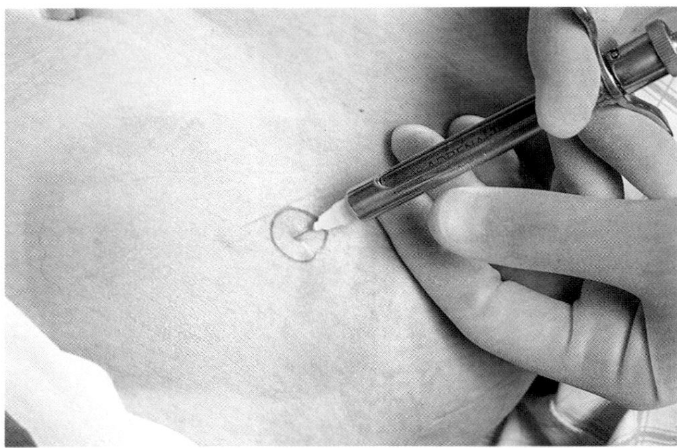

Fig. 14.13 Abdominal paracentesis; after preliminary skin antisepsis, local anaesthetic is infiltrated through the skin, down to peritoneum.

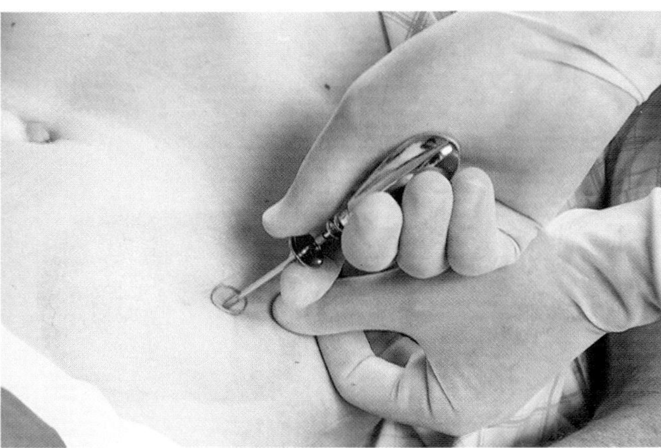

Fig. 14.14 Insertion of trocar and cannula.

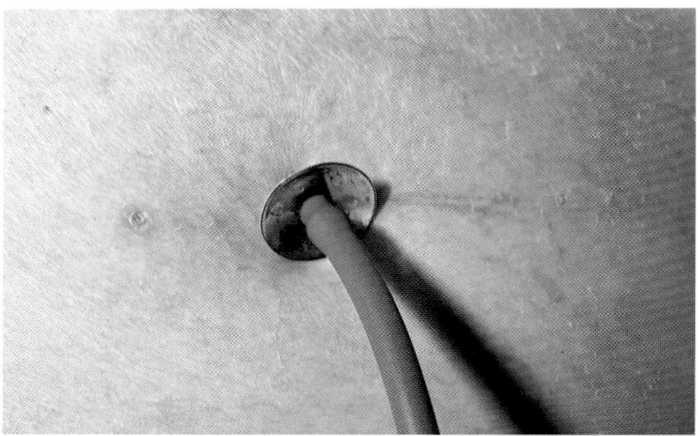

Fig. 14.15 The trocar is withdrawn, and the cannula connected to rubber tubing to a drainage bag.

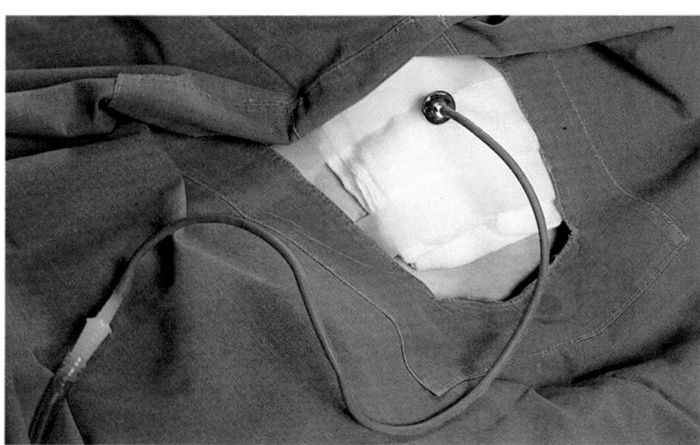

Fig. 14.16 Rubber tubing is connected to urine drainage bag.

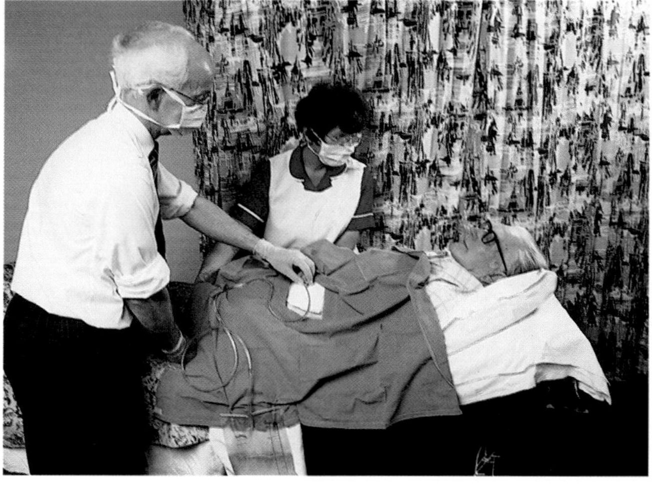

Fig. 14.17 Abdominal paracentesis. A procedure which may readily be performed in the patient's home.

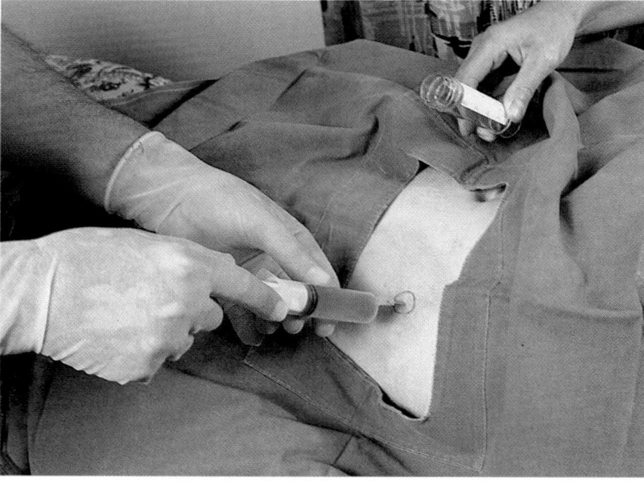

Fig. 14.18 Abdominal paracentesis; diagnostic aspiration. Fluid may then be sent for analysis and cytology.

be emptied merely by opening the drainage tap into a basin beneath. If the rate of flow via the cannula is too rapid, it may be slowed by the application of an adjustable screw clamp to the rubber tubing (Fig. 14.16). Throughout the procedure, regular checks on the patient's pulse and blood pressure should be made.

Once sufficient fluid has been withdrawn to alleviate pressure effects, nausea, dyspnoea, discomfort and tightness, the cannula should be withdrawn, a self-adhesive dressing applied, and if thought necessary, a many-tailed abdominal bandage applied. Unless an excessive volume of fluid has been withdrawn this is probably unnecessary.

The patient should then remain in the bed for the next twelve hours to allow the circulation and blood pressure to reach equilibrium, should they need to get out of bed for any reason they should be accompanied.

The immediate relief of symptoms is generally followed by a gradual weakening of the patient, and on average it is rarely necessary to have to repeat an abdominal paracentesis more than three times.

The procedure for diagnostic 'tap' is exactly the same as for paracentesis, except that a 20 ml syringe attached to a 21 SWG × 1½″ (0.8 mm × 40 mm) needle is used instead of the trocar and cannula (Fig. 14.18).

If preferred, a size 14 SWG (2 mm) intravenous cannula (Abbocath T) 14 may be used in place of the traditional trocar and cannula; this gives equally good results, and is probably slightly easier to insert, but a Luer type adaptor is necessary to connect to the tubing.

14.9 ASPIRATION OF PLEURAL EFFUSIONS

The majority of general practitioners will probably not need to aspirate pleural effusions, the main indication is diagnostic cytology; carcinoma of the lung is now replacing tuberculosis and empyema as the main indication for aspiration. A chest X-ray is desirable whenever possible, this will help to decide the best site for aspiration. With modern chemotherapeutic agents, radiotherapy, diuretics and surgery, the need for large volume aspiration is far less than in previous years.

Instruments required

- 10 ml syringe filled with 1% Lignocaine and 1:200 000 adrenalin
- 1 25 SWG × ⅝″ (0.5 mm × 16 mm) needle
- 1 2-way tap with Luer connectors
- 1 21 SWG × 2½″ (0.8 mm × 63 mm) needle
- sterile universal containers

Careful clinical examination and a recent chest X-ray will determine the best site for aspiration; this will usually be an intercostal space towards the back. A preliminary intravenous injection of pethidine (Demerol) 50 mg and Diazepam 5–10 mg may be offered if the patient is unduly apprehensive.

The overlying skin is painted with Povidone-iodine in spirit (Betadine alcoholic solution) and a small amount of Lignocaine injected intradermally with the 25 SWG (0.5 mm) needle to raise a wheal. The needle is then changed for the longer 21 SWG (0.8 mm) needle and two-way tap and the subcutaneous tissues, intercostal muscles and pleura infiltrated with local

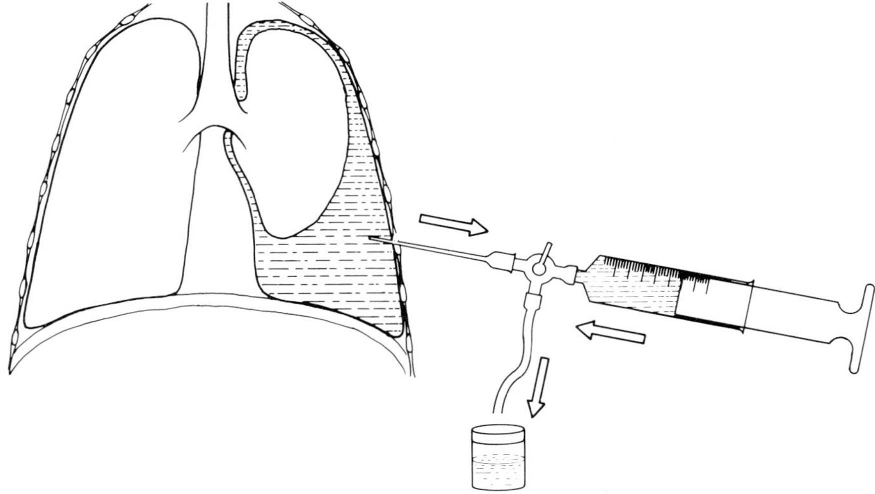

Fig. 14.19 Aspiration of pleural effusion.

anaesthetic. As with abdominal paracentesis, the local anaesthetic should be given very slowly, injecting a little before advancing the needle, and allowing time for the area to become anaesthetized. The doctor should be fully conversant with the working of the two-way tap and should test it before use; it should be possible to inject local anaesthetic through the needle, aspirate fluid back, and by turning the tap, isolate the needle in the pleural cavity while injecting the aspirated fluid into the universal container. It is essential that air is not accidentally allowed into the chest.

Normally the practitioner can feel the various layers through which the aspirating needle is passing; as soon as the pleural cavity is entered, fluid should be withdrawn into the syringe and transferred to the universal container (Fig. 14.19). If it is intended only to withdraw a small quantity of effusion for cytology, the two-way tap may be omitted and a 20 ml sterile syringe with 21 SWG × $2\frac{1}{2}$″ (0.8 mm × 63 mm) needle used instead. In this case, just 20 ml of fluid are taken and the needle and syringe are withdrawn. A collodion dressing is immediately applied.

14.10 NEEDLE BIOPSY

Histological diagnosis of certain tumours may be obtained by needle biopsy. Its use in general practice is limited, but it has a particular place for swellings in the breast which the practitioner feels are probably cystic and which, when aspiration is attempted, produce no fluid and feel hard, indicating the possibility of a tumour. By applying strong traction to the syringe plunger to create a vacuum and at the same time rotating the syringe and needle in a clockwise and anticlockwise direction as the needle is slowly withdrawn, a small piece of tissue will be left in the needle (Fig. 14.20).

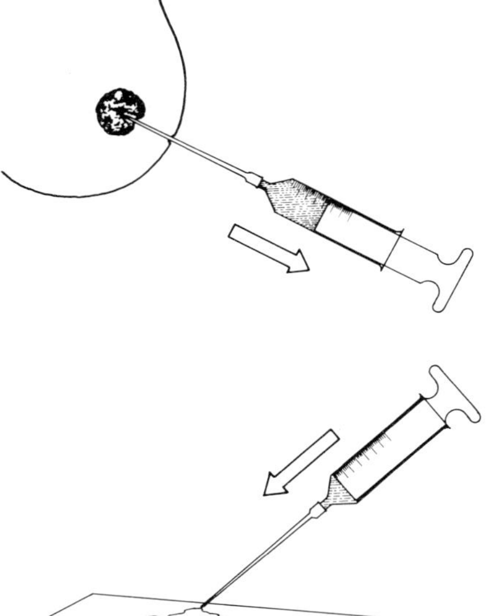

Fig. 14.20 Needle aspiration of breast lump.

By carefully 'blowing' the contents of the needle on a microscope slide, fixing with preservative (the fixative used for cervical cytology is suitable) a sample may be sent for histological or cytological examination. Although not giving 100% positive accuracy, nevertheless a diagnosis may be made correctly in about 90% of needle biopsies. Obviously a swelling with a negative needle biopsy should still be referred to the surgeons for excision, but a swelling with a positive diagnosis on needle biopsy enables the patient and surgeon to plan the most appropriate treatment. Biopsy specimens may also be taken using a Tru-Cut biopsy needle; this is manufactured as a sterile disposable unit in various lengths and diameters (Fig. 14.21).

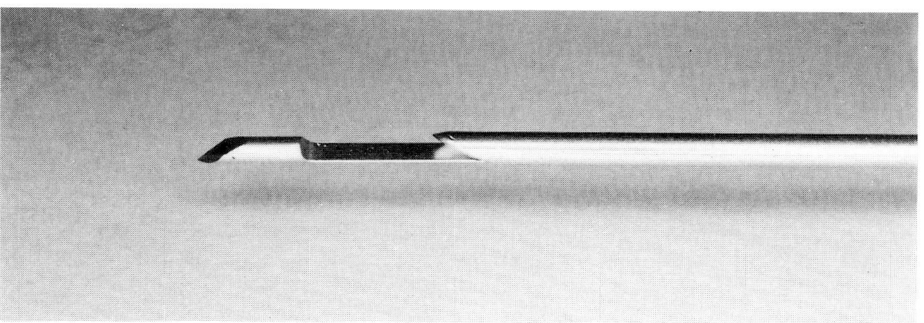

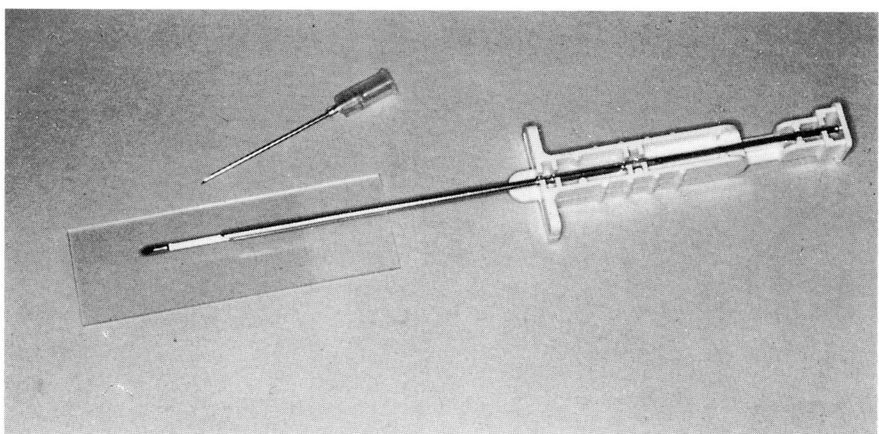

Fig. 14.21 The tru-cut biopsy needle (Travenol Laboratories Inc.).

FIFTEEN

Incision of abscesses

'Recent wounds if inflammation has set in, will result in fever with chills and throbbing. One should induce suppuration as soon as possible and not let the pus be blocked up. The flesh should be lacerated by the weapon. After that new tissue sprouts up'

(Hippocrates, 460–377 BC)

Instruments required

- scalpel handle size 3
- scalpel blade no. 11
- 1 malleable probe
- 1 pair sinus forceps
- assorted small drains
- Fucidin Caviject
- sterile dressings
- wide-bore aspirating needle and syringe.

It is only within one generation that we have witnessed a dramatic reduction in the numbers of bacterial infections; largely thanks to antibiotics. The image of the family doctor taking out his 'lancet' from his pocket to open a 'boil' is still in living memory! Large necrotic abscesses, so familiar in the last century, are now fortunately rarer, and in one year, the general practitioner will need to open only a few. Common sites for abscesses are the perineum, infected operation scars, and fingers. Small abscesses probably require little other than a dry dressing.

Spreading cellulitis and induration with lymphangitis is best treated

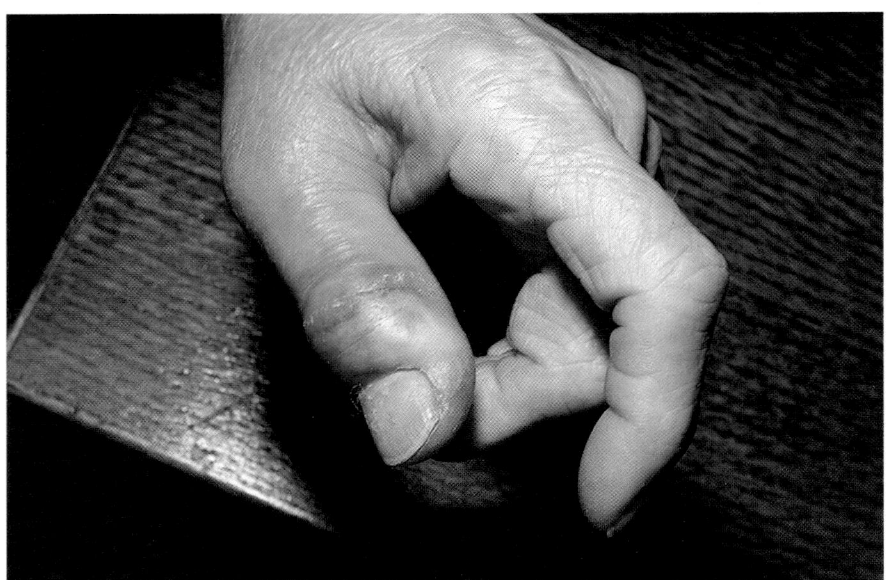

Fig. 15.1 Paronychia thumb; simple incision and dressing is all that is required.

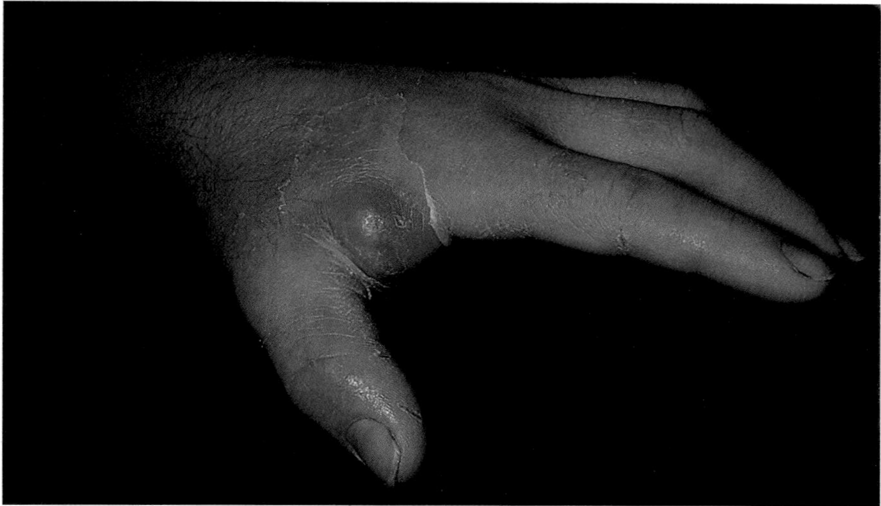

Fig. 15.2 Web-space abscess; incision and dressing required.

with antibiotics, but once pus has collected it should be released, usually by incision. If the abscess is superficial and distending the overlying skin which has become thinned, incision using a pointed no. 11 scalpel blade on no. 3 handle is all that is necessary. Deeper abscesses, recognized by fluctuation, pain, fever and rigors with leucocytosis will require incision, but because of the pain, will require some form of anaesthetic; this may best be managed with a general anaesthetic, but occasionally, where a general anaesthetic is considered inappropriate, careful local anaesthesia may suffice. However, even this causes pain, is not always effective, and increases the risk of spreading the infection.

Having incised the abscess, the pus should be expelled by pressure, a bacterial swab taken for culture of the organisms, and a suitable drain inserted to prevent premature closure of the wound.

Recently good results have been obtained by incising the abscess, curetting the lining, and instilling Fucidin Caviject. No drain is necessary, a dry dressing is applied, healing occurs rapidly and recurrence is rare. In some cases, even primary closure is possible.

Aspiration alone, using a wide bore needle, often results in a cure, particularly with Bartholin's abscesses (see Chapter 20) and may avoid the need for more radical surgery.

SIXTEEN

Warts and verrucae

'Regardless of this, small morbid swellings arise in the skin such as myrmicia (flat warts) achrocordones, psydraces, and epinytides (herpes zoster). . . . All of these are well-known diseases'

(Galen of Pergamum, AD 129–199)

Warts and verrucae are extremely common; they affect children and young adults primarily, are caused by the wart virus and are therefore infectious. They may be single or multiple, painless or painful, slowly growing or rapidly growing, disappear spontaneously after a few weeks, or remain stubbornly resistant to all treatments for years, the multiplicity of treatments and so called 'cures' gives an indication of how ineffective most are! They can cause despair in doctor and patient alike! Fortunately, practically all warts and verrucae eventually disappear spontaneously, never to return, but as this may take several years, most patients seek treatment in an attempt to cure them in a shorter time. Some treatments are undoubtedly harmless and worth trying – others definitely carry certain well recognized risks and may leave permanent scarring. In a self-limiting condition, therefore, the practitioner must not let his or her surgical enthusiasm inflict a treatment which is worse than the original condition. Neither should the treatment be painful as the majority of sufferers will be young children unlikely to forget or forgive.

Treatments for warts and verrucae fall into two categories: medical and surgical. No apology is made for including a selection of medical treatments before considering a surgical approach.

16.1 MEDICAL TREATMENTS FOR WARTS AND VERRUCAE

16.1.1 Psychological therapy

Although warts are known to be caused by a virus infective agent, they can be made to disappear by psychological treatments. This fact was known for centuries by the 'Wart Charmers' and in recent years by hypnotherapists. If a patient believes that their warts are going to disappear as a result of any treatment, a significant proportion do in fact regress and disappear!

16.1.2 Monochloro-acetic acid

Solitary warts or verrucae respond well to a saturated solution of monochloro-acetic acid pricked into the wart using a sharp-pointed wooden applicator (Fig. 16.1).

One drop of acid is placed on the surface of the wart, and with a wooden applicator is pricked through the horny outer layer. Often the acid appears to soak into the wart very much like absorbent paper. Further drops of acid are applied and pricked into the wart until no more will soak in. It is most

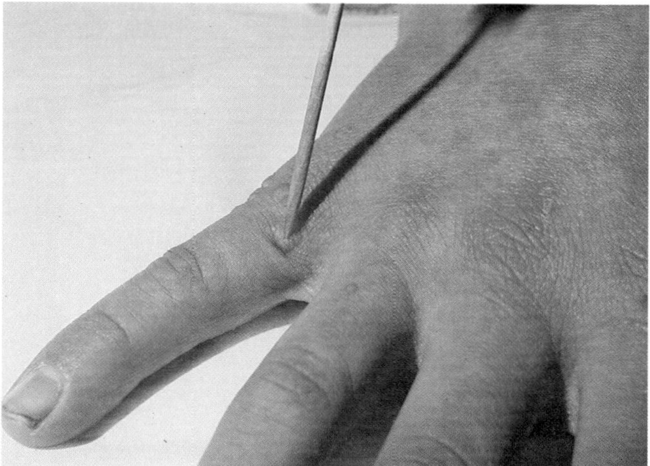

Fig. 16.1 Solitary warts may be effectively treated with a saturated solution of monochloro-acetic acid, pricked in with a wooden applicator until no more is absorbed.

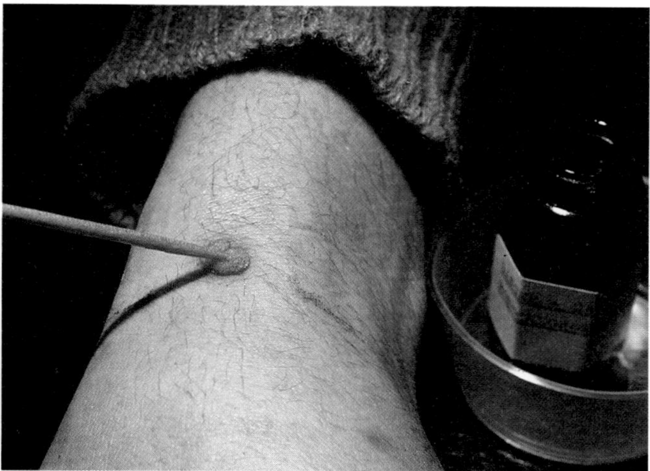

Fig. 16.2 Monochloro-acetic acid acid being applied to solitary wart on wrist.

important not to allow any acid on the surrounding skin or a painful burn will result. Should any spread from the wart, it should be immediately removed with a soft paper tissue.

Following the application of monochloro-acetic acid, there is normally a reddening of the skin over the next four or five days, and signs of healing after eight days. One application is often successful, and the treatment may be repeated if necessary. Ointments containing Podophyllin and/or salicylic acid are equally effective.

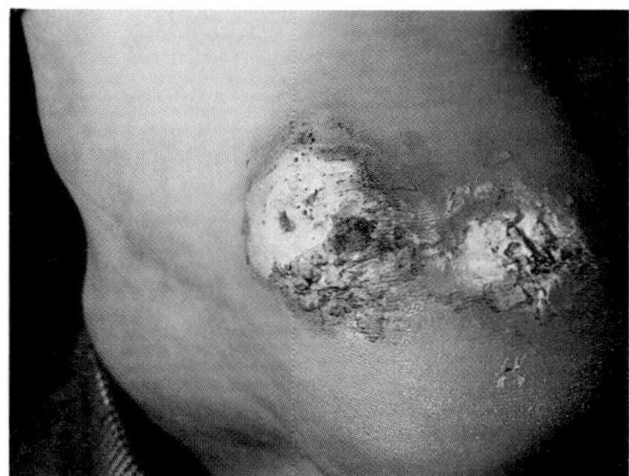

Fig. 16.3 Over enthusiastic treatment of verrucae with podophyllin and salicyclic acid.

16.1.3 Podophyllin and/or salicylic acid

The risk of podophyllin is over-enthusiastic treatment in a desperate attempt to cure the verruca; this results in painful burns to the surrounding skin, often the verruca is cured, but at the expense of considerable discomfort (Fig. 16.3). If using podophyllin and salicylic acid ointment (Posalfilin) only enough to cover a pin-head should be used; this should be placed in the centre of the verruca, covered with a plaster dressing and repeated daily until cured. A simple way by which the patient can tell if the verruca is cured is by compressing the skin on either side of the verruca: if painful it is still present, if painless, it is cured (Fig. 16.4).

Plasters with 40% salicylic acid are an effective means of dealing with multiple plantar warts; they macerate the top layers of skin, including the wart.

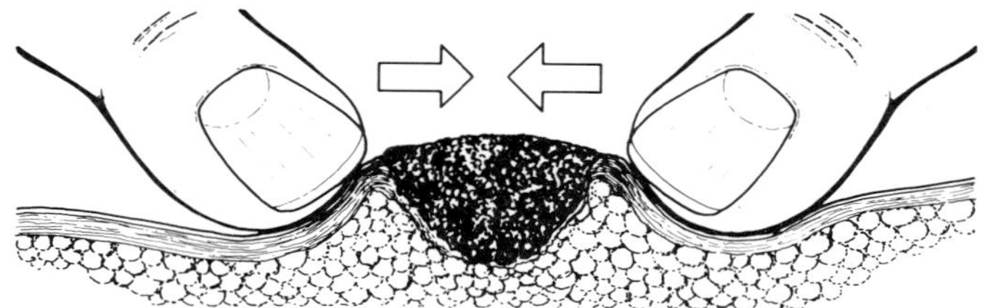

Fig. 16.4 A simple method to determine whether a wart or verruca is cured: compress laterally between finger and thumb, if no pain – cured!

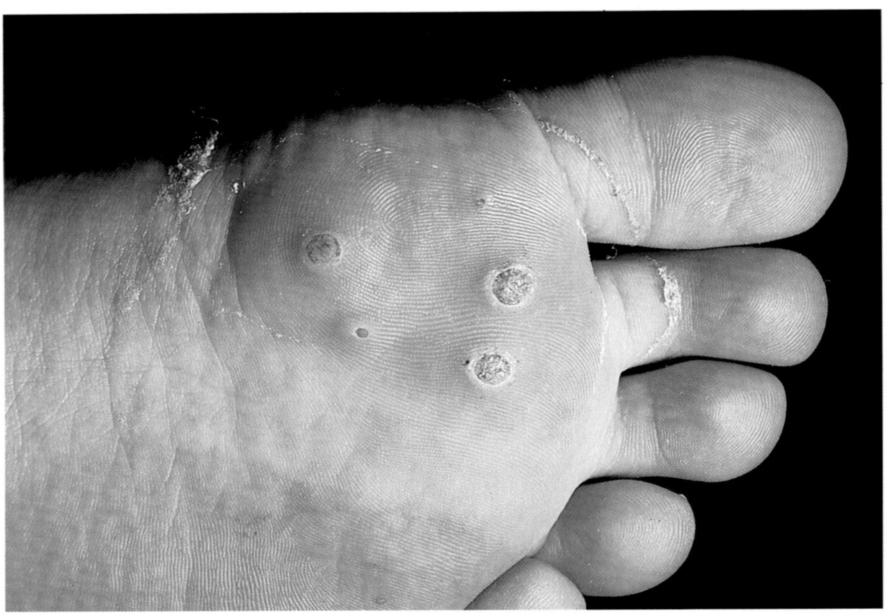

Fig. 16.5 Multiple verrucae; best treated medically with salicyclic acid or formalin.

16.1.4 Aqueous formalin or glutaraldehyde solution

Multiple verrucae may also be treated by soaking the whole foot in 20% aqueous formalin solution for 10 min each day. The skin becomes hard and like leather, and liable to crack, particularly between the toes if the solution is not washed off. Using a similar principle, glutaraldehyde solution may be applied just to the wart or verruca daily until it is cured.

16.1.5 Venereal warts

Venereal warts (condylomata acuminata) are more susceptible to treatment than the ordinary hard wart; in this case the treatment of choice is podophyllin in spirit or tinct. benz. co. applied *very* carefully to each wart. Traditionally 25% podophyllin was recommended, unfortunately this often burned the surrounding skin, and a trial using 0.5% podophyllin resin in 70% ethanol [18] applied twice daily for three days gave equally good results.

16.2 SURGICAL TREATMENTS OF WARTS AND VERRUCAE

There are as many surgical as there are medical treatments for warts and verrucae, indicating again that no one treatment offers more than a reasonable chance of cure. Treatments involve burning, freezing, curetting and excision. There are various instruments which will destroy warts or verrucae by heat, the simplest is the standard electrocautery, by which a platinum electrode is heated to red heat by the passage of an electric current. It is first necessary to infiltrate the base of the wart with local anaesthetic (Lignocaine 1% with or without adrenalin depending on the site), the wart may then be destroyed using the electrocautery.

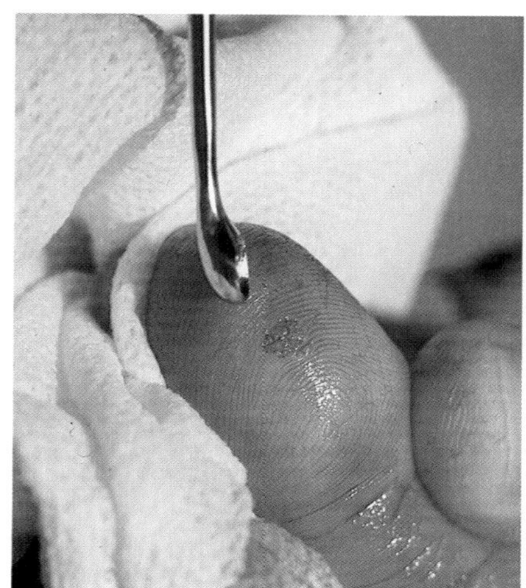

Fig. 16.6 Solitary wart on thumb; present for one year and painful. Curette and cautery offers high chance of permanent cure.

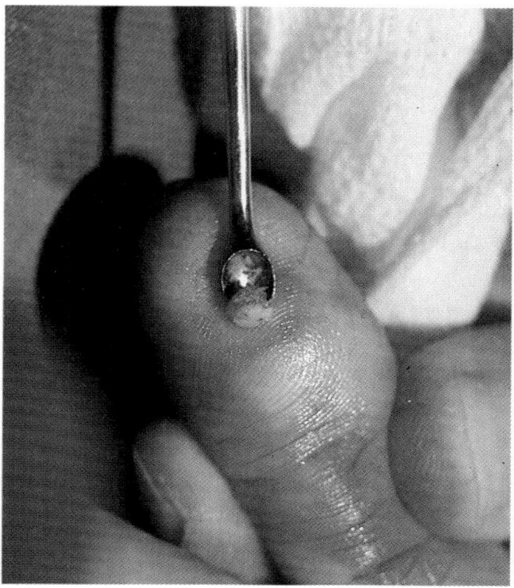

Fig. 16.7 Wart being curetted out. A tourniquet and ring block prevents bleeding at this stage.

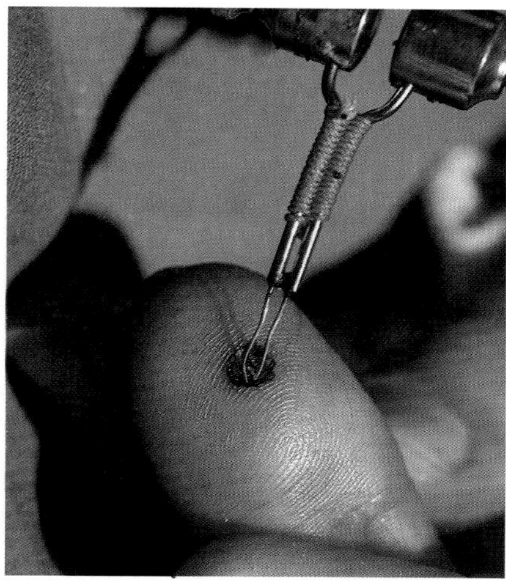

Fig. 16.8 The base of the wart is now cauterized with the electrocautery.

Another method of producing heat within tissues is by passing a high-frequency electric current through it; this is used regularly for coagulating bleeding vessels in the operating theatre; a large pad is strapped to the patient's thigh and connected to one side of the output of the machine while the other output lead is connected to a small pointed instrument such as a pair of artery forceps. This is a bi-polar diathermy apparatus. Similar portable diathermy machines are now available which use just one electrode and these are the unipolar diathermy machines, or hyfrecators. In use, the needle electrode is inserted in the centre of the wart and the electric current switched on. The heat generated within the wart destroys it; normally a local anaesthetic is used to infiltrate the base of the wart before applying the electrode. No further treatment is required apart from a sterile dry dressing.

16.2.1 Curetting and cautery

Most solitary warts can be removed with a curette and this is probably the treatment of choice (Figs 16.7 and 16.8).

Instruments required

1 dental syringe and 30 SWG needle (0.3 mm)
1 cartridge of 2% Lignocaine with 1:80 000 adrenalin
OR
1 2 ml syringe
1 25 SWG × $\frac{5}{8}$" (0.5 mm × 16 mm) needle
1 ampoule 1% Lignocaine with 1:200 000 adrenalin

1 Volkmann double-ended sharp-spoon curette
1 electrocautery and pointed burner or unipolar diathermy
histology container
dry dressing
Povidone-iodine in spirit (Betadine alcoholic solution)

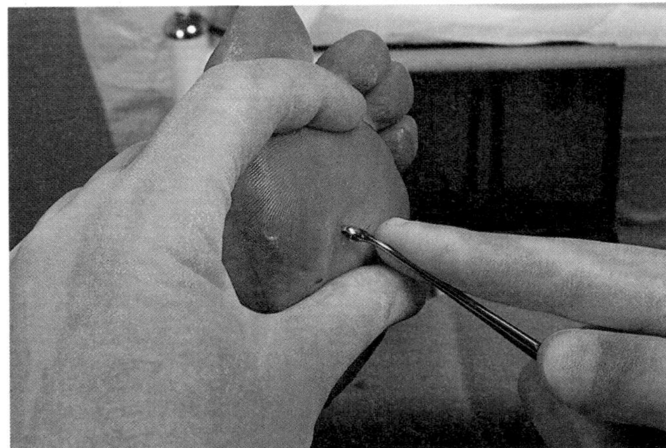

Fig. 16.9 Verruca on sole of foot. Anaesthesia by posterior tibial nerve block.

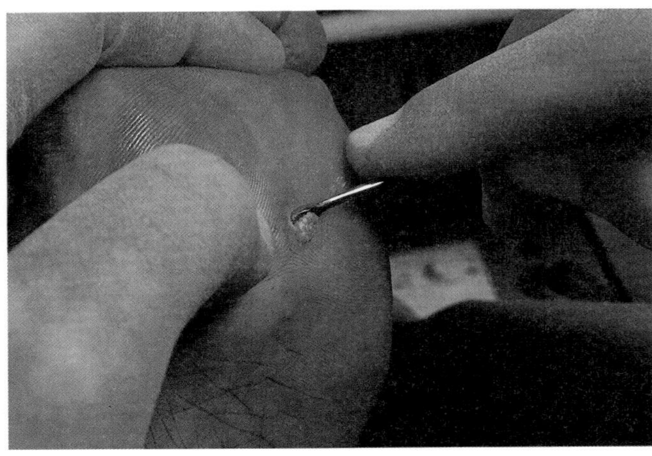

Fig. 16.10 Showing technique of using curette to remove verruca; firm pressure and a rotating action.

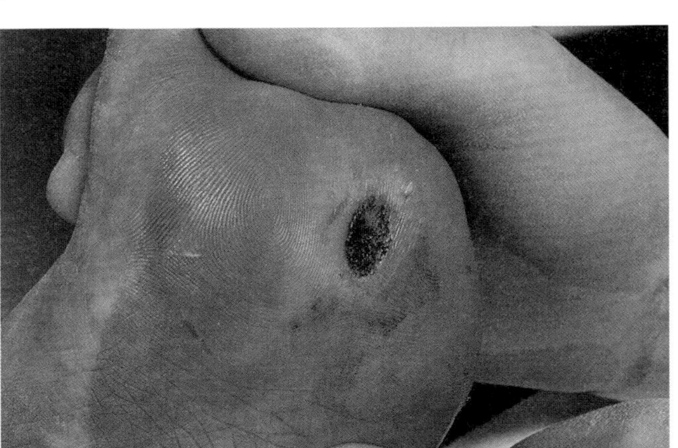

Fig. 16.11 After removing the verruca, the base is cauterized with the electrocautery.

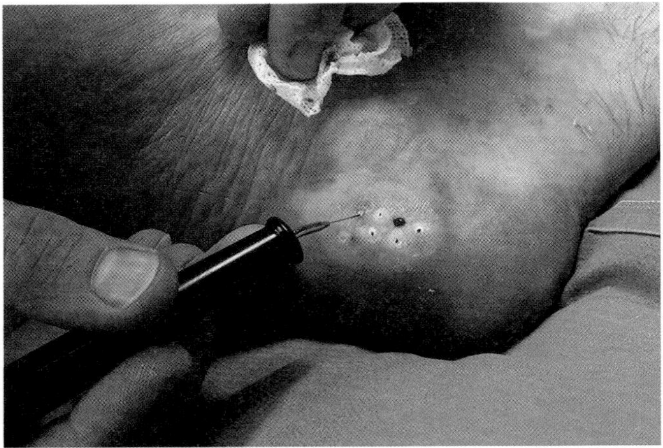

Fig. 16.12 A cluster of stubborn verrucae being individually treated with the hyfrecator needle after preliminary paring of any hard skin.

The wart and adjacent skin is painted with Povidone-iodine in spirit (Betadine alcoholic solution). Using the dental syringe and 30 SWG needle or the 2 ml syringe with 25 SWG (0.5 mm) needle the base of the wart is infiltrated with local anaesthetic. It is now possible to curette the wart easily from the skin; this is best achieved by holding the handle of the curette firmly, perpendicular to the skin, pressing the curette firmly, against the edge of the wart, and then by a rotating action, shelling out the wart. When the correct tissue plan is reached the wart or verruca will readily separate leaving a neat circular hole which bleeds easily despite the adrenalin in the local anaesthetic mixture. To control this bleeding the vessels are coagulated using the electrocautery, which additionally destroys any remaining fragments of wart. A dry dressing is applied; healing is usually complete in three weeks with freedom from pain after two days.

16.2.2 Excision of warts

Excision of warts is appropriate in certain sites such as the face where a neat scar is desirable, but as the majority of warts will disappear spontaneously without leaving a scar, excision should only be considered as a last resort.

Instruments required for excision of warts

1 10 ml syringe
25 SWG × $\frac{5}{8}$" (0.5 mm × 16 mm) needle
21 SWG × $1\frac{1}{2}$" (0.8 mm × 40 mm) needle
1 scalpel handle size 3
1 scalpel blade size 10
1 pair toothed dissecting forceps
1 pair stitch scissors
1 Kilner needle holder
1 suture: Mersilk Ethicon. Ref. W533
1 ampoule 10 ml 1% Lignocaine with adrenalin 1:200 000
dressings
Povidone-iodine in spirit (Betadine alcoholic solution)

The wart and surrounding skin is painted with Povidone-iodine in spirit (Betadine alcoholic solution) and the base anaesthetized using first the 25 SWG (0.5 mm) needle, followed by the 21 SWG (0.8 mm) needle. An ellipse of skin is removed with the wart in the centre; this is sent for confirmatory histology and the wound closed using fine, interrupted mersilk sutures. These are removed between five and ten days depending on the site of the original lesion.

16.2.3 Cryotherapy for warts and verrucae

As well as destruction by heat, tissues can be destroyed by freezing, and in many situations this method offers a better treatment, free from pain, with an excellent cosmetic result. The different equipment and modes of use are described in Chapter 30, but there are three different machines, using carbon dioxide, nitrous oxide and liquid nitrogen, in ascending order of efficiency. Liquid nitrogen gives the lowest temperature and has the highest success, carbon dioxide has only limited uses, while the nitrous oxide cryoprobe is valuable for superficial lesions. The technique is as follows:

The wart or verruca is moistened with water soluble jelly or glycerine and the cryoprobe applied. As freezing progresses, the probe becomes frozen to the wart, which may now be lifted a few millimetres from subcutaneous tissues by gentle traction on the probe. When the wart is frozen solid, the probe is warmed, detached, and the wart allowed to thaw. The procedure is repeated as this second freeze appears to give improved results.

Immediately following freezing little can be seen, and the wart appears exactly as before treatment; slight throbbing is experienced during the next few hours, to be followed over the ensuing days by painless necrosis, and healing. It is the absence of pain and the very acceptable end result which makes cryotherapy so attractive.

Condylomata acuminata are easily treated with nitrous oxide cryoprobe. Larger warts are better treated with liquid nitrogen using a spray applicator (see Chapter 30).

SEVENTEEN

Intradermal lesions

'Naevi Materni are those marks which frequently appear on the bodies of children at birth and which originate from impressions made on the mind of the mother during pregnancy'

(Encyclopaedia Brittanica, 1797)

Almost all intradermal lesions can be removed in the surgery by a general practitioner, the two exceptions being any lesion which is too large to permit skin closure and the malignant melanoma. Facilities for histological examination are essential, and it is good practice to send every specimen excised for histological examination; not only does this improve the doctor's diagnostic acumen, it avoids the pitfall of inadvertently removing an amelanotic malignant melanoma, and provides a permanent record of the tissues and pathology removed. Most of the lesions to be described can be removed leaving a neat inconspicuous scar; where the doctor anticipates otherwise the patient should be advised in advance.

One instrument set will be suitable for all the lesions described and the technique with slight variations is applicable to each.

Instruments required

- 1 scalpel handle size 3
- 1 scalpel blade size 10
- 1 Volkmann double-ended-sharp-spoon curette
- 1 Kilner needle holder $5\frac{1}{4}''$ (13.3 cm)
- 1 pair standard stitch scissors 5″ (12.7 cm) pointed
- 1 pair toothed dissecting forceps 5″ (12.7 cm)
- 1 pair Halstead mosquito artery forceps curved 5″ (12.7 cm)
- Povidone-iodine in spirit (Betadine alcoholic solution)
- 1 10 ml syringe
- 1 25 SWG × $\frac{5}{8}''$ (0.5 mm × 16 mm) needle
- 1 23 SWG × 1″ (0.6 mm × 25 mm) needle
- 1 21 SWG × $1\frac{1}{2}''$ (0.8 mm × 40 mm) needle
- 1 ampoule 10 ml 1% Lignocaine with or without added adrenalin 1:200 000
- skin closure strips (Steri-strips) 6 mm × 75 mm. Ref. 3M GP41
- sterile braided silk suture metric gauge 2 (formerly 3/0) 45 cm long (black) with 25 mm super cutting curved needle. Ref. Ethicon W 533
- 1 electrocautery with platinum tip burner or equivalent unipolar diathermy for coagulation

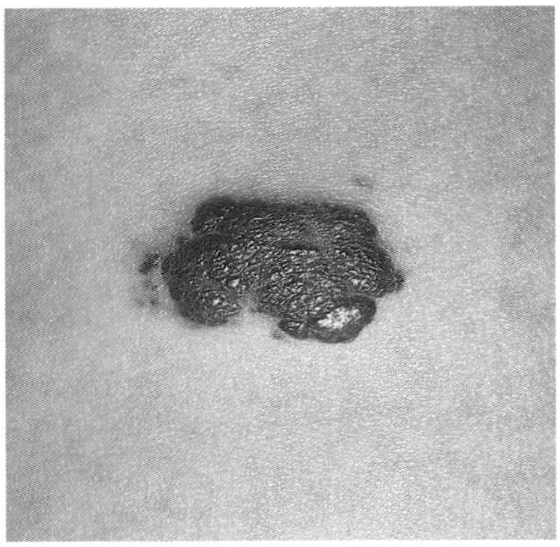

Fig. 17.1 The 'strawberry naevus' which will disappear completely without any treatment; it should never be excised or cauterized.

17.1 GENERAL TECHNIQUE FOR EXCISION

The first consideration with any intradermal lesion is a provisional diagnosis, secondly, does it need to be removed? Lesions such as the

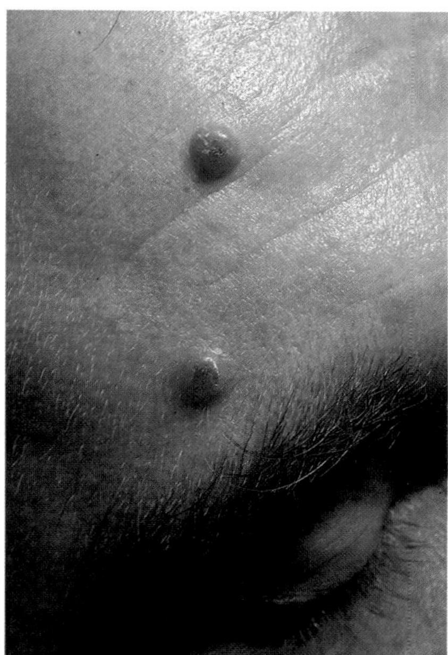

Fig. 17.2 Two solitary lesions of molluscum contagiosum. May be either left alone, curetted and cauterized, or treated with phenol or iodine pricked through the 'dimple' in the spot.

infant's strawberry naevus should be left alone as it always resolves completely (Fig. 17.1). Similarly many warts and molluscum contagiosum may well regress spontaneously and be better left to nature (Fig. 17.2). The third consideration, once it has been decided to remove any intradermal lesion, is to decide the line of the final scar, bearing in mind that scars in the line of skin creases and wrinkles are much neater, as are transverse scars across joints, and scars which lie at right angles to the direction of pull of underlying muscles (see Chapter 8). Picking up the skin and squeezing the lesion between finger and thumb will demonstrate skin creases and also help to assess whether excision will result in too much skin tension. The fourth consideration is the method of removal – is this lesion better excised, or curetted and cauterized, desiccated, fulgurized, treated with the diathermy or cryoprobe, or is the diagnosis such that a preliminary skin biopsy should be taken?

Assuming excision is the method of choice, the lesion and surrounding skin is liberally painted with Povidone-iodine in spirit (Betadine alcoholic solution) and the area anaesthetized using infiltration of local anaesthetic. For small lesions, a skin bleb of Lignocaine is raised at either end of the proposed scar using either a 30 SWG needle and dental syringe or a 25 SWG × $\frac{5}{8}$" (0.5 mm × 16 mm) needle (Fig. 17.3). The needle is then changed for a larger one, either 23 SWG (0.6 mm) or 21 SWG (0.8 mm) and inserted through the skin bleb, infiltrating the underlying skin in a fan shape distribution from either end. A sterile 'lithotomy type' drape is put over the skin, leaving just the intradermal lesion exposed. After washing and scrubbing the hands thoroughly with Chlorhexidine in detergent (Hibiscrub) they are dried, and a pair of sterile surgical gloves applied.

From now on, a completely aseptic technique must be used, preferably no-touch, with the minimum of tissue trauma and handling. The wearing of a face-mask is optional – provided the operator does not cough, sneeze or talk continuously over the wound, it is probably not essential. However, wearing a mask does protect the patient from droplet infection, and does enable the doctor to hold a conversation with the patient, explaining the procedure. Similarly if the patient has any upper respiratory infection, or is liable to cough, sneeze, or talk, he or she should likewise wear a mask, as should any assistant.

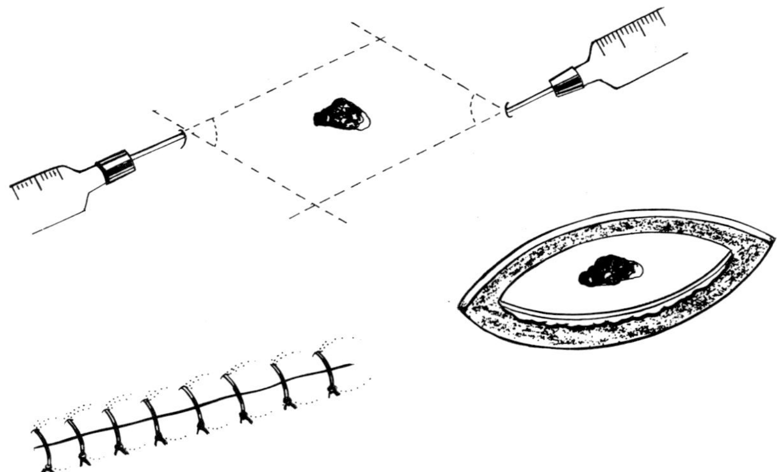

Fig. 17.3 Illustrating method for infiltrating skin with local anaesthetic for excision of intradermal lesion, and skin closure with interrupted sutures.

The lesion is now excised using an elliptical incision through skin and subcutaneous tissues, attempting to excise a triangular wedge of tissue rather than leaving a flat base. Any small bleeding points can be controlled with pressure alone using a sterile gauze swab. The excised wedge/ellipse of tissue is placed immediately in a histology container and covered with 10% formol-saline as preservative. This container should be promptly labelled with the patient's name, date, and nature of specimen, and if appropriate, which side or digit. The resulting wound is generally much bigger than expected due to retraction of the skin edges; bleeding vessels usually stop spontaneously, any brisk bleeding can be controlled by artery forceps.

It is a good idea at this stage to ascertain whether the skin edges will approximate without undue tension. If they can be brought together easily, the wound may be stitched forthwith, if tension is present, it is worth under-cutting the edges with a scalpel so that the skin will slide over the subcutaneous tissues, and then suturing the wound.

The two reasons for poor healing are dead spaces and undue skin tension. Dead spaces fill with blood and serum and produce a subcutaneous haematoma which can become infected, while undue tension on skin edges produces ischaemia, non-union and necrosis.

Both dead spaces and skin tension can be dealt with by the judicious use of absorbable subcutaneous sutures such as catgut or dexon, but only the minimum number necessary should be used as too many act as foreign bodies and increase the risks of infection.

Generally the wound is best closed using interrupted mersilk sutures, spaced closely together, supported if necessary by the application of self-adhesive skin closure strips (Steri-strips). When inserting sutures, the aim should be to slightly evert the skin edges; this can be achieved by taking slightly more of the subcutaneous tissue in the bite of the needle than skin. If the skin edges still tend to invert despite this manoeuvre, the suture should be passed through the skin 1 mm from each edge (Vertical mattress). This is an excellent stitch, but can be difficult to remove. Depending on the site of the scar, the sutures may be removed on the 5th to 10th day, leaving the Steri-strips to give additional external support.

All that remains is the application of a dry sterile dressing and the instructions to the patient to leave the dressing completely undisturbed

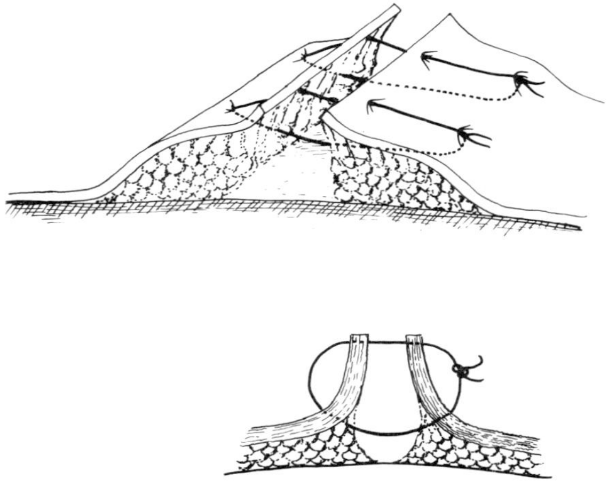

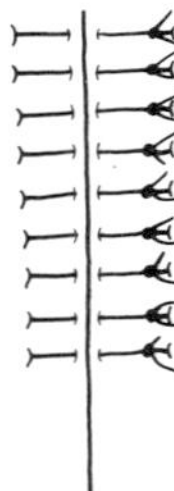

Fig. 17.4 Showing method of skin closure to avoid inversion of the skin edges (Vertical mattress suture).

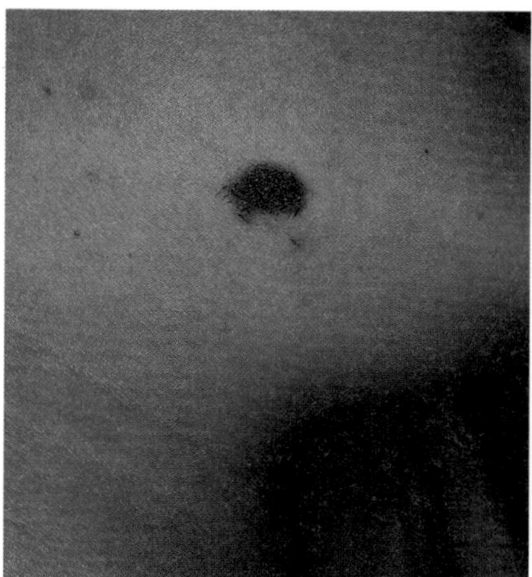

Fig. 17.5 Pigmented intradermal naevus which bled regularly after shaving.

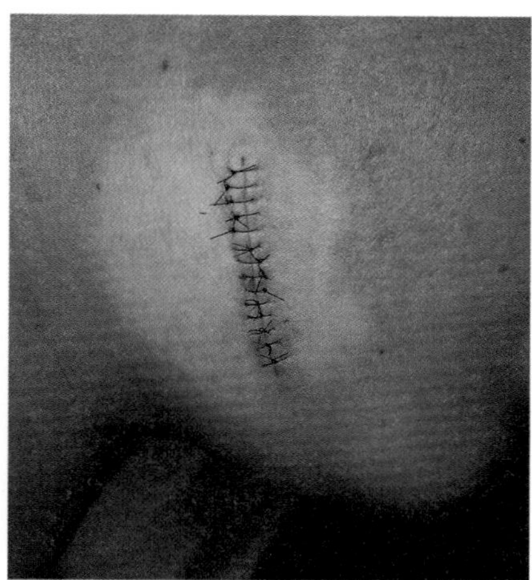

Fig. 17.6 Excised; closure with fine, interrupted sutures. (Blanching of surrounding skin is from adrenalin in local anaesthetic.)

until the sutures are removed, unless there is a specific reason to inspect the wound earlier. It is also helpful to rest the limb or part of the body containing the scar for at least 48 hours to initiate healing. Thereafter, gentle activity is beneficial.

17.2 CURETTE AND CAUTERY

As an alternative to surgical excision, many lesions may successfully be removed with a sharp-spoon Volkmann curette, afterwards cauterizing the base with the electrocautery to control bleeding. The technique is exactly as described under the section on warts and verrucae (see Chapter 16). As with warts, it is important to find the correct plane of cleavage when using the curette; it is also helpful to have a selection of curettes of various sizes corresponding to the size of the lesion.

17.3 INTRADERMAL NAEVI

Pigmented naevi are lesions with melanocytes and neural elements in the dermis; they can be divided into flat lesions, slightly raised lesions, verrucous lesions, dome-shaped lesions, and pigmented hairy lesions. The main indication for removal is any suspicion that it may be turning malignant, as suggested by sudden enlargement, alteration in the pigment, ulceration or bleeding. Most patients request removal for cosmetic reasons, or because the lesion is catching on clothing or razors when shaving. Surgical excision is the treatment of choice for all pigmented naevi.

17.4 HISTIOCYTOMA

This is a fairly common tumour found commonly on the legs, cause unknown but may be related to trauma. It occurs in the dermis and presents as a smooth firm nodule. They are benign, commonly multiple, and the treatment is surgical excision.

17.5 CYLINDROMA (TURBAN TUMOUR)

This is a rare tumour, also benign, occuring commonly on the scalp and initially may be mistaken for a sebaceous cyst until excision is attempted, when a firm granular adherent lesion is found. Treatment is surgical excision.

17.6 SOLAR KERATOSIS

As the name implies these lesions are found in areas of skin exposed to light; they are discrete and raised with a crumbling surface. As they are purely epidermal, they may be treated with curettage and electrocautery or cryotherapy, using a nitrous oxide or liquid nitrogen cryoprobe.

17.7 KERATOACANTHOMA

These are not uncommon lesions which can be mistaken for basal and squamous cell carcinomata; they present as a small papule which grows rapidly in size over a period of two or three months. The edges are rolled over with a central depression and a thickened keratin plug. Interestingly they gradually involute over a period of six months. The cause is still unknown. Treatment is by curettage and cautery (Figs 17.7, 17.8, 17.9 and 17.10).

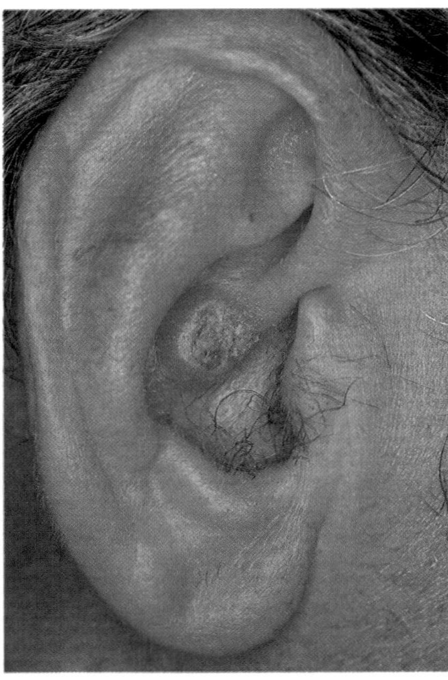

Fig. 17.7 Typical keratoacanthoma inside ear; present for three months, enlarging rapidly.

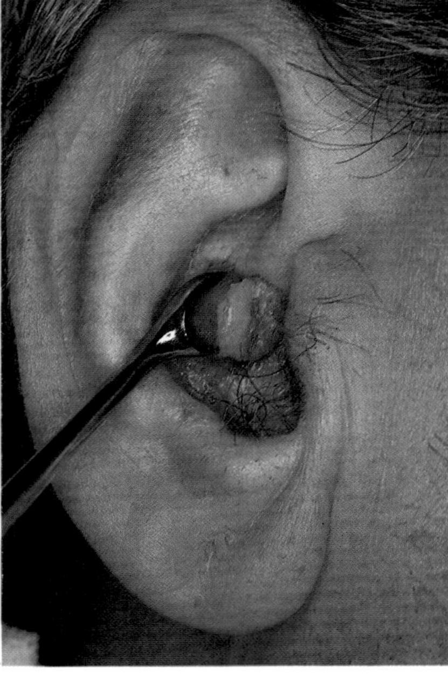

Fig. 17.8 Keratoacanthoma. Easily curretted with sharp-spoon curette.

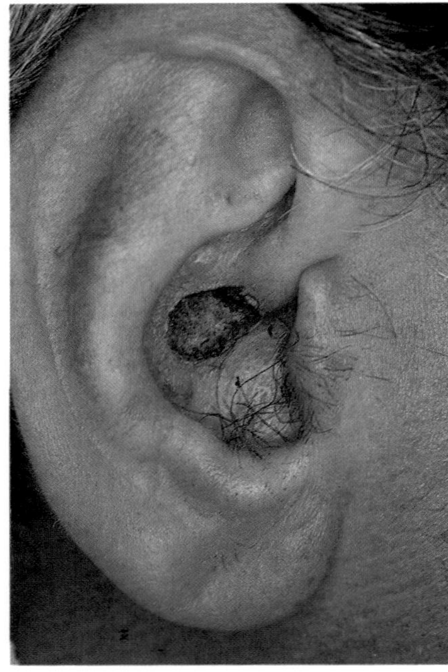

Fig. 17.9 The base of the lesion is cauterized with the electrocautery.

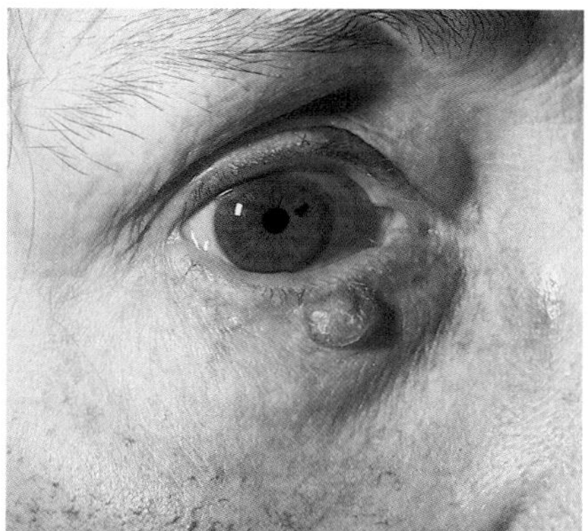

Fig. 17.10 An atypical keratoacanthoma; this could have been mistaken for an early basal-cell carcinoma.

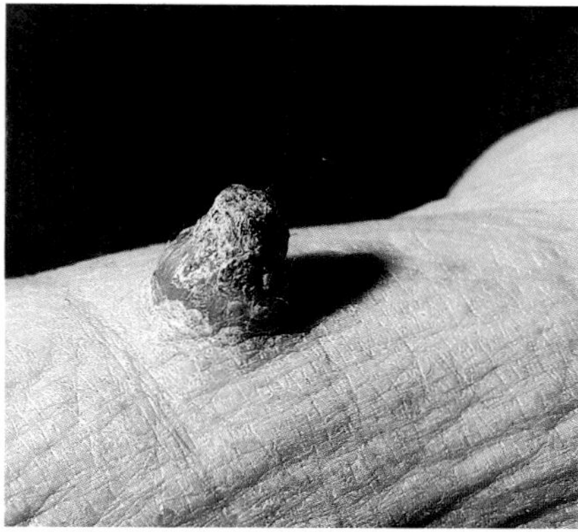

Fig. 17.11 Another typical keratoacanthoma; easily curetted and base cauterized.

17.8 GRANULOMA PYOGENICUM

This is a type of haemangioma, so called because it was originally thought to be due to infection by a staphylococcus. It presents as a solitary raised swelling, bright red in colour, and bleeds profusely. The most effective treatment is curettage and cautery under local anaesthesia.

17.9 SPIDER NAEVI

These are common vascular lesions typified by a very small central red papule from which radiate fine superficial blood vessels. The most effective treatment is electrocautery to the central papule without anaesthetic, or inserting the needle electrode of the hyfrecator into the papule, also without anaesthetic.

17.10 MOLLUSCUM CONTAGIOSUM

This is a viral tumour of the skin, commonly seen in children. They have a typically pearly appearance with an umbilicated centre. Treatment is either pricking each lesion with a pointed stick soaked in phenol, or destruction using the electrocautery or diathermy.

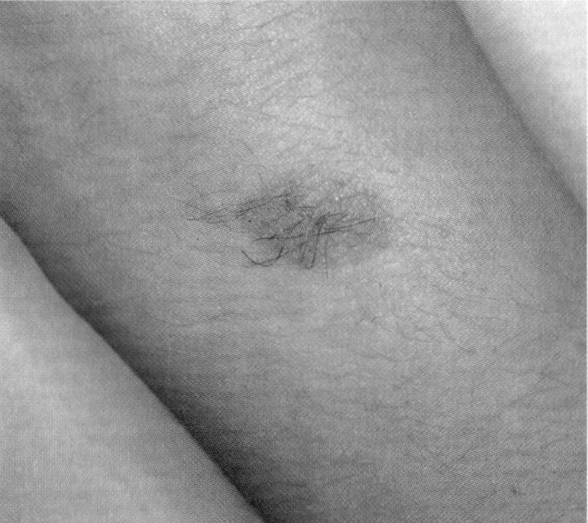

Fig. 17.12 Pale, pigmented hairy naevus on wrist, slowly enlarging and darkening.

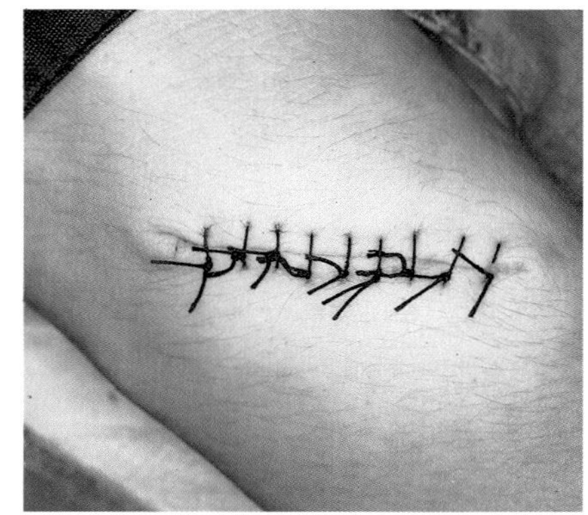

Fig. 17.13 After excision. Closure with interrupted fine braided silk sutures. (Blanching due to adrenalin in anaesthetic.)

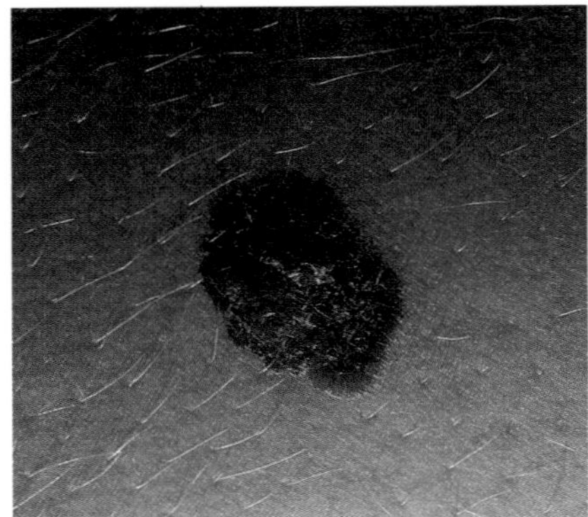

Fig. 17.14 The dreaded malignant melanoma. **Never** a minor surgical procedure. Always refer to hospital urgently.

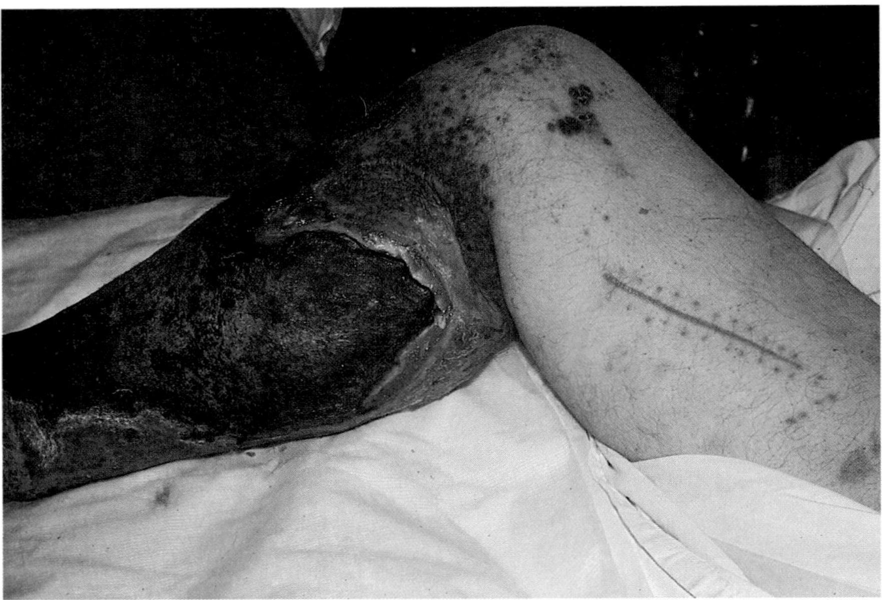

Fig. 17.15 Malignant melanoma. Six months after Fig. 17.14. Despite wide excision in hospital and chemotherapy, metastatic spread. (Patient died 3 months later.)

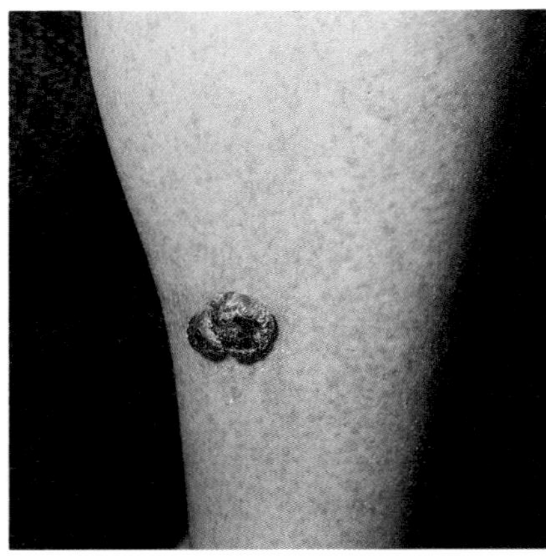

Fig. 17.16 Another malignant melanoma on the leg. Widely excised; patient still alive 20 years later.

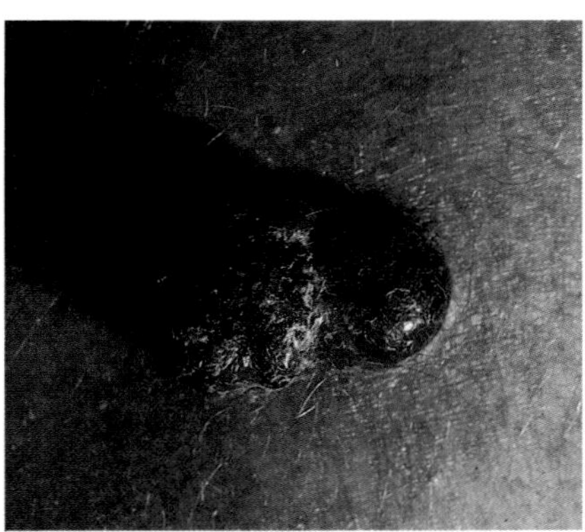

Fig. 17.17 Close-up of same malignant melanoma. Prognosis totally unpredictable.

17.11 REMOVAL OF TATTOOS

Many patients request the removal of tattoos which have been self-inflicted or professionally performed; small tattoos are excised exactly as any intradermal lesion,larger tattoos are better referred to a plastic surgeon or treated with the laser.

17.12 JUVENILE MELANOMA

This is a pigmented naevus which appears in childhood and grows rapidly. Histologically they resemble malignant melanomata, but they are always benign. (Pigmented naevi do not undergo malignant change before puberty.) Treatment, therefore, is surgical excision.

17.13 THE MALIGNANT MELANOMA (Figs 17.14, 17.15, 17.16 and 17.17)

This is the one nightmare of any doctor practising minor surgery. Fortunately they are relatively rare and most are recognizable. It is usually pigmented, has recently increased in size, and has an alteration in the pigment with a possible pigmented 'halo' or satellite lesions, and may have recently ulcerated or bled. The prognosis is not uniformly fatal, but is completely unpredictable. Treatment is by wide surgical excision and should not be undertaken by the general practitioner.

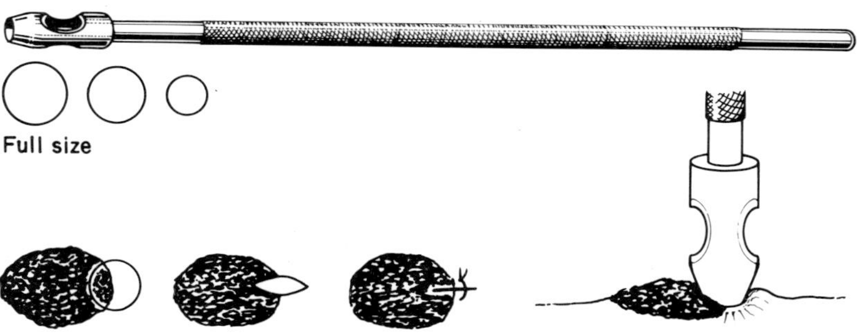

Fig. 17.18 Skin Biopsy: the Hayes Martin skin punch biopsy instrument (Chas F. Thackray Ltd) with three interchangeable heads. Closure is usually with just one stitch.

17.14 BASAL CELL CARCINOMA (RODENT ULCER)

This is the commonest malignant tumour of the skin, usually occurring on the face and appears to be induced by exposure to ultra-violet light. It starts as a small papule which spreads, leaving a central ulcer. The edges are pearl-coloured with fine telangiectasia; left alone they slowly increase in size but never metastasize. Treatment is by radiotherapy (95% cure), surgical excision (95% cure) or curettage and cautery (80% cure). Small basal cell carcinomata are easily treated by the general practitioner and although curettage and cautery gives a lower cure rate than radiotherapy, it gives a better cosmetic result.

17.15 SQUAMOUS CELL EPITHELIOMA

This, too, is thought to be due to over-exposure to ultraviolet light. They can occur anywhere on the body and can affect the mucous membranes, particularly lips and tongue. Unlike the basal cell epithelioma, squamous celled carcinomata have the ability to metastasise, but nevertheless if treated early the prognosis is excellent. Treatment is by surgical excision, radiotherapy or both.

17.16 SKIN BIOPSY

One of the advantages of general practitioner minor surgery is the ability to establish a rapid diagnosis of any suspect skin lesion by a simple biopsy. The technique is not difficult and, where histology facilities exist, a firm diagnosis is possible in a matter of days. The object is to choose a representative lesion, including the margin, together with a piece of adjacent healthy skin, and to remove a narrow ellipse, closing the wound with one or two fine interrupted mersilk sutures (Fig. 17.18). Neater results may be obtained by the use of a skin punch-biopsy instrument (Downs Surgical). These are manufactured in different sizes and consist of a sharpened steel tube mounted on a handle. They may be disposable (Stiefel Laboratories) or re-usable (Downs Surgical and Chas Thackray Ltd).

After choosing a representative area, which is then anaesthetized, the skin is stretched taut, and the punch pressed firmly against the skin. By rotating the handle a core of skin and subcutaneous tissue is obtained. Closure is usually with just one stitch.

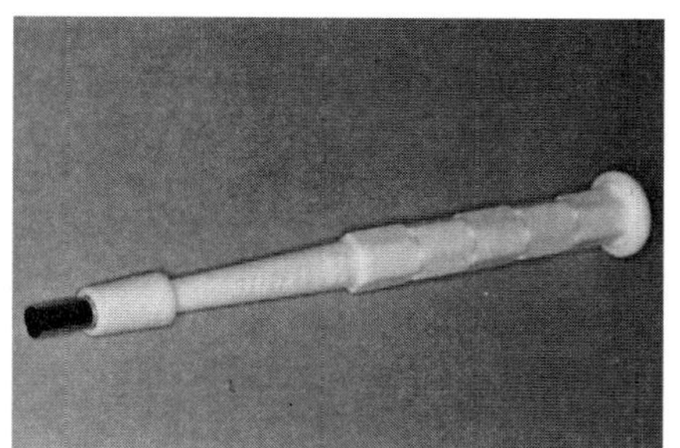

Fig. 17.19 Disposable, sterile skin biopsy punch (Stiefel Laboratories).

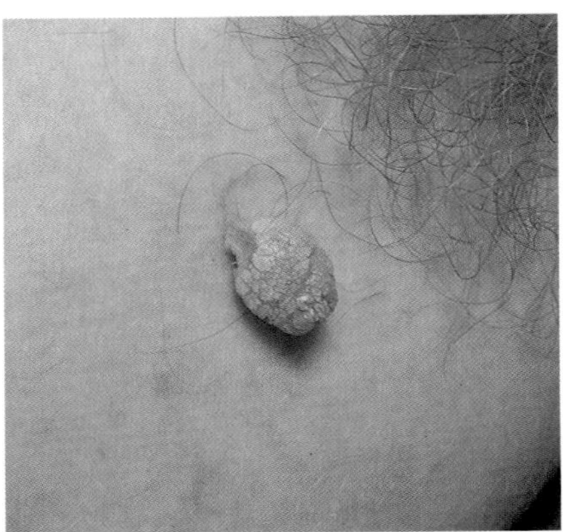

Fig. 18.1 Typical squamous papilloma; easily removed with the electrocautery.

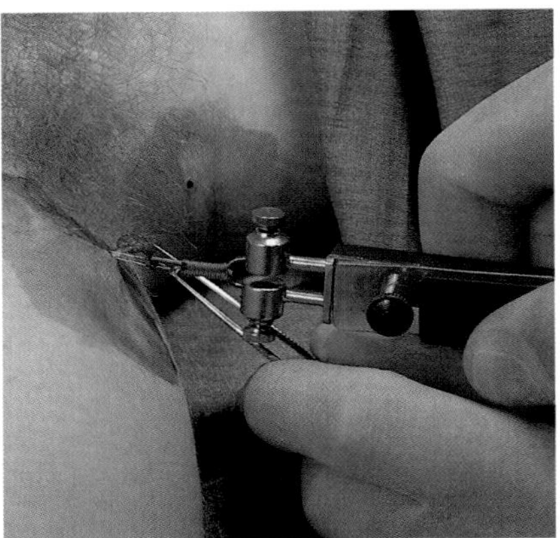

Fig. 18.2 Numerous small skin tags in axilla. Easily removed with the electrocautery.

EIGHTEEN

Skin tags and papillomata

'Polypi are pendulous fleshy indolent tumours, so-called from their supposed resemblances to the animal of that name. A ligature is passed round it and daily tightened till the tumour drops off'

(Encyclopaedia Brittanica, 1797)

It is surprising how many patients have lived with their assorted skin tags and squamous papillomata, feeling they were too trivial a condition to seek medical advice; yet they have caused much anxiety and embarrassment. The majority are easily removed in a matter of minutes, the diagnosis confirmed histologically, and the patient's anxiety allayed.

Instruments required

- 1 5 ml syringe
- 1 25 SWG × $\frac{5}{8}$″ (0.5 mm × 16 mm) needle
- 1 ampoule 1% Lignocaine with 1:200 000 adrenalin
- 1 pair toothed dissecting forceps 5″ (12.7 cm)
- electrocautery with pointed platinum tip burner
- Nobecutane spray or equivalent
- small adhesive plaster dressings
- histology container with 10% formol-saline

Very small skin tags may be picked up with the toothed dissecting forceps and separated at the base using the electrocautery. No bleeding occurs, the procedure takes one second, a small adhesive dressing is applied, the specimen can be sent for histology, and healing takes a matter of days.

Larger skin tags or papillomata can still be removed with the electrocautery but it is better to infiltrate the base with local anaesthetic first (Figs 18.1, 18.2, 18.3 and 18.4). Where the base of the lesion is very broad, and particularly where a neat cosmetic result is desired, it is preferable to excise

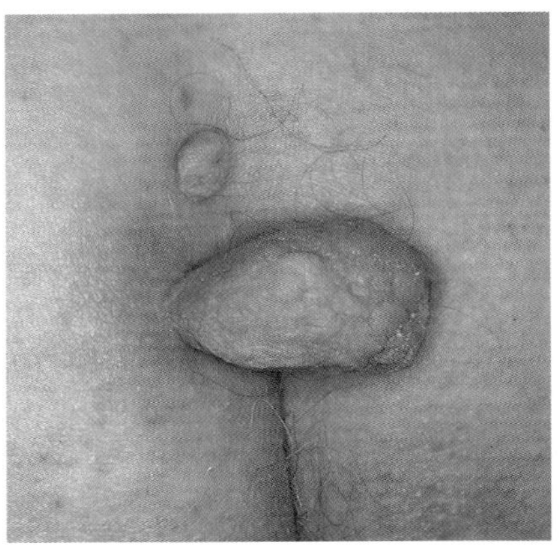

Fig. 18.3 Large fleshy fibro-lipoma, base of back. Narrow base; easily removed just with electrocautery.

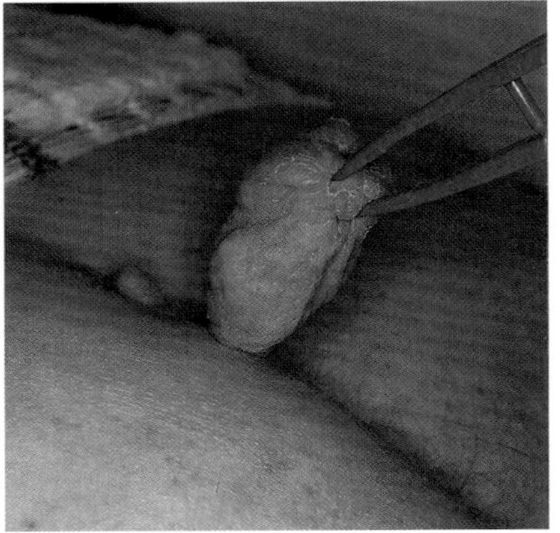

Fig. 18.4 Fibro-lipoma. Base infiltrated with local anaesthetic and removed with the electrocautery.

the papilloma under local anaesthesia, using an elliptical incision, and suturing the skin edges.

As an alternative method, if the practitioner does not possess an electrocautery, most small skin tags and papillomata may be tied off using a fine thread and allowed to drop off. This is perfectly acceptable but separation can take one or two weeks.

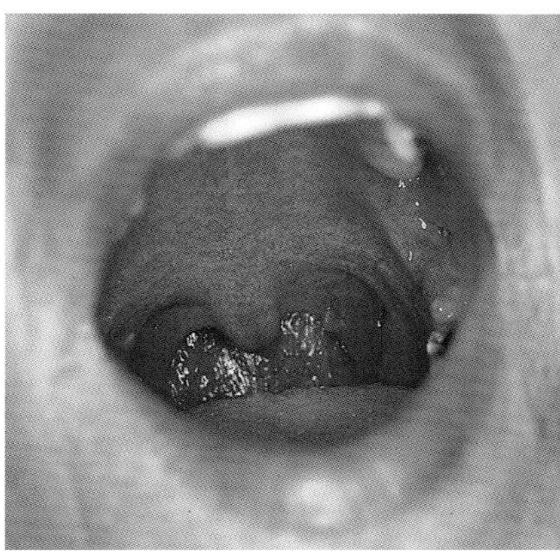

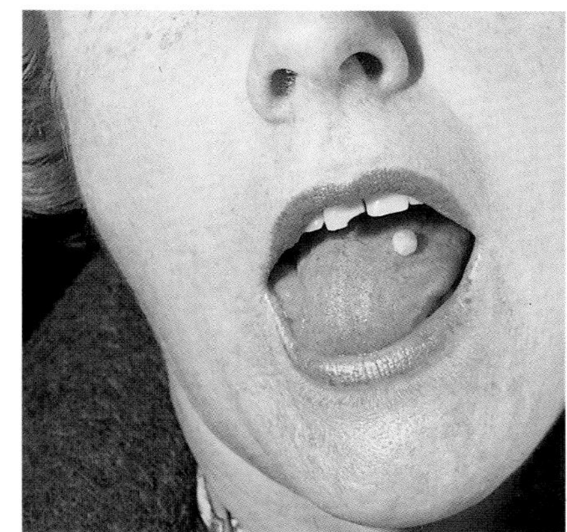

Fig. 18.5 Squamous papilloma on the posterior pillar of the fauces.

Fig. 18.6 Squamous papilloma on the tongue. Curetted and base cauterized after local infiltration anaesthetic.

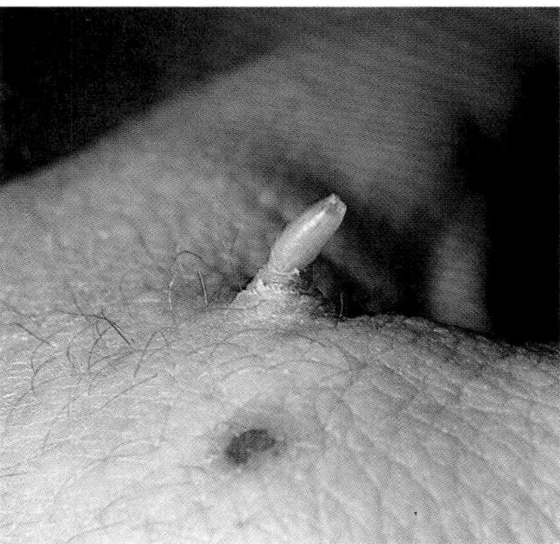

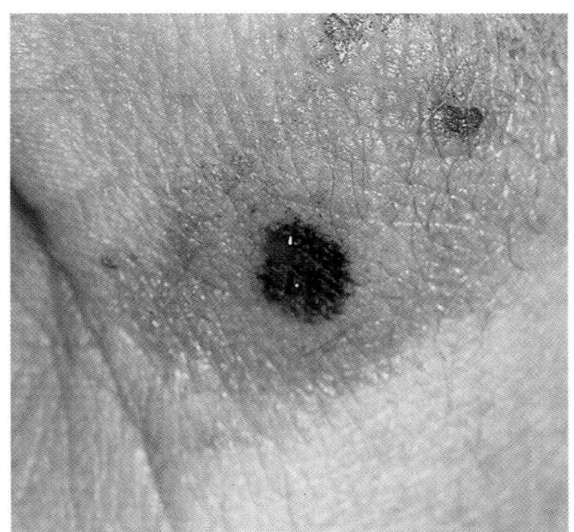

Fig. 18.7 Small cutaneous 'horn'. Easily curetted and base cauterized.

Fig. 18.8 After removal: base cauterized with the electrocautery, rapid healing.

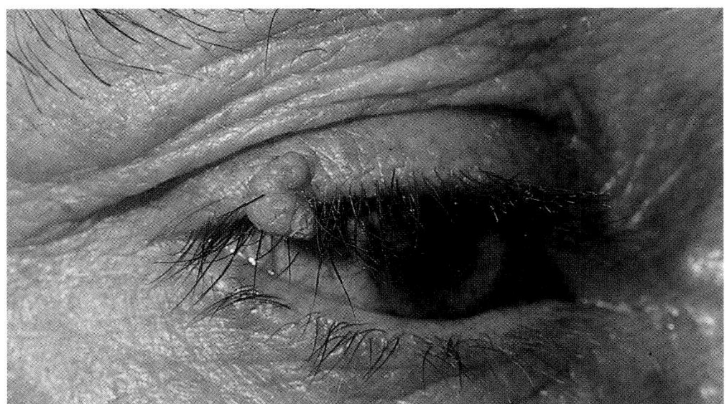

Fig. 18.9 Small warty papilloma on upper eye-lid removed with small curette and base cauterized.

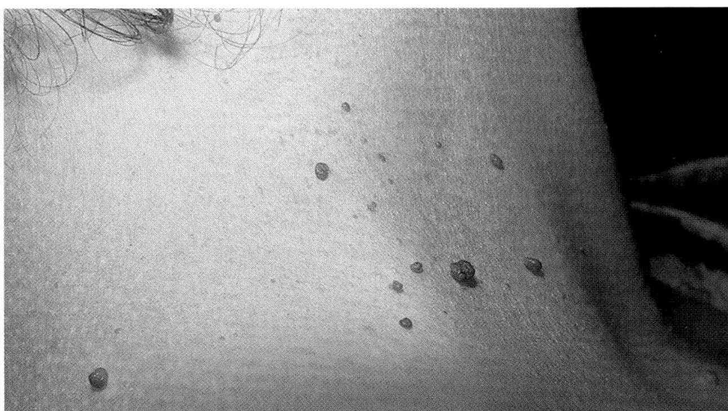

Fig. 18.10 Numerous filiform 'warts' on neck. Very common. Can be easily picked up with forceps and removed using just the electrocautery.

NINETEEN

Varicose veins

'Marius, Roman Consul, having both his legs full of great tumours, and disliking the deformity, determined to put himself in the hands of an operator. When, after enduring a most excessive torment in the cutting, never flinching or complaining, the surgeon went to the other, he declined to have it done saying "I see the cure is not worth the pain".'

(Plutarch's Lives, 155–86 BC)

Varicose veins are one of the commonest problems encountered in general practice, it has been estimated that one person in five in the population either has, or will develop varicose veins of the legs. Women are affected more than men, and the most frequent reasons for seeking advice and treatment are discomfort, fear of ulceration, and appearance.

As far as minor surgery is concerned, there are two successful treatments, sclerotherapy and multiple ligations. However, not all varicose veins are suitable for treatment – indeed in some, treatment might even be contra-indicated or give very poor results.

19.1 ANATOMY

There are two sets of veins in the leg: deep and superficial, being separated from each other by the fascia, and being connected to each other by perforating veins. The perforating veins have valves which allow blood to pass from the superficial veins to the deep veins, but not the reverse.

The long saphenous vein is the longest vein in the body – it starts at the medial dorsal end of the venous arch on the dorsum of the foot, lying 2 cm in front of the medial malleolus, and passing up the leg to join the femoral vein about 3 cm below the inguinal ligament.

The short saphenous vein starts behind the lateral malleolus as an extension of the dorsal venous arch, it passes up the back of the calf in the mid-line, to join the popliteal veins. Valves are frequent throughout the course of the superficial veins, most notably at the junction of the long saphenous and femoral vein, and it is incompetence of these valves which result in varicosities.

By the action of the calf muscles, blood is actively pumped from the feet to the abdomen; and during exercise, pressures up to 250 mm Hg have been recorded in these veins. If valvular breakdown occurs in the perforating veins, blood at this pressure is forced outwards into the superficial veins causing varicosities and eventual ulceration secondary to capillary stasis.

Varicose veins may conveniently be classified into three categories.

19.1.1 Type I varicose veins (Fig. 19.1)

These veins are dilated, but have competent valves; there is no oedema, but the patient may be troubled with attacks of superficial thrombophlebitis; they are common in men.

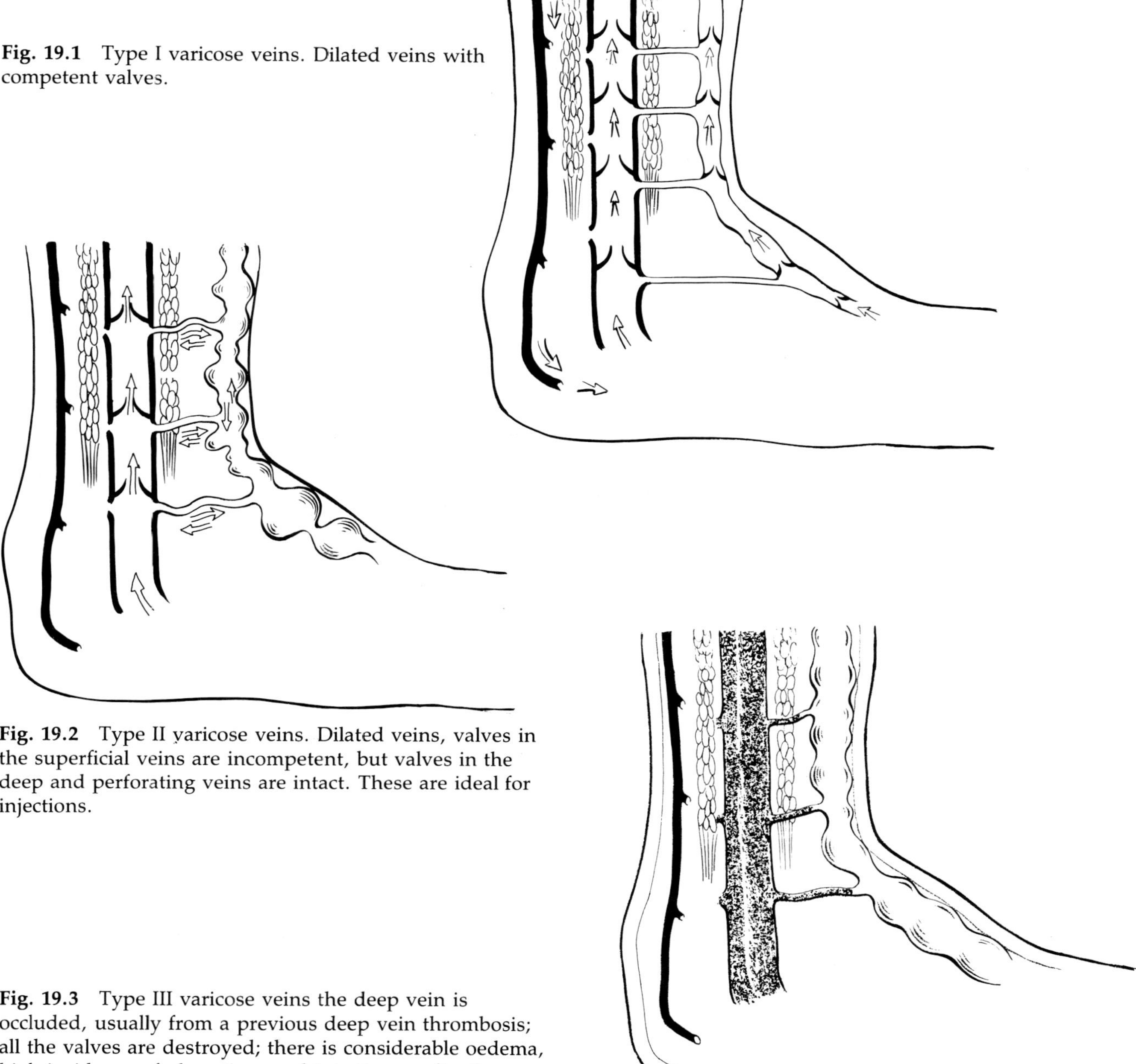

Fig. 19.1 Type I varicose veins. Dilated veins with competent valves.

Fig. 19.2 Type II varicose veins. Dilated veins, valves in the superficial veins are incompetent, but valves in the deep and perforating veins are intact. These are ideal for injections.

Fig. 19.3 Type III varicose veins the deep vein is occluded, usually from a previous deep vein thrombosis; all the valves are destroyed; there is considerable oedema, high incidence of ulceration, and injections or ligations are *contra-indicated*.

19.1.2 Type II varicose veins (Fig. 19.2)

These veins are dilated; the valves in the superficial veins are incompetent, but the valves in the deep and perforating veins are still intact. These veins are therefore ideal for treatment.

19.1.3 Type III varicose veins (Fig. 19.3)

In type III varicose veins, the deep vein is occluded, usually from a previous deep vein thrombosis, all the valves are destroyed, there is considerable oedema, distention of the superficial veins and a high incidence of venous ulceration. As the limb is now relying on the superficial veins to maintain a venous circulation, treatment by ligation or sclerotherapy is **contra-indicated** and will make the situation worse. In many instances, the patient only seeks help when varicose ulceration has occurred; this is still not too late to commence treatment of the veins, as by reducing the superficial venous pressure, healing of the ulcer will be facilitated.

19.2 SELECTION OF PATIENTS

A simple selective procedure will improve results and avoid unnecessary treatment for unsuitable cases.

1. A careful history should be obtained to exclude any serious systemic disease.
2. A past history of deep vein thrombosis in the affected leg is an absolute contra-indication to sclerotherapy.
3. Veins which are confined to below the knee are most suitable for sclerotherapy. Those above the knee are difficult to bandage effectively and are better ligated.
4. Current medication is noted; patients taking the combined contraceptive pill or oestrogens for any other reasons should be asked to stop medication for one month before treatment if this is practicable.
5. If ulceration is present, check the arterial system and test the urine for sugar.
6. A test of sapheno-femoral incompetence is made as follows. The patient lies down and the leg is raised to 30° to empty the superficial veins. A narrow tube is applied as a tourniquet around the upper thigh, the leg is lowered, and the patient asked to stand up. If just the sapheno-femoral valve is incompetent, the superficial veins will fill slowly over 30 seconds from below upwards. If the perforating veins at a lower level are leaking, the superficial veins will fill rapidly, in which case other tourniquets may be applied progressively at lower levels until the site of leakage is identified. A second simple test is to apply a tourniquet around the leg at the level of the tibial tubercle and ask the patient to walk around for one minute. If the perforating vein valves are competent, the superficial veins empty.
7. As the recommended treatment involves daily periods of walking by the patient, it is not advisable to offer injections if for any reason the patient cannot walk at least three miles each day.
8. Patients with obese legs should be advised to lose weight before offering a course of injections.
9. Any known allergic reactions to STD is a contra-indication to sclerotherapy.

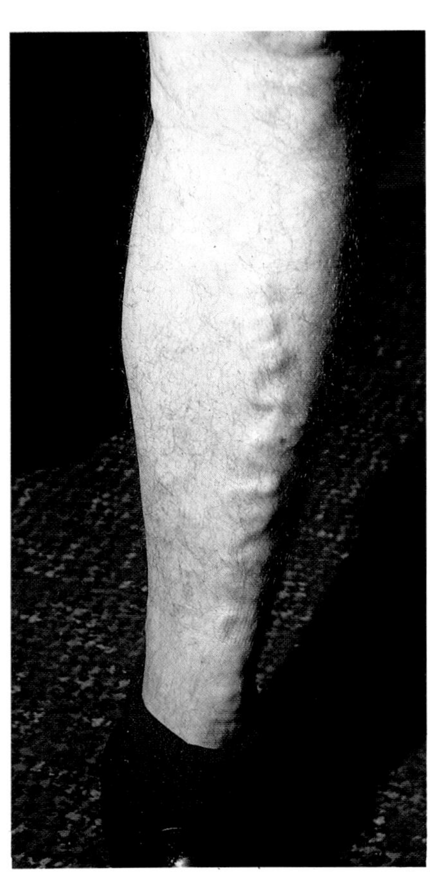

Fig. 19.4 Varicose veins affecting the short saphenous vein below the knee; ideal for sclerotherapy.

19.3 SCLEROTHERAPY

The object of sclerotherapy is to obliterate the lumen of the vein by injecting an irritant solution directly inside it, and compressing the inflamed surfaces together. Current interest in the technique was revived by Professor

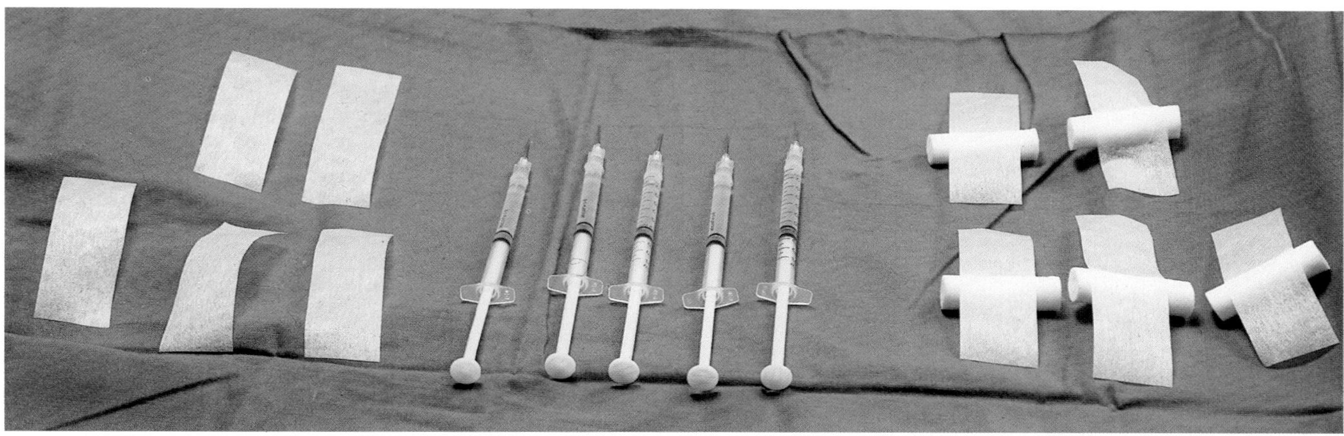

Fig. 19.5 Syringes with 3% STD adhesive tapes and cotton wool rolls in readiness for sclerotherapy.

Fegan in Dublin [19, 20] and provided suitable patients are selected carefully, i.e. Type I or II veins, below the knee, the results of treatment are very good.

Instruments required (Fig. 19.5)

- 6 × 1 ml sterile syringes
- 6 × 25 SWG × $\frac{5}{8}$″ (0.5 mm × 16 mm) needles
- 1 vial 30 ml 3% STD solution (sodium tetradecyl sulphate)
- elastic web bandage 3″ (7.6 cm) × 5 m
- tubular elastic stockinette (Tubigrip)
- size E 8.75 cm × 1 m or
- size F 10 cm × 1 m
- sorbo rubber pads or large cotton dental rolls
- adhesive tape (Micropore) 1″ (2.5 cm)

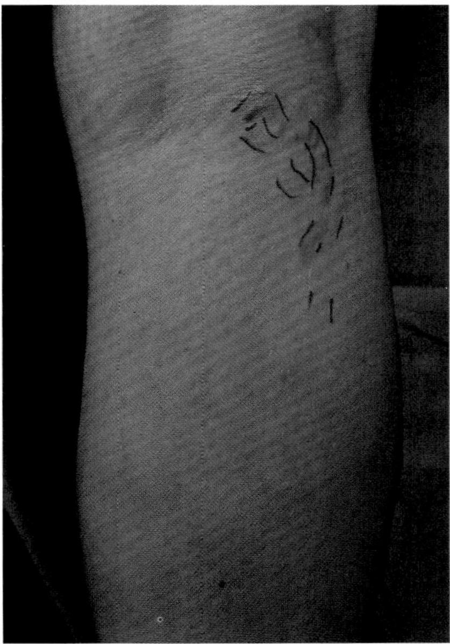

Fig. 19.6 The veins to be injected are first marked with a felt-tip pen, with the patient standing.

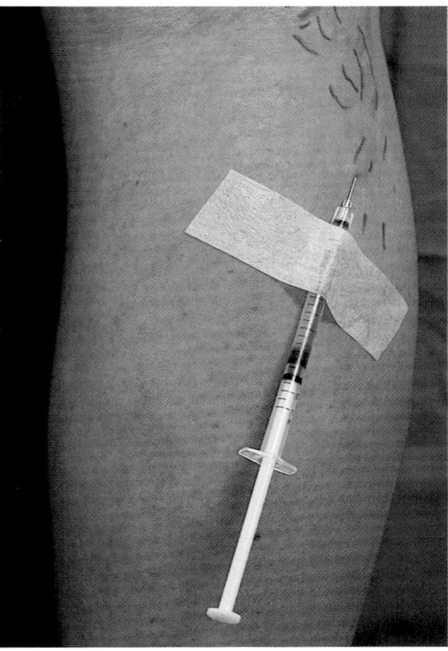

Fig. 19.7 With the patient standing, the first syringe is taped in position with the needle inside the vein.

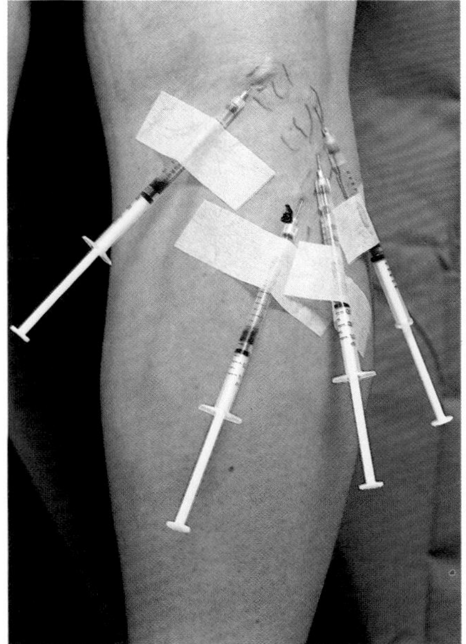

Fig. 19.8 Other syringes are now taped in position after placing the needle inside the vein.

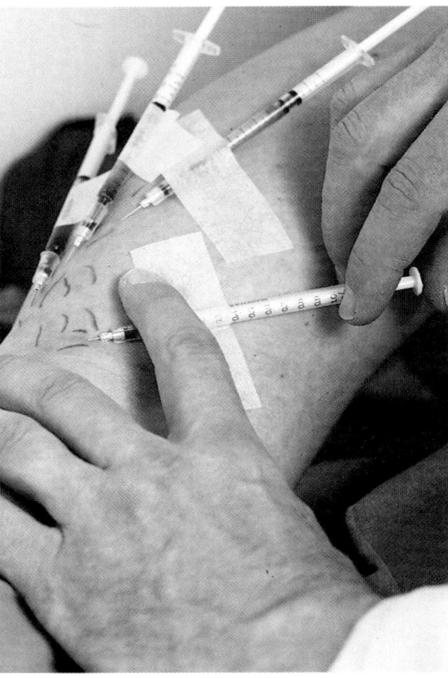

Fig. 19.9 With pressure on either side of the injection site, 0.5 ml 3% STD is injected into isolated segment of vein.

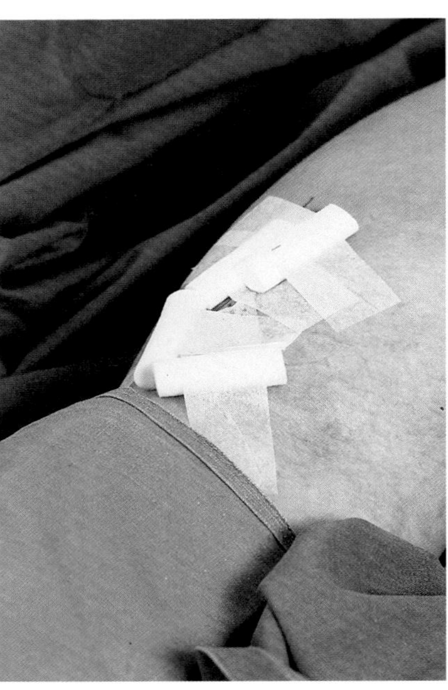

Fig. 19.10 Cotton wool rolls or sorbo-rubber pads are now placed over each injection site.

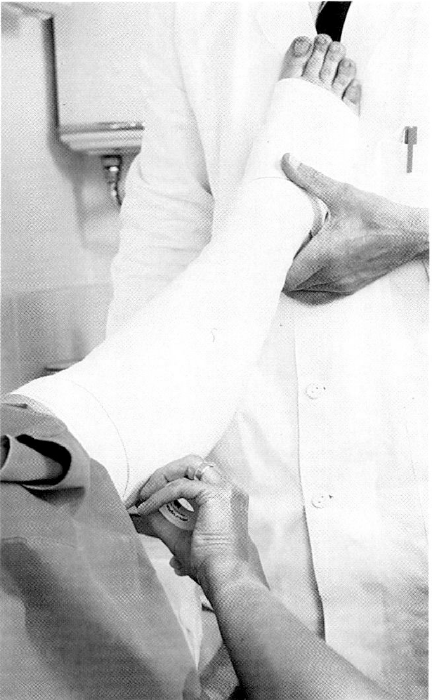

Fig. 19.11 An elastic web bandage (3″) is now applied from the toes to the knee.

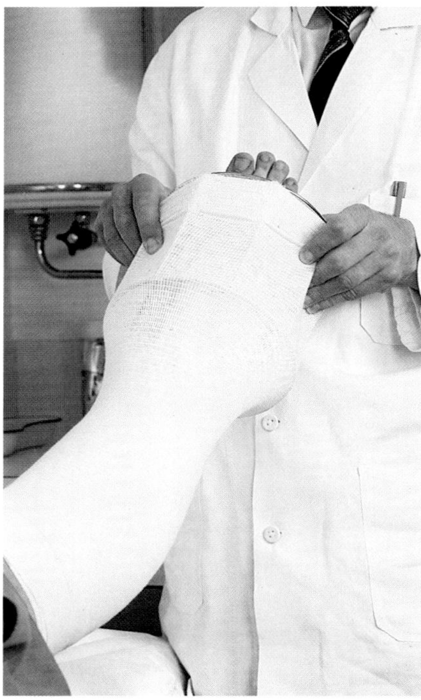

Fig. 19.12 An elasticated tubular bandage (Tubigrip) is now applied over the bandage, folding itself back to give two layers.

Good illumination is essential. The number of injections likely to be given is noted, and the same number of syringes filled with 3% STD solution; usually 0.7 ml per syringe is sufficient. One strip of adhesive tape, 1″ × 4″ (2.5 cm × 10 cm) per syringe is stuck to the glass shelf of the instrument trolley in readiness, and a second strip 1″ × 4″ (2.5 cm × 10 cm) with a large cotton dental roll, per syringe, also attached to the shelf.

With the patient standing on a low stool the veins to be injected are identified using a felt-tip marker (Fig. 19.6). Still with the patient standing, and the doctor kneeling, the needle of the pre-loaded syringe is inserted in the vein and the plunger very slightly withdrawn (Fig. 19.7). Dark blood enters the syringe, confirming that the needle is in the correct place.

Without moving the syringe or needle at all, they are carefully taped in position using the first strip of adhesive (Micropore) tape. The second injection is performed in exactly the same way, taping the syringe in place as before. Several injections may be given at one session, but the total volume of STD should not exceed 4 ml.

With all syringes taped in position, the operator carefully helps the patient to lie down on the couch or operating table and elevates the leg to about 30° from the horizontal. With an assistant holding the leg, the doctor now applies finger and thumb over the segment of vein to be injected, thus isolating this short strip of vein. With the other hand the contents of the syringe are injected into this segment, and a compression pad applied before removing the needle (Figs 19.9 and 19.10). It is important to keep the sclerosant in the empty and isolated segment for at least 30 seconds. If possible, an assistant maintains pressure over the injected site while the operator proceeds to inject the remaining sites.

When all sites have been injected, an elastic web bandage is applied from the toes to the knee, and this is then covered with an elasticated tubular bandage (Tubigrip E or F) doubled back on itself to produce two layers of compression. The patient is given an instruction sheet, advised to walk at least three miles every day for the next three weeks when the bandages and pads are removed. It is wise to warn the patient that they may experience severe pain in the leg during the first 48 hours, but that this will subside. They may reapply the bandages themselves if too tight, but should not disturb the compression pads.

19.3.1 Complications of sclerotherapy

Pain is a common accompaniment of injection treatment and this generally settles in a few days. Occasionally, extravasation of the sodium tetradecyl solution results in severe pain, followed by an area of necrosis that may slough and produce an ulcer. A dry dressing is all that is required, and healing may take very many months leaving a permanent depressed scar, and a depressed patient! Under these circumstances it may be prudent to excise the ulcer and close the wound by primary suture.

Accidental intra-arterial injection would result in immediate, severe, burning pain over the distal distribution. Should this occur, the needle should be left in the artery and heparin and Lignocaine slowly injected; this is obviously the most potentially serious complication in a technique which is otherwise remarkably free of complications.

19.4 LIGATION OF VARICOSE VEINS

Ligation of varicose veins is easily possible in a general practice setting, but as with sclerotherapy, careful selection of suitable patients is necessary to ensure that the ligation actually controls the underlying problem.

Instruments required

1 scalpel handle size 3
1 scalpel blade size 15
1 surgical suture mersilk. Reference Ethicon W533 (or equivalent)
2 pairs artery forceps, straight 5″ (12.7 cm)
1 10 ml syringe
1 25 SWG × $\frac{5}{8}$″ (0.5 mm × 16 mm) needle
1 23 SWG × 1″ (0.6 mm × 25 mm) needle
10 ml 1% Lignocaine with adrenalin 1:200 000
Povidone-iodine (Betadine) alcoholic solution

The technique is as follows: with the patient standing, suitable veins are identified and marked; the patient now lies down, and the area is painted with betadine alcoholic solution; 1% Lignocaine with adrenalin is carefully infiltrated in the overlying skin, and a small 5 mm incision is made over a marked site. The vein is lifted out, grasped on each side with the haemostats and divided. Each end may then be 'winkled' and a significant length of vein ligated and removed, leaving a cosmetically acceptable scar [21].

TWENTY

Minor surgical procedures in gynaecology

'If thou examinest a woman suffering in her abdomen so that the menstrual discharge cannot come away from her . . . apply Frankincense and incense between her two loins and cause the smoke thereof to enter her flesh'

(Edwin Smith, Surgical Papyrus, 3000–2500 BC)

As well as all the usual intradermal lesions which can effect the skin over the perineum and vulva, several lesions of the cervix, vagina and labia can be effectively treated with the minimum of instruments and equipment. Also included is cervical cytology and the insertion of intra-uterine contraceptive devices, together with repair of episiotomy following delivery.

20.1 CERVICAL CYTOLOGY

During the last decade most general practitioners have learned to take routine cervical smears for cytology. The procedure itself is quite straightforward, using a vaginal speculum (preferably not lubricated with jelly) the cervix is visualized. Good illumination is essential, whether external spotlight, integral fibre-optic illumination, or tungsten-filament bulbs. The cervix is first inspected, and any unusual features such as excessive discharge, bleeding, erosions, polypi, etc. noted. The purpose-designed wooden cervical spatula is placed at the entrance to the external cervical os, and rotated through 360 degrees, thus obtaining cells from the whole area. These are then transferred to a microscope slide by wiping the spatula on the glass in one direction only, followed by immediate fixation with suitable preservative. The slide is then labelled with the patient's name and the appropriate request form completed. Bacterial swabs may also be taken at the same time if necessary (Fig. 20.1).

20.2 ENDOMETRIAL CELL SAMPLERS

These are now also available by which the secretions inside the uterine cavity can be aspirated by gentle suction and sent for cytological examination; this will often obviate the need for a diagnostic D and C.

20.3 CAUTERIZATION OF CERVICAL EROSIONS

The popularity of cauterizing every cervical 'erosion' has waned in recent years with the realization that many so called erosions were not causing any symptoms and were not a sign of disease.

Where an erosion is giving symptoms such as a heavy discharge,

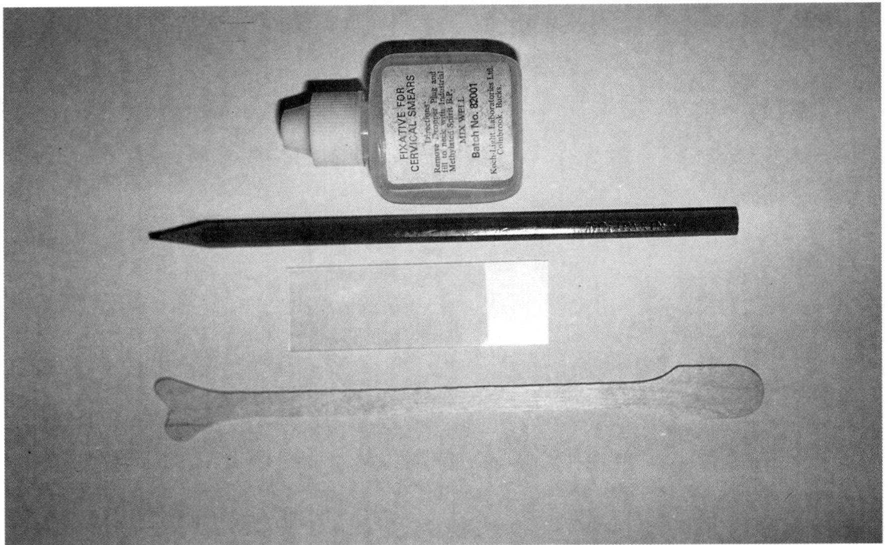

Fig. 20.1 All that is needed to take a cervical smear.

repeated infections and discomfort, it may be effectively treated with any one of these methods of cautery: Silver Nitrate, cryotherapy, electrocautery and diathermy. Silver Nitrate is still the simplest, cheapest, and quickest means of treating a moderate erosion and disposable applicators with a Silver Nitrate bead are readily available (see Chapter 28).

20.3.1 Technique of Silver Nitrate application

The cervix is visualized, and any cervical smears or bacterial swabs taken. The silver nitrate is now applied to the cervix, including the external cervical os; the area treated immediately turns white. The patient should be warned to expect an increased watery, sometimes blood-stained discharge for several weeks. A topical antiseptic or antibiotic cream may be given during this time to reduce risks of secondary infection.

20.4 CRYOTHERAPY FOR CERVICAL EROSIONS

A nitrous oxide or liquid nitrogen cryoprobe is ideal for cauterizing troublesome cervical erosions. Treatment is quick, simple to apply, and has a high success rate and patient acceptability (see Chapter 30).

20.4.1 Technique

Good visualization of the cervix is essential; one hazard of using the cryoprobe is that it can adhere to adjacent vaginal walls if they accidentally touch the probe tip or side and result in a small 'burn'. The cone shaped applicator is placed on the cervix *before* starting to freeze; this enables it to be accurately positioned. Once in position the nitrous oxide or liquid nitrogen is switched on and freezing commences. The probe will become adherent to the cervix at this stage, generally 1–2 minutes is sufficient treatment time, and the probe either allowed to thaw out spontaneously or 'de-frosted' with the built-in defroster attachment. One treatment is normally all that is required, but a greater depth of penetration is obtained by giving a second freeze immediately following thawing if this is felt necessary. Follow-up is exactly as for Silver Nitrate.

20.5 ELECTROCAUTERY OF CERVICAL EROSIONS

As the cervical nerve endings are not sensitive to heat, any erosion may be cauterized using the electrocautery. Care must be taken if cauterizing the cervical os or cervical canal not to cause fibrosis, scarring and stenosis, likewise during treatment, if steam is produced which passes inside the uterus, pain is caused. To avoid the risk of stenosis, linear radial cauterization should be employed, using the standard V-shaped platinum wire electrode.

20.6 DIATHERMY OF CERVICAL EROSIONS

The use of standard bi-polar diathermy requires a general anaesthetic; unipolar high-frequency diathermy may be used successfully without any anaesthetic. The hyfrecator electrode is held a short distance away from the cervix, the current switched on, and a stream of sparks drawn from the electrode to the cervix (see Chapter 31). This fulgurization effectively cauterizes the cervix. As with all other methods of cautery, the patient should be warned to expect an increased watery blood-stained discharge for several weeks following treatment. An antiseptic or antibiotic cream may be applied during this time to reduce secondary infection.

20.7 VAGINAL VAULT GRANULATIONS FOLLOWING HYSTERECTOMY

Granulations in the vault of the vagina are relatively common following hysterectomy, they may cause a blood-stained discharge or even frank bleeding, both of which can cause anxiety to the patient.

Examination with a vaginal speculum reveals typical, messy, granulations, easily friable, and which bleed on the slightest touch. Treatment is simple, using Silver Nitrate to each granulation. Normally one application is sufficient to cure the condition.

20.8 TREATMENT OF CONDYLOMATA ACUMINATA

The treatment of genital warts can be both time-consuming and disappointing; the application of podophyllin in spirit is traditionally the treatment of choice; strengths as high as 10–40% were originally used – more recently equally good results have been obtained by using 0.5% podophyllin in spirit, applied by the patient to each wart twice daily for three days [22]. More stubborn warts may be individually treated with electrocautery, diathermy or cryoprobe, but recurrences are common.

20.9 REPAIR OF EPISIOTOMY

A good repair of an episiotomy or second degree tear following delivery can occasionally be quite difficult; however, time taken identifying each layer is well spent, makes the repair easier, and results in better more comfortable healing. As with any surgical procedure, good illumination is paramount; the patient should be supported in the lithotomy position and a small swab on a cord inserted to the top of the vagina; this helps to control oozing from the uterus as well as helping to identify the extent of the laceration in the posterior vaginal wall. The top of this laceration *must* be identified, and the first suture inserted in the posterior vaginal wall just above the laceration. Chromic catgut 2/0 (metric 3.5) is suitable for this stitch (Ref. Ethicon W 565). Using a continuous stitch, the posterior vaginal wall is closed. Next, one or two interrupted catgut sutures are placed in the muscle layer between posterior vaginal wall and skin. Finally the perineal skin is approximated using either interrupted braided silk suture Ethicon W 667 (metric 3, 2/0) on a curved reverse cutting needle, interrupted chromic catgut stitches, a subcuticular catgut, or dexon suture, depending on the preference of the operator.

20.10 BARTHOLIN'S CYSTS AND ABSCESSES

These can be extremely painful, some rupture spontaneously; those that do not may be treated either by aspiration, aspiration and injection of Fucidic acid gel, or marsupialization.

20.10.1 Aspiration

Although one would not expect aspiration alone to cure an abscess, nevetheless, it is found that many Bartholin's abscesses respond to a single aspiration using a wide-bore needle and syringe. As an added safeguard, injection of Fucidic acid gel (Fucidin Caviject) following aspiration seems to give improved results.

20.10.2 Marsupialization

Recurrent Bartholin's abscesses are best treated by marsupialization. This consists in creating a permanent sinus by incision, followed by suturing the lining of the cyst to the outside skin; it is very effective and normally results in a permanent cure.

20.11 IUCD INSERTION

As a method of contraception, intra-uterine devices have become popular in the last 20 years. There are now many different sizes, shapes and materials to choose from, and the practitioner will need to refer to the instruction leaflets provided with each device to determine the method of insertion.

20.11.1 Counselling

The patient and preferably her husband should discuss with the doctor the pros and cons of this method of contraception; they should realize that no coil is 100% effective, that the periods following insertion may be much heavier and longer than previously, that occasionally the coil is expelled spontaneously, and that she should report for regular check-ups and cervical cytology. Although it has been shown to be a far safer procedure than was originally forecast, nevertheless, resuscitation facilities should be available for the unexpected vagal attacks. Similarly the risks of introducing infection are very much less than was anticipated – however, a rigid no-touch technique should be used throughout.

20.11.2 Technique

Whether the patient is lying on her left side or on her back depends on the preference of the doctor, whichever position is used, it is essential to visualize the cervix clearly. Using vulsellum forceps, the anterior lip of the cervix is grasped, and downward traction applied; this has the effect of straightening the longitudinal axis of the uterus and makes insertion easier. A uterine sound may be used to ascertain the dimensions and shape of the uterus – however, it is not always necessary as the coil and introducer may serve as a sound during insertion and give just as much information (Fig. 20.2).

The coil is loaded in the introducer, which may be given a very slight bend at the tip using the fingers and thumb of the left gloved hand; this simple manoeuvre makes sounding and insertion much easier and is to be

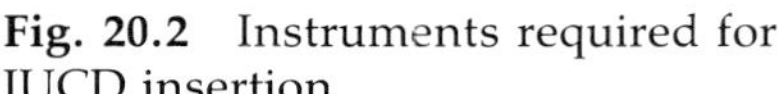

Fig. 20.2 Instruments required for IUCD insertion.

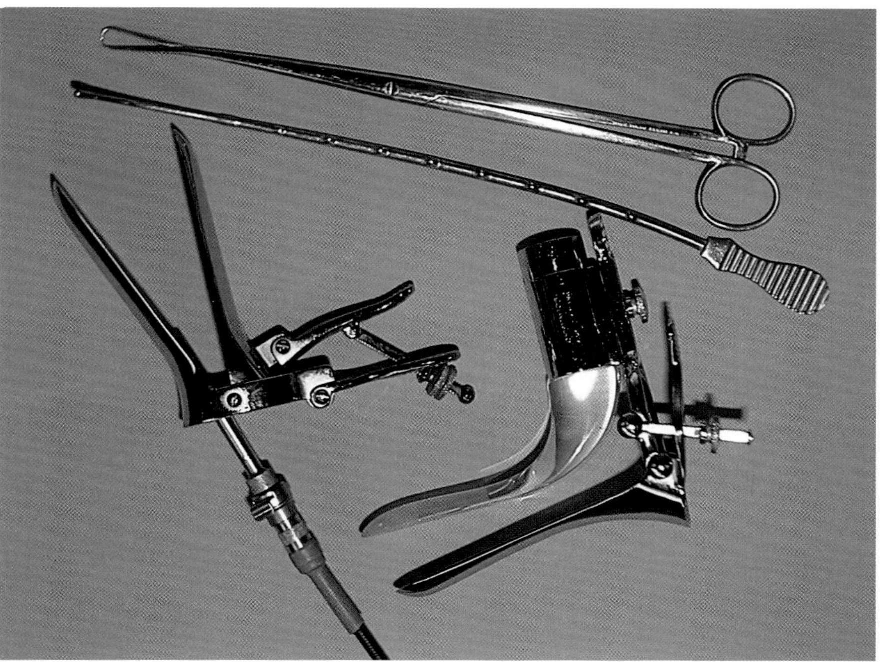

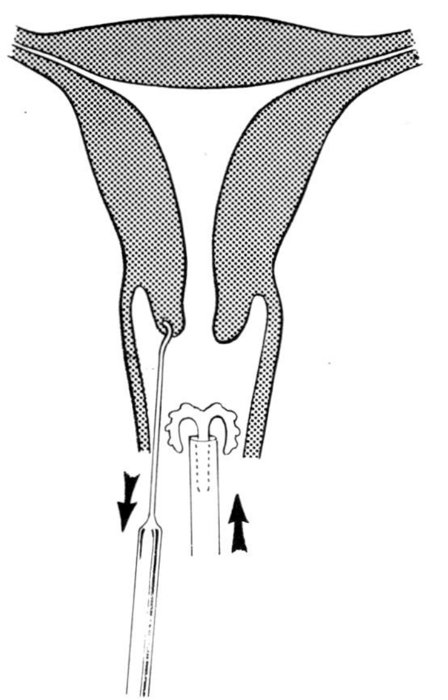

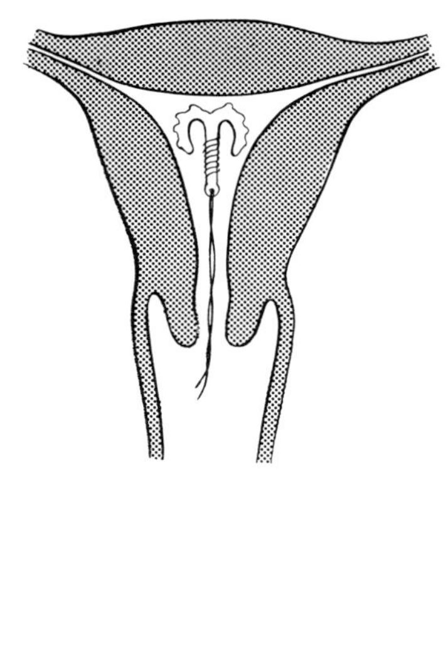

Fig. 20.3 IUCD insertion; the cervix is steadied by the application of a pair of vulsellum forceps, and slight traction applied. The IUCD is then inserted inside the uterine cavity.

recommended. Using gentle pressure, and if necessary slight rotation to 'feel' the direction of the cervical canal, the coil is introduced in the uterine cavity until it is felt to touch the fundus. The introducer is then withdrawn leaving the coil in position. The threads are then cut using McIndoe's curved 7″ (17.8 cm) scissors, and the vaginal speculum removed. The patient is requested to return for a coil check in four weeks and if all is well, annually thereafter. Copper containing coils have a limited life of 2–3 years and need to be changed after this interval. Generally the optimum time to insert a coil is at a six week post-natal examination, or at the end of a menstrual period. Nulliparous patients tend to have more abdominal cramps and side-effects.

TWENTY-ONE

Sebaceous cysts

'I made an incision in the scalp, and upon the side on which I stood, which was about three-fourths of its size, I with difficulty detached it from the skin. . . . The edges of the wound were brought together and lint and plaster applied. The King bore the operation well'

(Account by Sir Astley Cooper of the removal of a sebaceous cyst from the scalp of King George IVth, 1820)

True sebaceous cysts are very rare; epidermal and tricholemmal cysts are very common and usually referred to as sebaceous cysts (Fig. 21.1).

Epidermal cysts occur following implantation of epidermis, or from the epidermal lining of pilo sebaceous follicles and are filled with macerated keratin; they can occur anywhere on the body, commonly fingers, from implantation.

The cysts commonly seen on the scalp are tricholemmal (pilar) cysts which are derived from the hair follicle; they occur in families, being inherited as an autosomal dominant gene, and are often multiple. Both types of cyst are ideal for removal in the doctor's treatment room under local anaesthetic. For the remainder of the chapter the term 'sebaceous cyst' will be used as it is better known for both epidermal and tricholemmal cysts.

Instruments required

1 scalpel handle size 3
1 scalpel blade size 15
1 pair stitch scissors 5″ (12.7 cm)
1 pair McIndoe curved scissors 7″ (17.8 cm)
1 pair toothed dissecting forceps
1 pair Halstead mosquito forceps 5″ (12.7 cm) curved
1 Kilner needle holder $5\frac{1}{4}$″ (13.3 cm)
surgical sutures, braided silk, metric
gauge 2 (3/0) on curved cutting needle (Ref. Ethicon W 533)
1% Lignocaine with adrenalin 1:200 000
syringes and needles
Povidone-iodine in spirit (Betadine alcoholic solution)

21.1 TECHNIQUE FOR REMOVAL OF 'SEBACEOUS CYST' ON THE SCALP

The patient should preferably be lying down rather than sitting in a chair; even the most unlikely character is liable to faint, and it is embarrassing to have to complete the excision of a cyst on the floor!

Any overlying hairs are clipped with scissors (it is not necessary to shave large areas of scalp) and the overlying skin painted with Povidone-iodine in spirit (Betadine alcoholic solution).

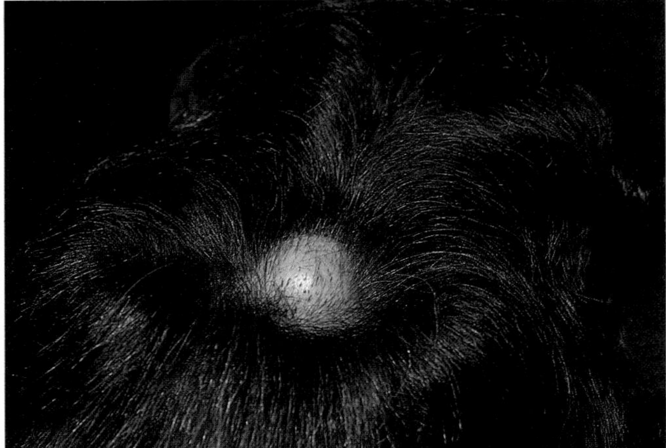

Fig. 21.1 Typical sebaceous cyst on scalp.

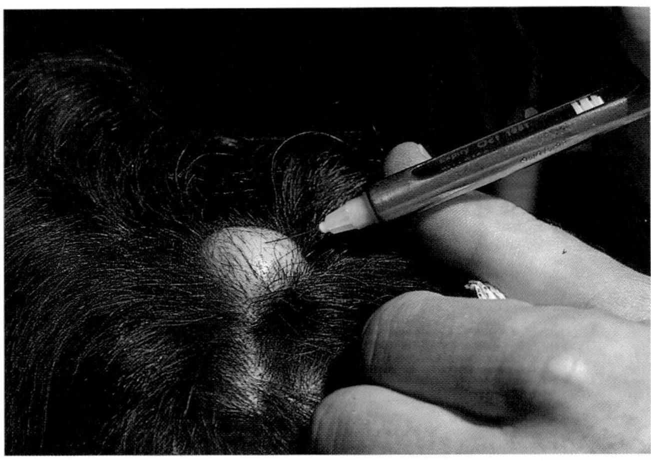

Fig. 21.2 The overlying skin is infiltrated with local anaesthetic and a small quantity injected to the base of the cyst.

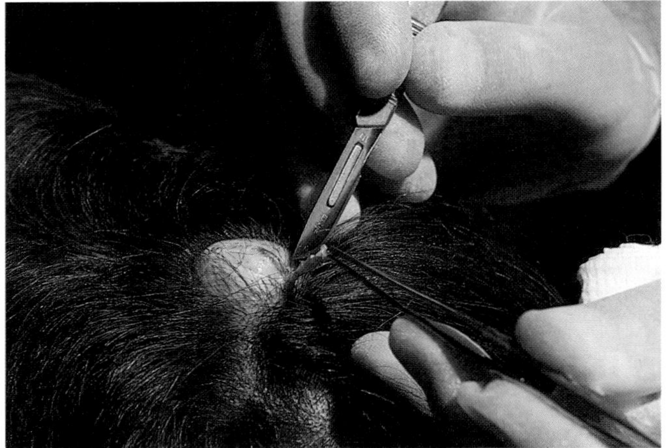

Fig. 21.3 An elliptical incision is made over the cyst exposing the underlying cyst.

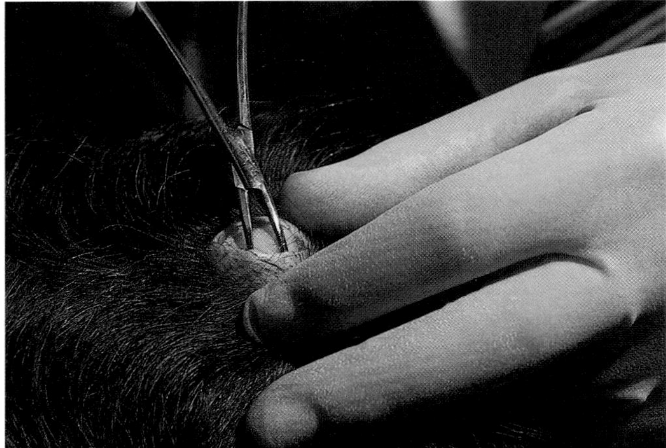

Fig. 21.4 Using curved mosquito forceps or curved McIndoe scissors, the cyst is dissected free.

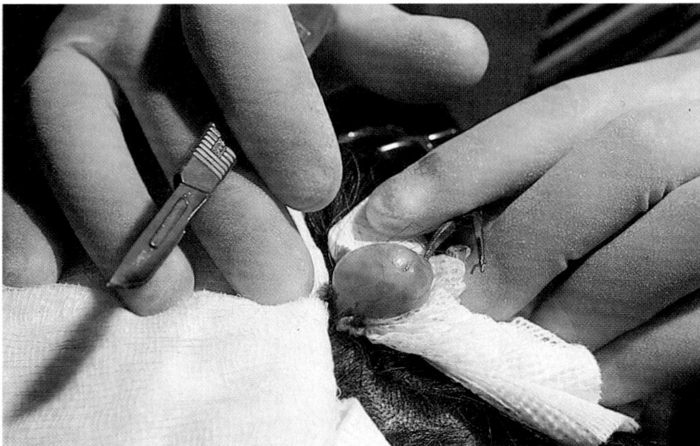

Fig. 21.5 With a little patience and careful dissection, the cyst may be removed complete.

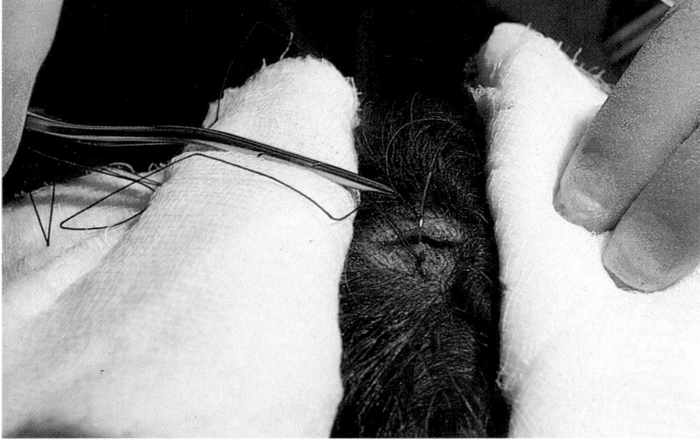

Fig. 21.6 Closure is with interrupted braided silk sutures.

With the finger and thumb of the left hand fixing the cyst, local anaesthetic is injected through the skin using a 25 SWG × $\frac{5}{8}$" (0.5 mm × 16 mm) needle, with the bevel flat against the skin. Keeping pressure on the syringe plunger, the needle is slowly advanced, until it reaches the tissue plane between skin and cyst. At this stage, there is a loss of resistance in the syringe plunger, and distention of the cyst may be felt with the palpating finger and thumb of the left hand. Further pressure on the syringe plunger spreads the Lignocaine and adrenalin around the cyst, causing the overlying skin to blanche (Fig. 21.2).

Done carefully, this technique separates the tissue planes and makes subsequent excision easier. One additional injection of local anaesthetic is made underneath the cyst before finally removing the needle. Occasionally the pressure of the local anaesthetic infiltration causes the cyst to eject some of its contents through the blocked punctum.

21.1.1 Incision

Very small cysts can be removed merely by a single incision and digital pressure, when the cyst will 'pop out'. Closure with one stitch is all that is required. Larger cysts require dissection, and the excision of an ellipse of redundant skin. The ellipse of skin should be chosen to include the central punctum; it may be excised exposing the underlying cyst. Using the blades of a curved McIndoe's scissors, the cyst is freed by gently inserting the closed blades and opening them. Any adhesions can be separated either by this method or cutting, using the same scissors (Figs 21.3, 21.4). At this stage the cyst may be grasped with the toothed dissecting forceps, traction applied, and the remaining adhesions divided. Bleeding is not usually a problem, except perhaps with cysts at the back of the neck; it can normally be controlled with firm pressure and usually stops when the edges of the wound are sutured. The aim should be to remove the cyst complete, although this is not always possible, particularly with thin-walled cysts where the centre has become infected. Where there is evidence of infection, the cyst should still be removed, but before closure, a small quantity of fucidic acid gel (Fucidin Caviject) should be instilled into the cavity and the skin then sutured in the usual way.

21.1.2 Closure

Interrupted braided silk sutures should be used which may be removed on the 8th–10th post-operative day. Where there is redundant skin which tends to invert on skin closure, the edges should be picked up in the stitch as shown in Fig. 21.7.

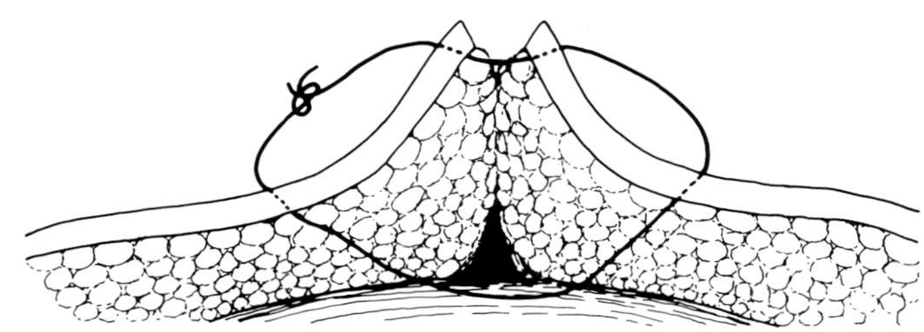

Fig. 21.7 Method of preventing skin edges inverting when suturing (Vertical mattress suture).

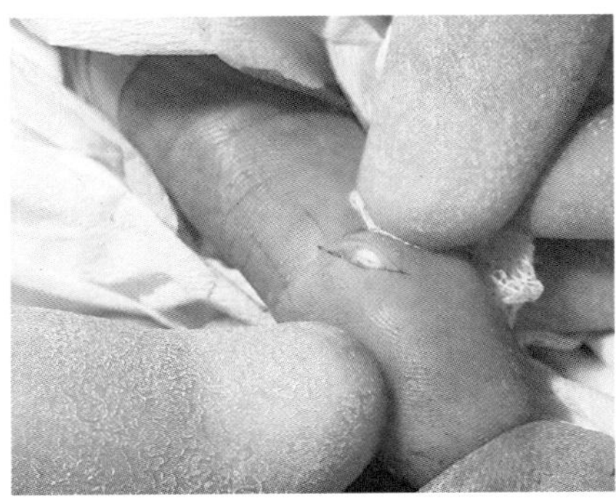

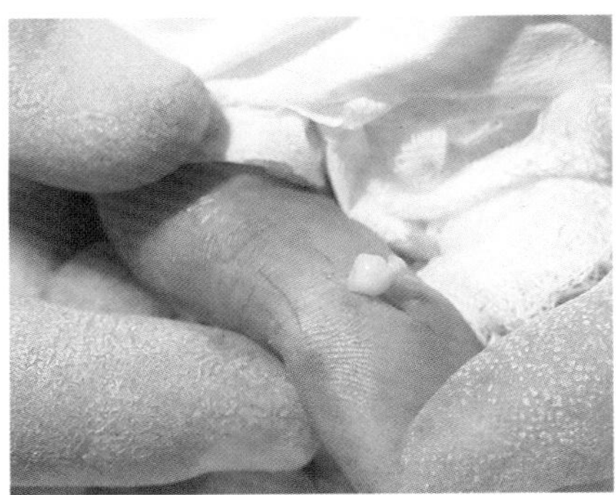

Fig. 21.8 Small inclusion or epidermal cyst in finger. Easily removed under ring-block and tourniquet.

Fig. 21.9 The same cyst being expressed by the application of finger-pressure on either side.

21.1.3 Alternative method of removal of sebaceous cysts

Some practitioners prefer to bisect the cyst, squeeze out the contents with a gauze swab, and then pull out the lining of the cyst with a pair of artery forceps. This is a much quicker procedure than dissection, but has the disadvantage of being messy, carries a slightly higher infection rate, and the contents of a sebaceous cyst have a slightly unpleasant, persistent, odour. Nevertheless, it is a perfectly acceptable method of removal.

21.1.4 Histology

As with all excised specimens, even the humble 'sebaceous cyst' should be sent for histological examination if at all possible; just occasionally an unsuspected squamous celled tumour, cylindroma or other rarity may be discovered.

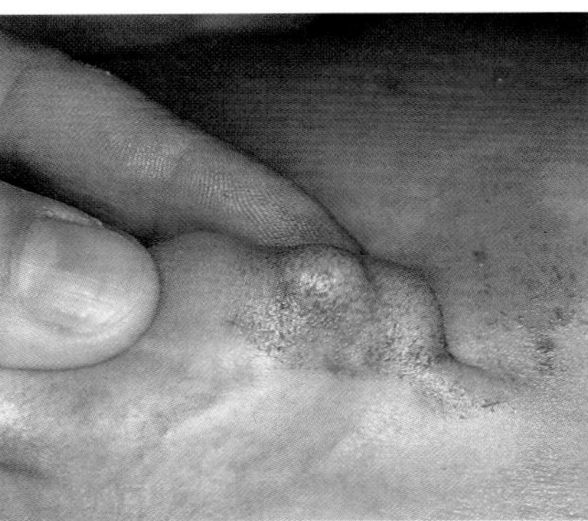

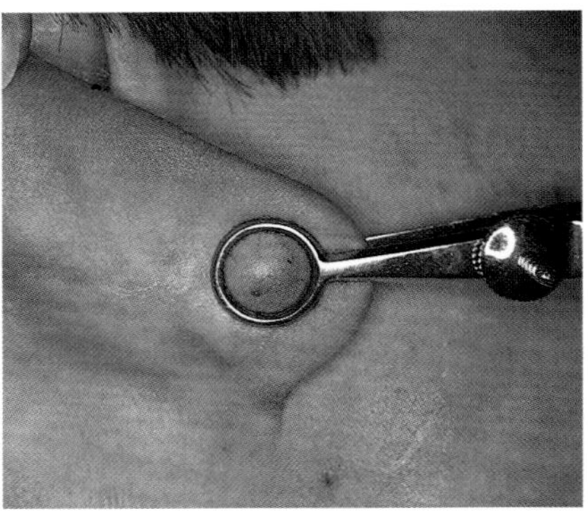

Fig. 21.10 Small ear-lobe cysts are very common.

Fig. 21.11 The application of ring forceps enables the cyst to be held and also controls bleeding.

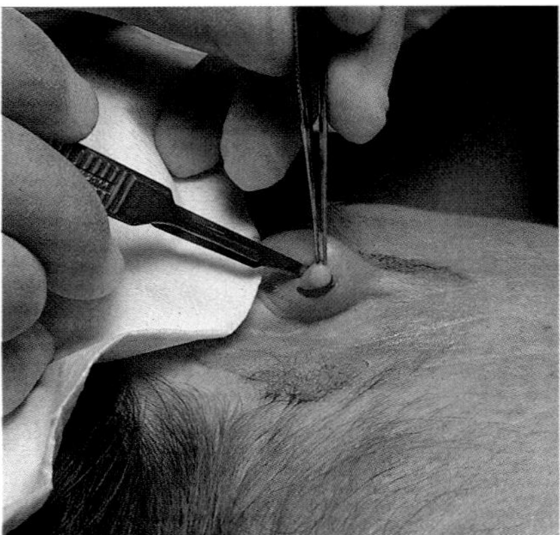

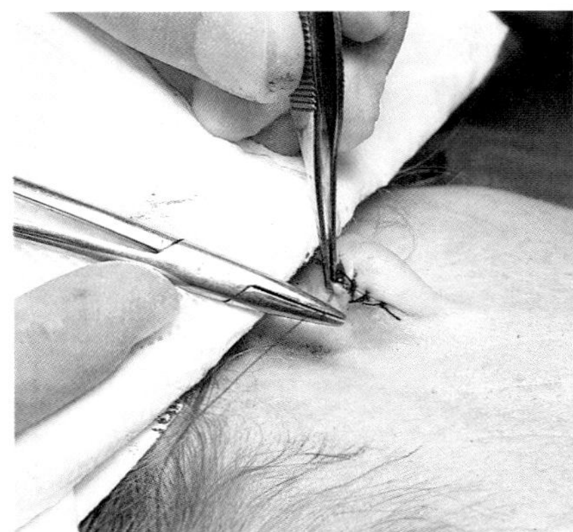

Fig. 21.12 Small epidermal cyst behind the ear; dissected free after infiltration with local anaesthetic.

Fig. 21.13 After removal of cyst, wound closed with fine interrupted braided silk sutures.

TWENTY-TWO

Lymph gland biopsy

'A Scrofula is an indurated gland, mostly forming in the neck, armpits and groins. . . . When the base of the scrofulous tumour runs out into a narrow point, we may cut it away readily'

(Paul of Aegina, 7th Century AD)

Although not a common minor operation in general practice, excision of an enlarged lymph node may give extremely valuable information, establish a diagnosis rapidly, and enable treatment to be commenced. Most patients are understandably anxious if they discover an enlarged lymph gland; if excision and histological examination can be arranged in a matter of days, much of the worry is allayed. Fortunately many lymph glands are situated superficially and may be excised simply under local anaesthesia.

22.1 SELECTION OF PATIENTS

Certain preliminary investigations will help to establish a diagnosis and may make the need for lymph node biopsy unnecessary. These include a full blood count, haemoglobin, differential white cell count and platelets, ESR, or plasma viscosity, serum proteins and electrophoresis, liver function tests, LE cells, auto-antibody screening, chest X-ray and possibly blood culture if pyrexial and bone marrow.

These tests, together with a careful clinical examination will establish a diagnosis in the majority of patients; those remaining will then be helped by excision of a gland for histological examination. Before embarking on surgery, a representative gland should be chosen; indeed if a Tru-cut biospy needle is available, a needle biopsy might give the pathologist sufficient material to make a diagnosis. If not, excision should be undertaken.

22.2 TECHNIQUE FOR EXCISION OF GLAND

Instruments required

1 scalpel size 3
1 scalpel blade size 10
1 toothed dissecting forceps 5″ (12.7 cm)
1 McIndoe's scissors, curved 7″ (17.8 cm)
1 Kilner needle holder $5\frac{1}{4}$″ (13.3 cm)
2 pairs Halstead mosquito artery forceps curved 5″ (12.7 cm)
surgical suture, braided silk metric 2 (3/0) on curved cutting needle, (Ref. Ethicon W 533)
Povidone-iodine in spirit (Betadine alcoholic solution) 10 ml 1%
Lignocaine with adrenalin 1:200 000
syringes and needles

The overlying skin is painted with Povidone-iodine in spirit (Betadine alcoholic solution) and the area anaesthetized by infiltration using 1% Lignocaine and adrenalin 1:200 000. An incision is now made down to the gland, which may be dissected free using the curved McIndoe's scissors and scalpel, holding the gland with the toothed dissecting forceps. Bleeding can be troublesome, but normally responds to firm pressure; should any small bleeding points not be controlled by pressure, they may be clipped and ligated (Figs 22.1 and 22.2).

Closure is by interrupted braided silk sutures to the skin, with chromic catgut to the deeper layers if a dead space has been left. The excised gland should be placed in 10% formol saline, immediately labelled and sent for histological examination.

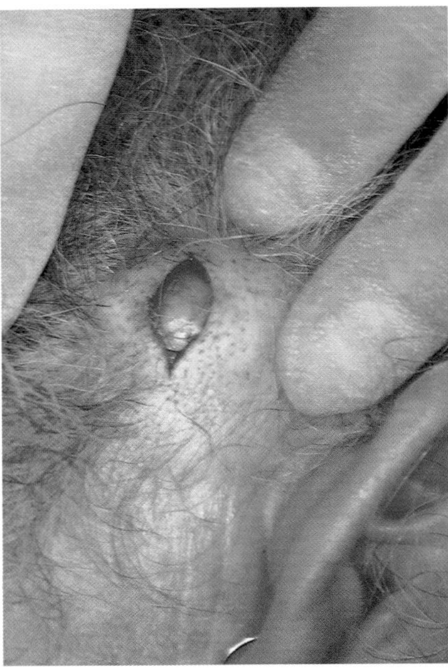

Fig. 22.1 Lymph-gland biopsy; technique similar to removal of sebaceous cyst.

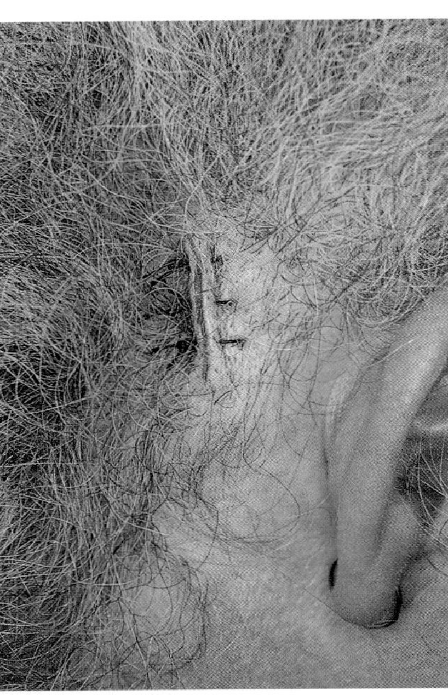

Fig. 22.2 Lymph-gland biopsy; closure with interrupted braided silk sutures.

TWENTY-THREE

Excision of lipoma

'When thou meetest a fatty growth, in the neck . . . then say thou 'He has a fatty growth in his neck – I will treat the disease with the knife, taking care of the blood vessels the while'

(Ebers Papyrus, 1500 BC)

A lipoma is a benign, fatty tumour which can occur anywhere on the body varying in size from a small marble to larger than a football. On palpation a lipoma feels lobulated and semi-cystic – smooth in outline, and generally painless. They may be solitary or multiple and the most commonly given reason for requesting removal is cosmetic, although in some sites, pressure effects may cause symptoms. Although appearing to be quite superficial, many lipomas extend deeper than expected, and the doctor should be aware of this fact before embarking on excision.

Many lipomata can be enucleated using a gloved finger; others are tethered by fibrous bands which give the lipoma its typical lobulated appearance; these bands need to be dissected free with the curved McIndoe's scissors.

Instruments required

- 1 scalpel handle no. 3
- 1 scalpel blade no. 10
- 1 pair McIndoe's scissors 7″ (17.8 cm) curved
- 1 pair toothed dissecting forceps
- 1 Kilner needle holder $5\frac{1}{4}$″ (13.3 cm)
- 1 Halstead's artery forceps 5″ (12.7 cm) curved
- Povidone-iodine in spirit (Betadine alcoholic solution)
- 10 ml 1% Lignocaine with 1:200 000 adrenalin
- syringes and needles

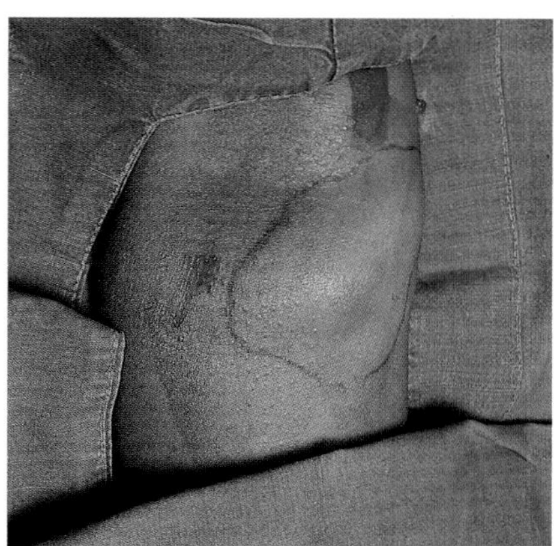

Fig. 23.1 Lipoma situated in antecubital fossa; the brachial artery is marked in red.

The size, shape and extent of the lipoma is first ascertained, and its relationship to any adjacent structures noted. The overlying skin is painted with Povidone-iodine in spirit (Betadine alcoholic solution) and the area infiltrated with 1% Lignocaine with adrenalin 1:200 000, remembering to include the deeper part of the lipoma (Fig. 23.1). An incision is made boldly through the skin directly to the lipoma which will bulge typically into the wound. At this stage a gloved finger can be inserted between skin and lipoma to see whether it will shell out; if not, further blunt dissection is carried out using the McIndoe's curved scissors and an opening action, dividing any fibrous bands tethering the lipoma to deeper tissues. With patience, the complete lipoma can be freed and removed; it is then sent for routine histological examination. Following removal of a large lipoma, a substantial 'dead' space is left which might collect blood and delay healing; in this case, it is advisable to close the space with interrupted catgut sutures. In excising larger lipomata, an ellipse of skin should also be removed to enable accurate closure with no redundant skin. Finally, skin

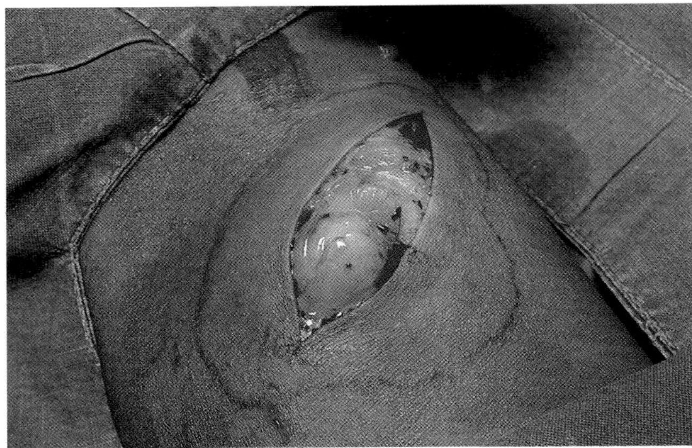

Fig. 23.2 Incising through the skin allows the lipoma to bulge through the wound.

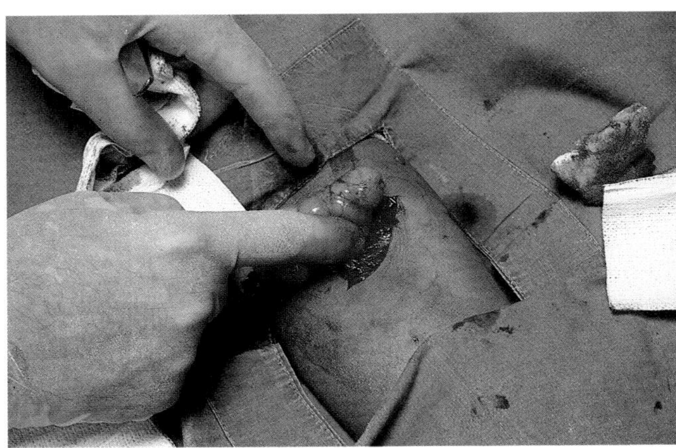

Fig. 23.3 Using finger dissection, the lipoma may be removed.

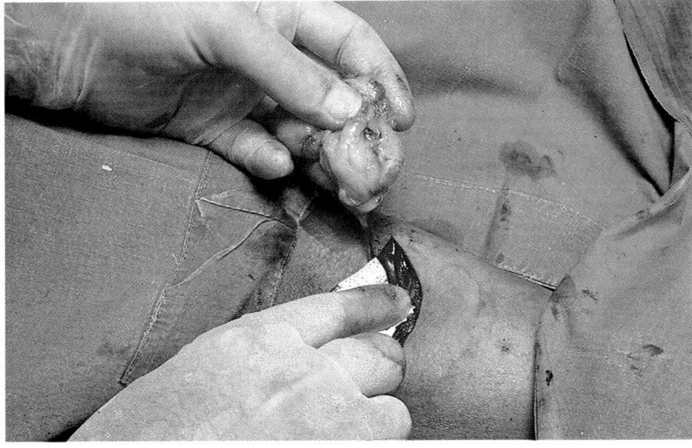

Fig. 23.4 Lipoma removed complete; any mild bleeding controlled with gauze swab.

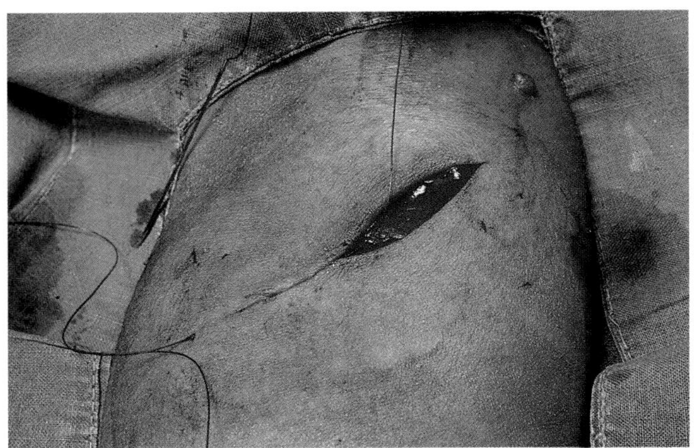

Fig. 23.5 Wound being closed with sub-cuticular nylon stitch.

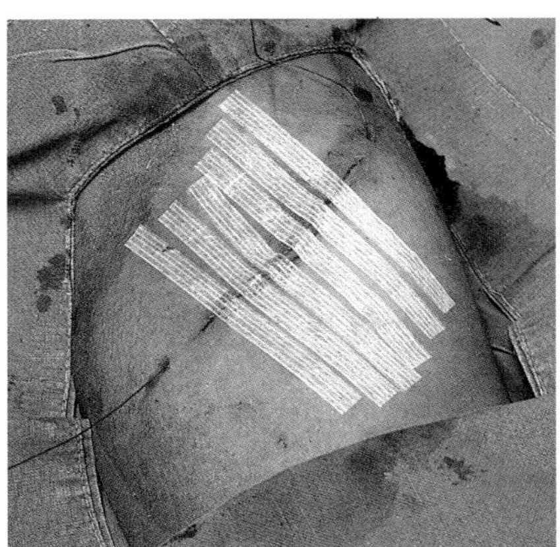

Fig. 23.6 Additional support may be given by the use of skin closure strips.

closure should be with either interrupted braided silk sutures, or a subcuticular nylon or dexon suture, the latter being probably more acceptable to the patient who requested removal on cosmetic grounds (Figs 23.2–23.6).

TWENTY-FOUR

Meibomian cysts

'Now one eyelid must be held open by the assistant, the other by the surgeon. Thereupon the surgeon passes a sharp hook, the point of which has been a little incurved under the edge of the pterygium and fixes the hook in it . . .'

(Celsus, AD 30)

Meibomian cysts (Tarsal cysts, Chalazion) are extremely common and lend themselves admirably for general practitioner minor surgery, taking only a few minutes to cure. When large, and situated in the upper lid, the patient may complain of blurred vision owing to distortion of the cornea produced by pressure of the cyst on it, resulting in a temporary astigmatism of up to 3 dioptres. Spontaneous resolution is likewise common, but may take many months, and as surgical treatment is so quick and simple, is to be preferred to waiting an indefinite time.

The diagnosis is usually straightforward; a small swelling can usually be seen on the outer surface of the affected eye-lid, eversion of this lid reveals a typical reddened spot with a paler centre, often pointing, and sometimes even discharging. The object of treatment is to incise the cyst, curette the cyst wall, and provide topical antibiotic cover until healing is complete, usually seven days (Fig. 24.1).

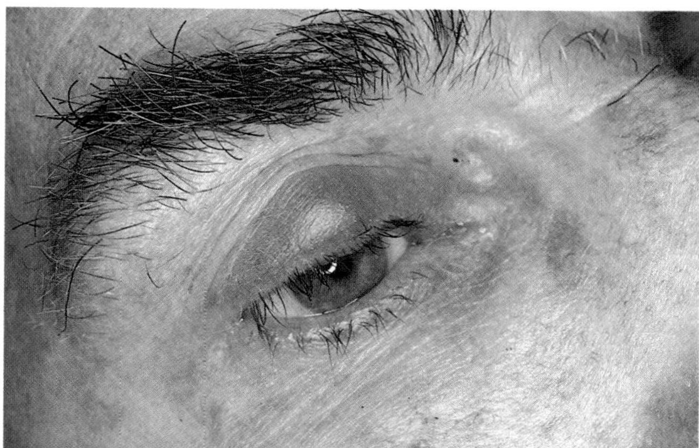

Fig. 24.1 External appearance of a meibomian cyst on the upper eye-lid.

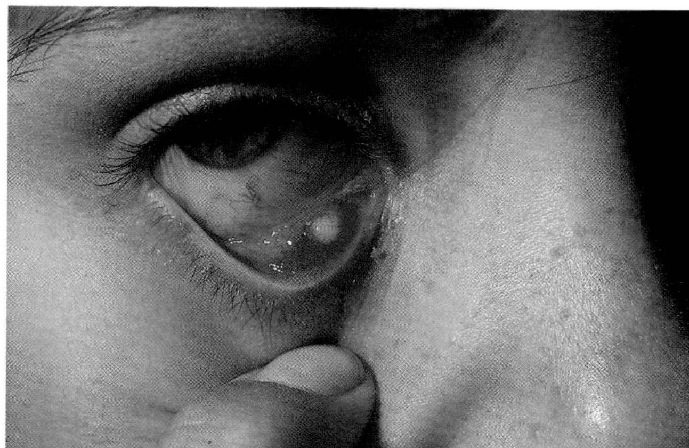

Fig. 24.2 A typical Meibomian cyst on the lower eye-lid.

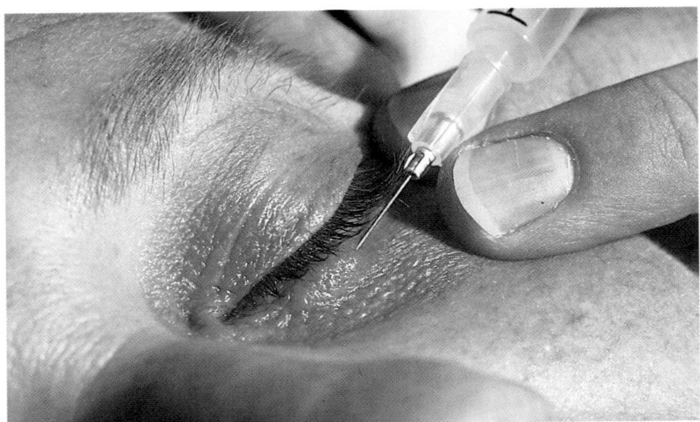

Fig. 24.3 After applying topical anaesthetic drops to the conjunctiva, the skin over the cyst is infiltrated with local anaesthetic, injecting a little into the cyst itself.

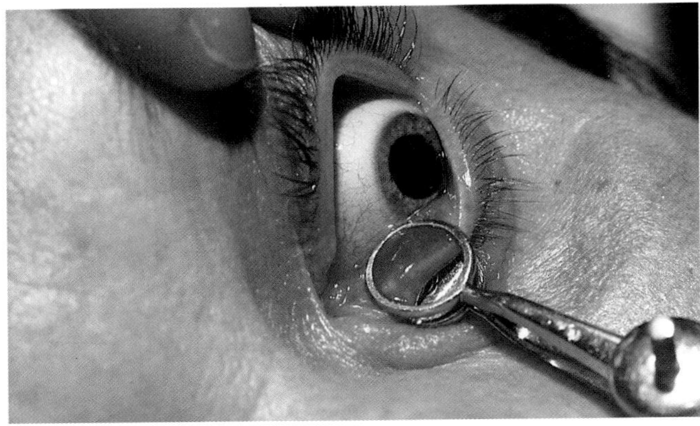

Fig. 24.4 The ring forceps are now applied so that cyst lies in the centre of the ring.

Instruments required

- 1 dental syringe
- 30 SWG (0.3 mm) needle
- 1 cartridge of Lignocaine 2% with 1:80 000 adrenalin
- anaesthetic eye-drops Amethocaine, Lignocaine or Minims Oxybuprocaine
- 1 chalazion ring forceps (blepharostat)
- 1 chalazion curette
- 1 pair iris scissors $4\frac{1}{2}$" (11.4 cm) curved
- 1 scalpel handle size 3
- 1 scalpel blade size 11
- 1 pair fine-toothed Adson dissecting forceps $4\frac{3}{4}$" (12 cm)
- chloramphenicol eye-drops and ointment
- 1 eye pad and bandage

The conjunctiva is anaesthetized using local anaesthetic eye drops; then with the fine 30 SWG (0.3 mm) needle, Lignocaine and adrenalin is injected into the skin over the cyst and a small quantity injected actually into the cyst itself. Next, the chalazion ring forceps are applied to the eye-lid with the ring on the conjunctival surface exactly over the cyst, and the circular flat blade over the skin of the eye-lid. By tightening the screw on the ring forceps, the cyst is not only fixed and any bleeding controlled, but also the eye-lid may comfortably be everted, exposing the bulging cyst in the centre of the ring clamp (Fig. 24.4). Using the pointed no. 11 blade, a vertical incision is made in the cyst and the gelatinous contents released. The cyst wall is then curetted using the small sharp-spoon chalazion curette, a small quantity of Chloramphenicol eye ointment applied, the ring forceps removed, and an eye-pad and bandage applied.

This eye-pad is removed after three hours when the topical anaesthetic has worn off, and the patient is advised to clean away any blood, secretions and eye ointment with warm water. The patient is advised to use Chloramphenicol eye-drops three times a day for seven days, when healing should be complete. Occasionally, in old cysts, most of the contents are fibrous and cannot be removed with the curette. In such cases the fibrous cyst should be grasped with a pair of fine toothed forceps introduced into the wound, and the mass removed using the curved iris scissors and scalpel.

TWENTY-FIVE

The use of the tonometer to detect glaucoma

'The eye be growne more solid and hard than it should be'
(Banister, describing 'absolute glaucoma' 1622)

Glaucoma is the most preventable cause of blindness in this country; if detected early, medical treatment is 90% effective in reducing the intra-ocular pressure. It is estimated that in the UK 300 000 people suffer from the disease, and it now accounts for 13% of all new blind registrations each year.

The intra-ocular pressure is measured in mm Hg; the normal pressure in patients over the age of 40 is considered to be 15 mm; above 21 mm requires referral to a consultant ophthalmologist for further investigation including charting of the visual fields.

Various instruments are available to measure the intra-ocular pressure; they vary in price from fifty pounds to several thousand pounds but the two most popular instruments in use are the Schiotz tonometer and the more recent Perkins applanation tonometer (Figs 25.1 and 25.3).

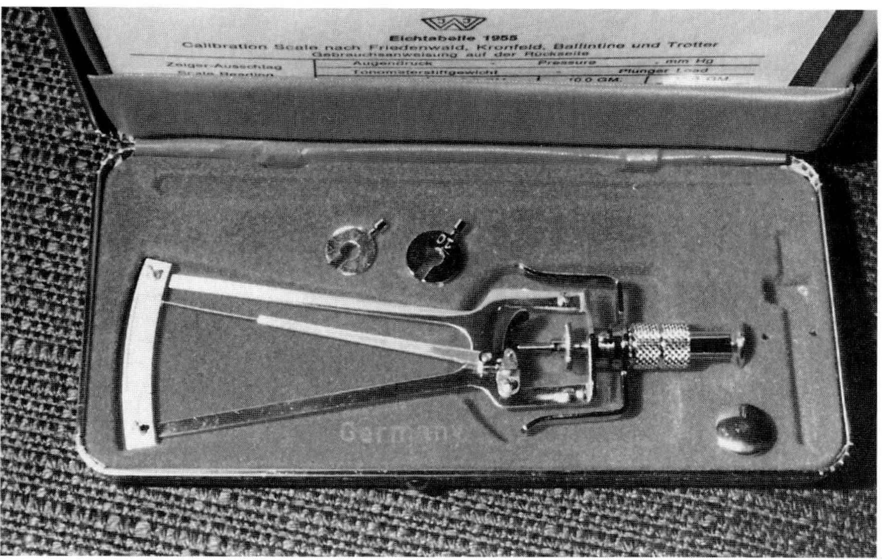

Fig. 25.1 The Schiotz tonometer; simple to use, and inexpensive.

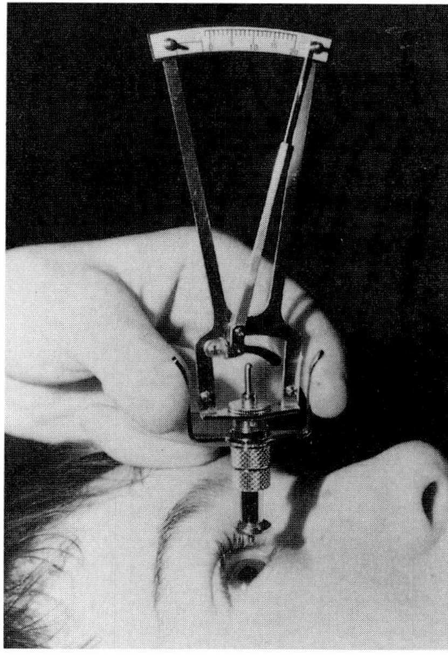

Fig. 25.2 Measuring the intraocular pressure with the Schiotz tonometer. After anaesthetizing the conjunctiva the instrument is gently lowered on the eye-ball and the reading on the scale noted.

As it is not always feasible to screen the whole population for glaucoma, certain groups can be identified as being at special risk as follows:

1. those patients over the age of 40;
2. patients with a family history of glaucoma;
3. patients with diabetes;
4. patients with a high degree of myopia;
5. patients with cardiovascular disease;
6. patients with a history of a bleeding episode requiring blood transfusion.

25.1 TECHNIQUE OF USING THE SCHIOTZ TONOMETER

With the patient lying flat on the couch, local anaesthetic drops are instilled in each eye (Minims Benoxinate 0.4% are suitable). Holding the tonometer as illustrated, the scale is calibrated against a stainless steel spherical surface to check that the instrument reads '0'. It is now gently lowered on the centre of the eye as shown in the illustration, and the reading on the scale noted. (The scale has an inverse ratio to the intra-ocular pressure, i.e. the higher the reading the lower the pressure, and vice-versa.) The same procedure is carried out on the other eye, and the reading noted (Fig. 25.2). Using the conversion scale supplied with the instrument, the readings are translated into mm Hg; the whole procedure taking less than one minute to perform.

Merely by using the criteria for screening as age – over 40 years – and a family history of glaucoma, the number of patients identified can be increased five-fold.

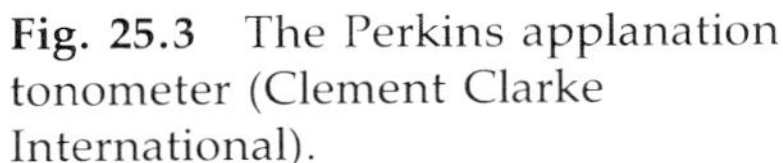

Fig. 25.3 The Perkins applanation tonometer (Clement Clarke International).

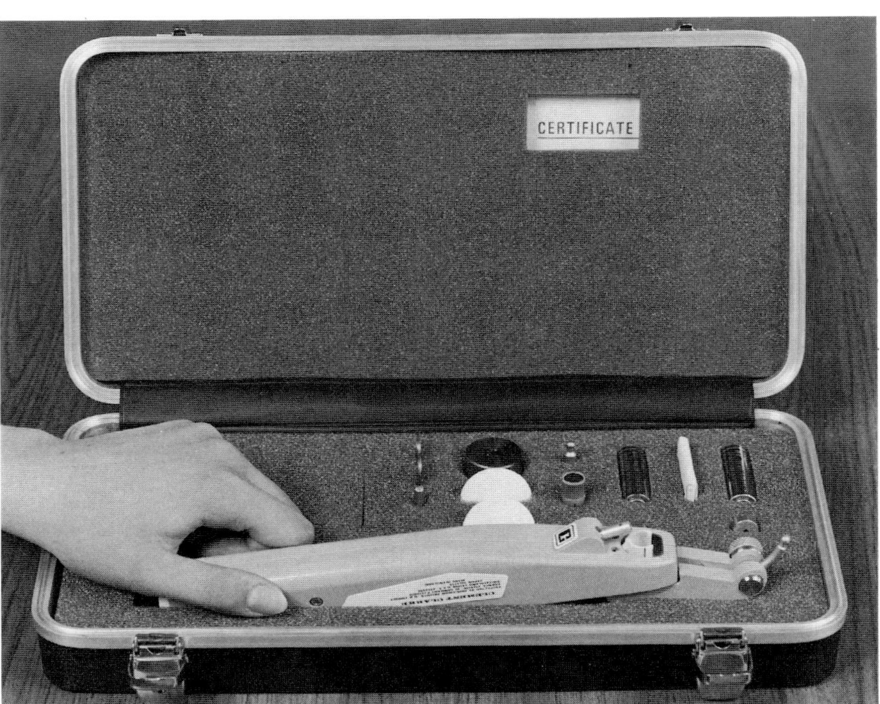

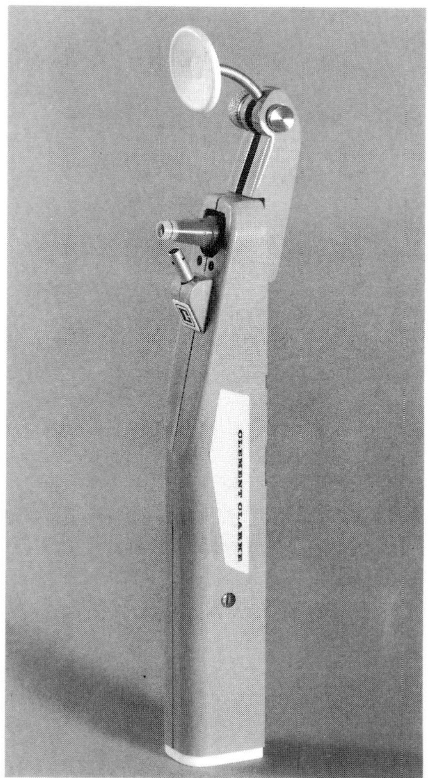

Fig. 25.4 To measure the intra-ocular pressure using the Perkins applanation tonometer, drops of Fluoroscein and Lignocaine are put in each eye, the instrument rested against the eye-ball, and the pressure read directly in mm Hg on the scale.

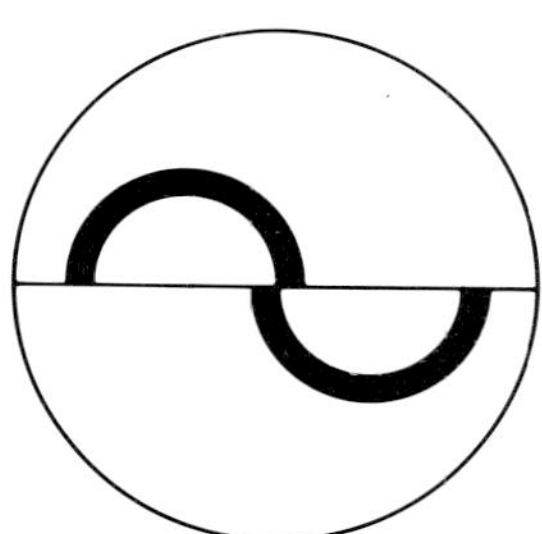

Fig. 25.5 Showing the positions of the fluorescein semi-circles when the pressure is correct.

25.2 THE USE OF THE PERKINS APPLANATION TONOMETER

This instrument is a hand-held tonometer, designed by Professor E. S. Perkins, and has the advantage that it can be used to measure the intra-ocular pressure with the patient in any position (Fig. 25.4). The principle is the same as that of the Goldmann applanation tonometer, in that an applanating surface is placed in contact with the cornea, and the force applied varied until a fixed diameter of applanation is achieved. A special doubling prism is used, through which the operator looks, and which rests directly against the cornea.

25.2.1 Method of use

The eyes are anaesthetized using eye-drops containing local anaesthetic and fluorescein. The Perkins tonometer should be held so that the thumb rests on the milled wheel which controls the internal spring as well as the switch for the illumination. The light is switched on by turning the wheel and the doubling prism gently pressed against the cornea, with the operator viewing through the prism. Two semi-circles of fluorescein are visible through the viewing lens, and the force adjusted by turning the thumb-wheel until the inner margins of the semicircles coincide (see Fig. 25.5). The tonometer is removed from the eye, and the reading noted on the sliding scale. Multiplying the reading by 10 gives the tension in millimetres of mercury (mm Hg).

The instrument is completely portable, can be held in the hand, has its own internal batteries and light, may be used in any position, and gives readings which are extremely reliable in less than one minute.

TWENTY-SIX

The treatment of ingrowing toe-nails

'To Heal the diseased Toes
Fennel Wax, Incense, Cyperus, Wormwood, Dried Myrrh, Poppy Plant, Poppy grain, Elderberries, Berries of the Uan tree, Resin of Acanthus, Dough of Acanthus, Resin of the Mafet tree, Grain of Aloes, Fat of the Cedar tree, Fat of the Uan-tree, fresh Olive Oil, Water from the rain of Heavens. Make into one poultice and apply for 4 days'

(Ebers Papyrus, 1500 BC)

Ingrowing toe-nails are extremely common, cause much discomfort and yet can be one of the most rewarding conditions to treat in general practice.

Surgical textbooks abound with scores of treatments, varying from quite minor procedures, often ineffective, to complete removal of the nail, ablation of the nail bed, and even amputation of the terminal phalanx – resulting in weeks of painful, messy dressings and much time away from school or work. The cause is still not known; ill fitting shoes, and incorrect cutting of the nails have both been incriminated, but many patients are seen in whom these certainly do not apply and as the condition largely affects the big toe-nail on either foot, and appears to be cured by permanently narrowing the width of the nail, it may be that the width of the nail is an important contributing factor.

Three types of ingrowing toe-nail are seen. The first group is commonly seen in young patients between the ages of 10 and 20. Here, the nail is entirely normal in contour but the skin is hypertropied, often with granulations in the nail fold (Figs 26.1 and 26.2). The second group is more likely to be seen in adults, here the nail has increased its convexity so that its edges press firmly on the shallow nail groove. In the third group, seen in all ages, the nail is incurving and ingrowing so that the nail plate has

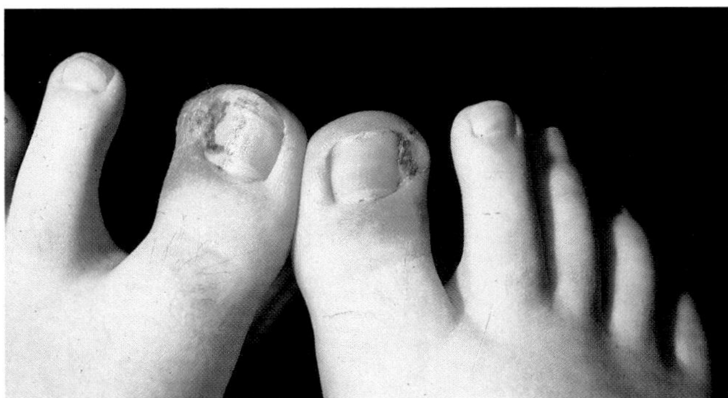

Fig. 26.1 Typical ingrowing toe-nails affecting the big toes on either foot.

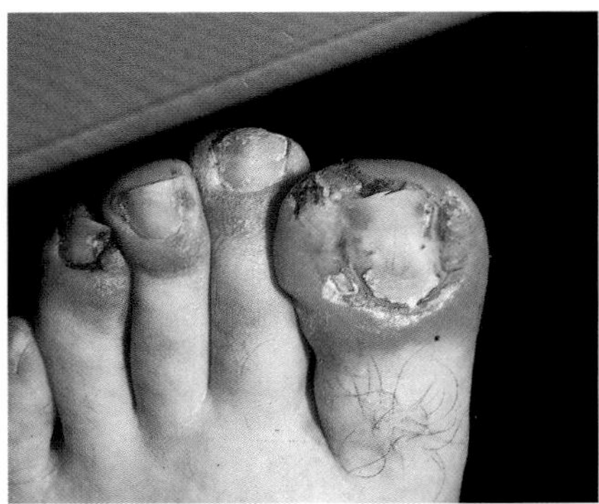

Fig. 26.2 A severely infected ingrowing toe-nail. Even one as bad as this can easily be cured with matrix phenolization.

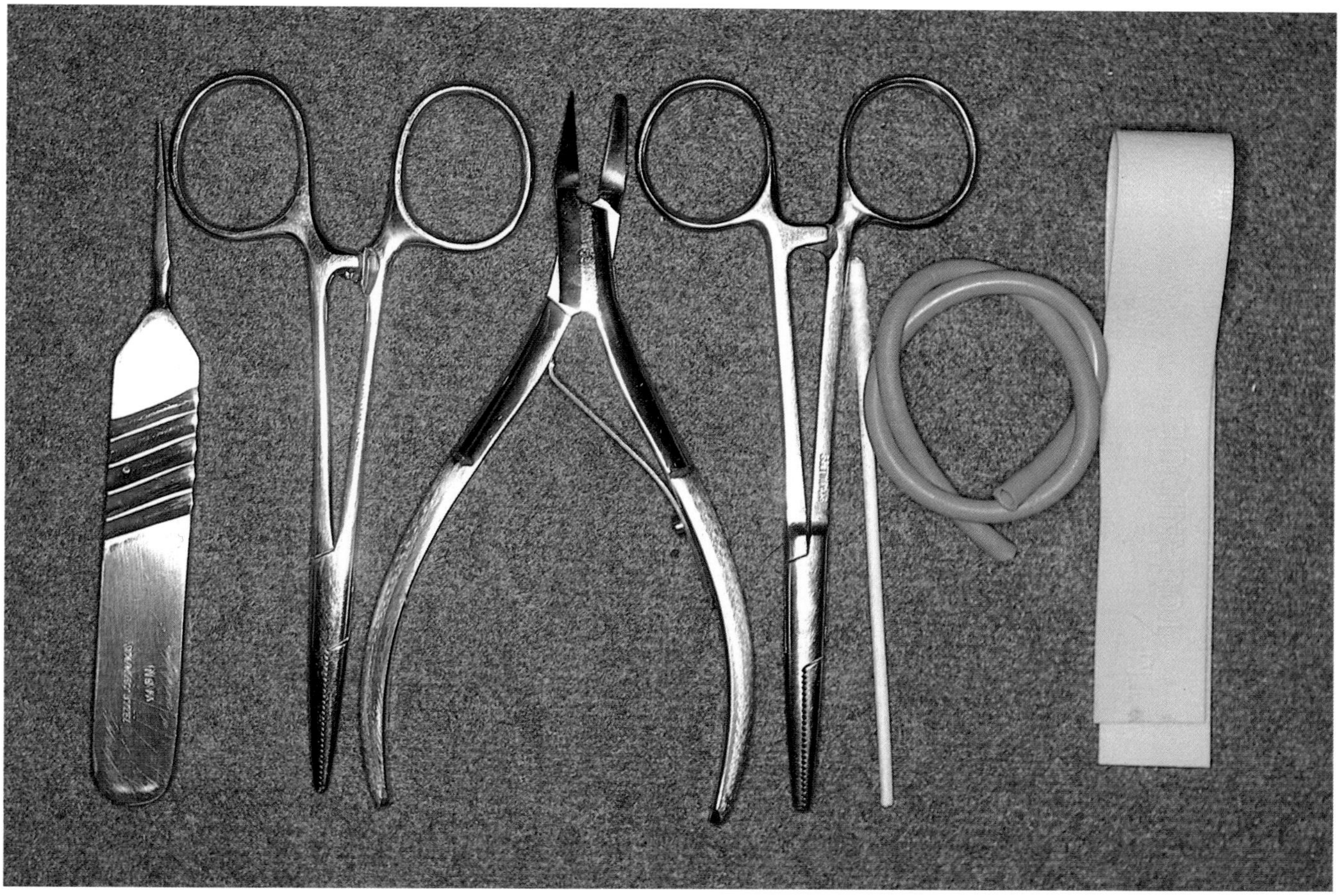

Fig. 26.3 Instruments required for ingrowing toe-nails; from left to right:
1 nail chisel (Nova); 1 artery forceps, straight; 1 Thwaites nail nipper; 1 artery forceps, straight; 1 wooden applicator; 1 rubber tube tourniquet.

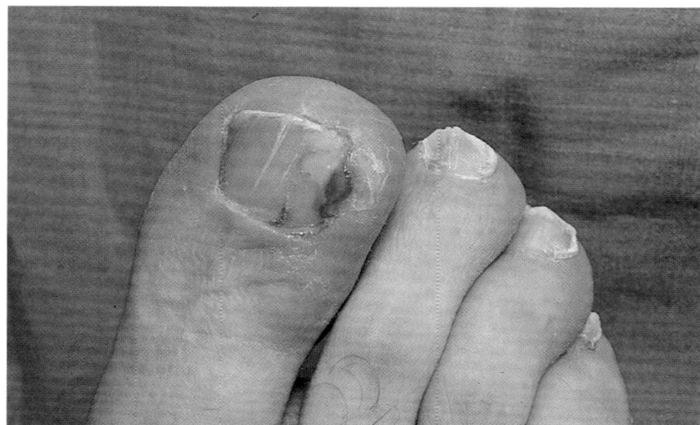

Fig. 26.4 Ingrowing big-toe-nail.

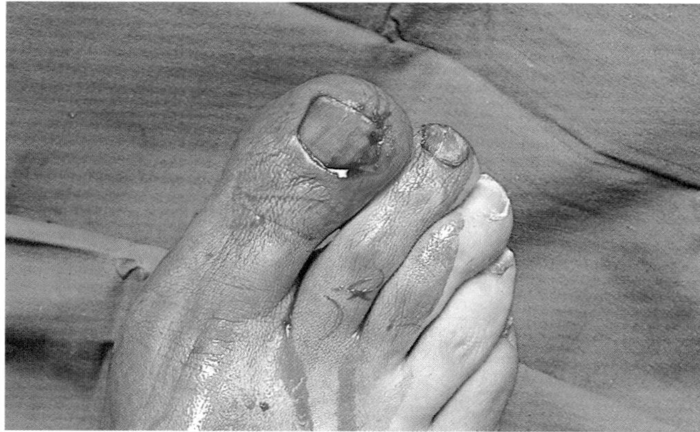

Fig. 26.5 The toe-nail and fore-foot is liberally painted with Povidone-iodine in spirit.

increased its convexity particularly at the lateral edges so that the edge of the nail has curved through almost 180° and is digging into the lateral edge of the nail groove.

Before embarking on surgery, medical treatments may be tried; one of the simplest for mild, early, ingrowing toe-nails is the application of Sofradex drops (Dexamethasone 0.005% Framycetin Sulphate 0.5% and Gramicidin 0.005%) four times daily for one week. If by the end of the time there has not been an obvious improvement, surgical treatment is indicated, offering nearly 100% cure.

The operation of choice is one which has been used by chiropodists for many years [23, 24, 25, 26], correctly described as nail matrix phenolization, and consists of removing a narrow strip of nail together with nail matrix on the affected side, and the application of liquefield phenol to cauterize the germinal epithelium. It is highly effective and gives rapid, painless healing, with virtually no recurrence.

Phenol appears to have a three-fold action. First, it destroys the nail matrix and prevents that portion of nail re-growing. Secondly, it destroys the nerve-endings, which explains the absence of pain during the healing phase. Thirdly, it destroys all pathogenic organisms resulting in a sterile cauterized area.

In the UK pure liquefied phenol containing 80% w/w in water is used; in the USA, liquefied phenol USP containing not less than 89% w/w in water is used. The higher strength used in America is unlikely to make any significant difference to the results, but it should be stored in brown glass bottles, ideally with a glass stopper as the solution changes from colourless to pink or brown when exposed to light, and the phenol can affect plastic caps and washers. Although it appears that phenol which has changed colour is nonetheless effective, it is probably wise to use a relatively fresh and colourless solution.

Wooden applicators with a wisp of cotton wool tightly wound around the tip are the best way of applying the phenol. They must be narrow enough to be easily inserted into the matrix cavity, and only enough phenol to saturate the space should be used, avoiding spilling the solution on adjacent skin.

26.1 NAIL MATRIX PHENOLIZATION

Instruments required (Fig. 26.3)

- syringes and needles
- local anaesthetic **without** adrenalin
- Povidone-iodine in spirit (Betadine alcoholic solution)
- Paraffin tulle with 0.5% Chlorhexidine (Bactigras.)
- 2″ Kling bandage (5 cm)
- 1 Thwaites nail nipper or sharp-pointed stitch scissors 5″ (12.7 cm)
- 2 pairs straight artery forceps 5″ (12.7 cm)
- 1 nail chisel (Nova Instruments)
- wooden applicator sticks
- 1 Volkmann sharp-spoon curette
- rubber strip tourniquet
- rubber tube tourniquet
- pure liquefied phenol (BP) (USP)

It is helpful to advise the patient to arrange transport home and to bring a large shoe or slipper to accommodate the bandaged toe. Povidone-iodine in spirit (Betadine alcoholic solution) is liberally applied to the toe (Fig. 26.5) extending proximally at least 1″ beyond the interdigital clefts. A ring block or digital nerve block is performed using **plain** Lignocaine or Prilocaine: under **no** circumstances should adrenalin or any other vasoconstrictor be added to the local anaesthetic, otherwise ischaemia and possible necrosis could occur (Fig. 26.6).

For greatest comfort, and particularly in children, a 30 SWG (0.3 mm) needle should be used with a dental syringe and cartridge. Unfortunately most dental anaesthetic cartridges contain adrenalin, but Prilocaine 4% (Citanest) containing 40 mg/ml is manufactured in 2 ml cartridges (maximum adult dose prilocaine 400 mg). Failing this, a standard 5 ml syringe with 25 SWG × $\frac{5}{8}$″ (0.5 mm × 16 mm) needle may be used with 1% Lignocaine.

The digital nerves to the toe lie on the plantar side of the coronal plane; each should be infiltrated with 0.5 ml local anaesthetic, followed by a 'bridge' of solution across the dorsum of the toe, plus a similar bridge on the plantar surface, producing a complete ring block (Fig. 26.7).

Toes which are very reddened and inflamed are more difficult to anaesthetize, but it is well worth taking additional time and effort to achieve complete anaesthesia before operating.

A sterile gauze swab is now wrapped around the toe and over this is applied a rubber strip tourniquet or 1″ cotton non-stretch bandage to exsanguinate the toe. (The rubber strip included in the butterfly intravenous cannulae kits makes an ideal tourniquet for fingers and toes.) Next, a fine rubber tube tourniquet is tied tightly around the base of the toe, and fixed with one of the pairs of artery forceps (Figs 26.8, 26.9 and 26.10). The rubber strip and gauze swab are now removed, leaving a bloodless, anaesthetic toe (Fig. 26.11).

More Povidone-iodine in spirit is applied, and a sterile paper drape is placed over the foot, with the toe protruding through a small hole cut in the paper.

Using the Thwaites nail nipper or pointed stitch scissors, the operator cuts a thin strip of nail adjacent to the granulations, approximately 2–3 mm away from the nail fold, and extending to the base of the nail (Fig. 26.12). This cut is then extended to the nail matrix or germinal epithelium using a special nail chisel which splits the nail, using firm pressure, until resistance is encountered (Fig. 26.13).

The chisel is removed, and the strip of nail is grasped with a pair of straight artery forceps and gently removed using a combination of traction and rotation, making sure not to tear the base of the strip, nor leave any fragments in the groove. Any excess granulations are now removed with the curette, although most can be left, and the phenol applied with the wooden applicator using a massaging action to ensure complete absorption, particularly in the matrix cavity (Fig. 26.14). The phenol is applied for exactly 3 min; if less than this, recurrence is likely. Sufficient is used to cauterize the groove formerly occupied by the strip of nail, but care is taken not to use too much which might spread over the adjacent skin and delay healing (Figs 26.16, 26.17 and 26.18). After 3 min, a dry swab is used to mop away any surplus phenol; earlier accounts of the technique described the use of 5% Chlorhexidine in spirit to 'neutralize' the phenol, this is now thought not to be necessary.

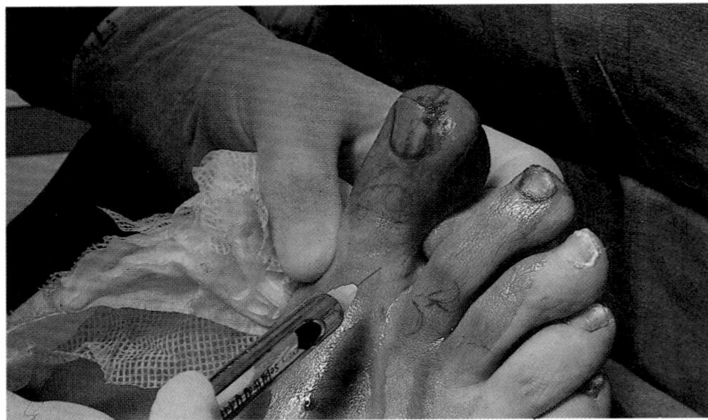

Fig. 26.6 The digital nerves are blocked with local anaesthetic (**never** use added adrenalin).

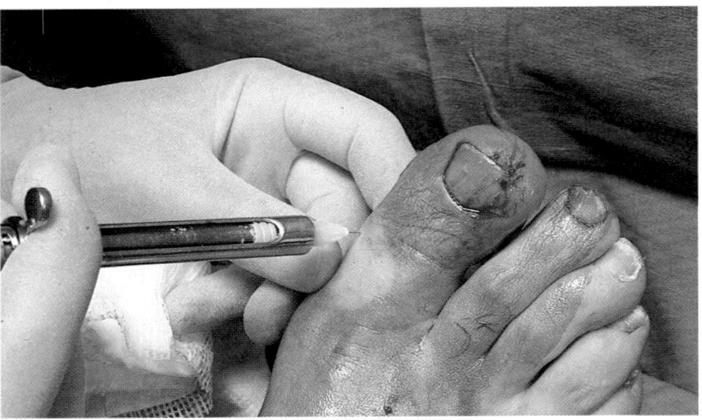

Fig. 26.7 A complete ringblock anaesthetic is performed.

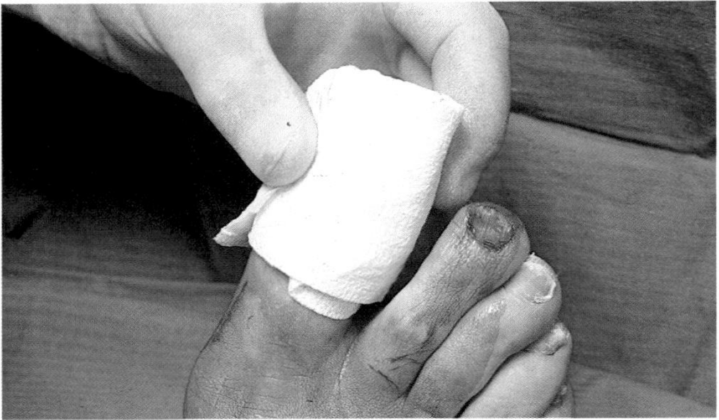

Fig. 26.8 A sterile gauze swab is wrapped around the toe.

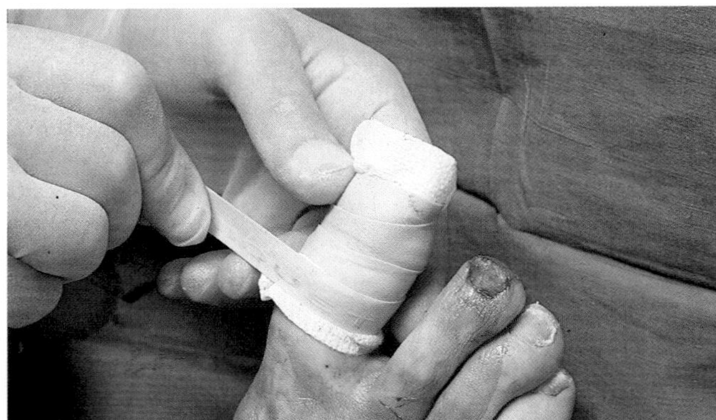

Fig. 26.9 A rubber strip tourniquet is wrapped over the gauze swab to exsanguinate the toe.

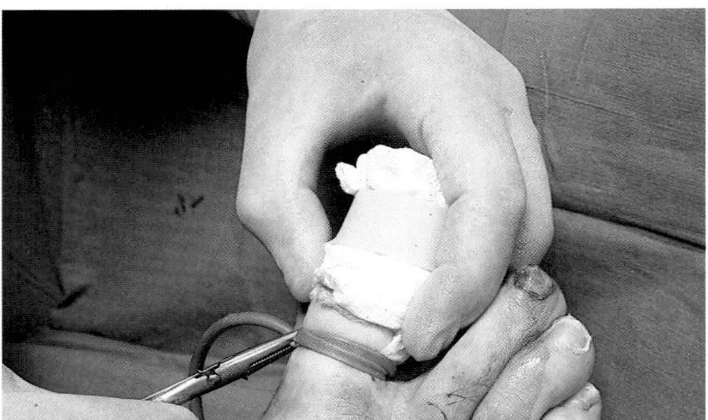

Fig. 26.10 A rubber-tube tourniquet is tied round the base of the toe and secured.

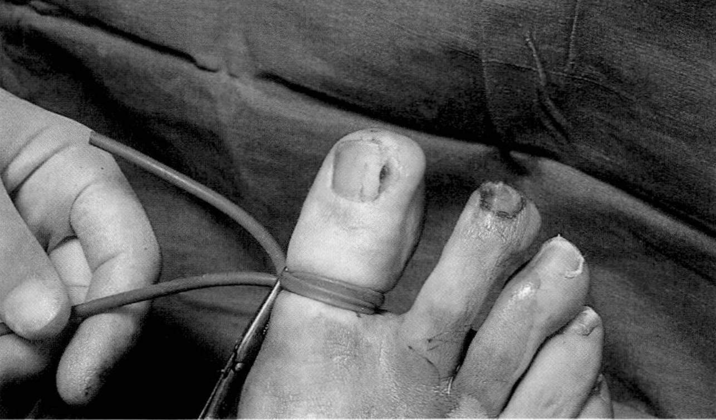

Fig. 26.11 The rubber strip and gauze swab are removed, and more Povidone-iodine applied.

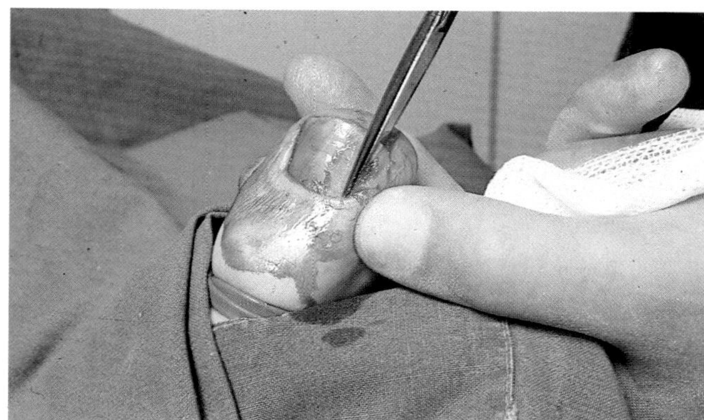

Fig. 26.12 Using either stitch scissors or Thwaites nail nippers a strip of nail is cut out as shown.

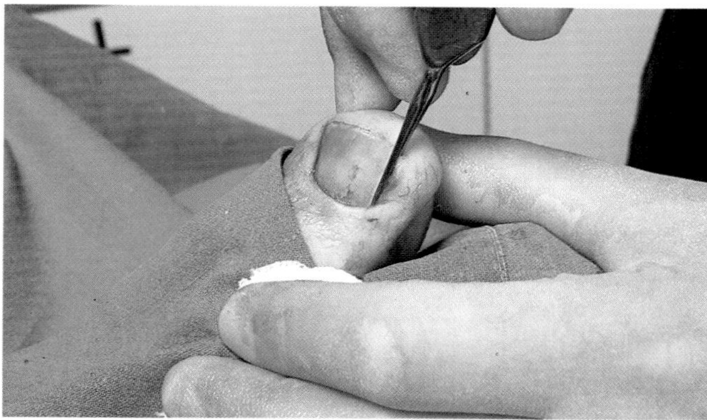

Fig. 26.13 The cut is deepened using the nail chisel, pushing it firmly down to the nail root.

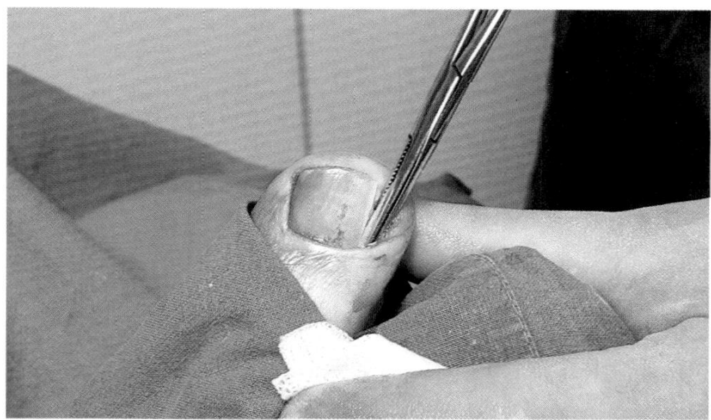

Fig. 26.14 The strip of nail is grasped with artery forceps and removed.

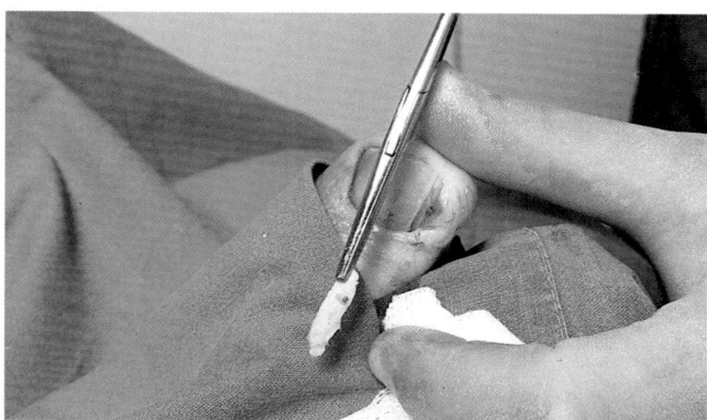

Fig. 26.15 Showing the strip of nail which has been removed.

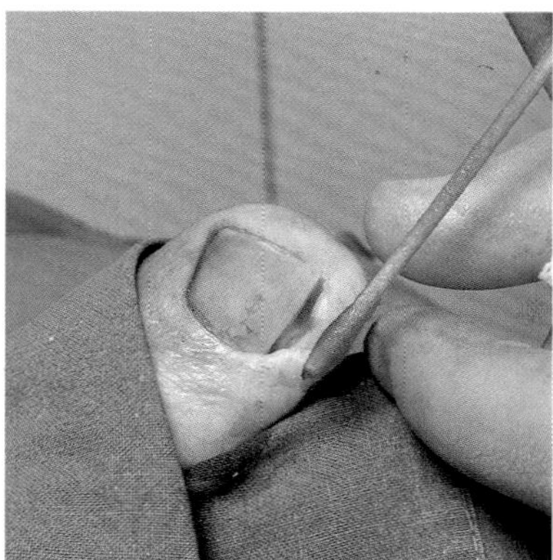

Fig. 26.16 Pure phenol is now applied, using a wooden applicator and cotton wool.

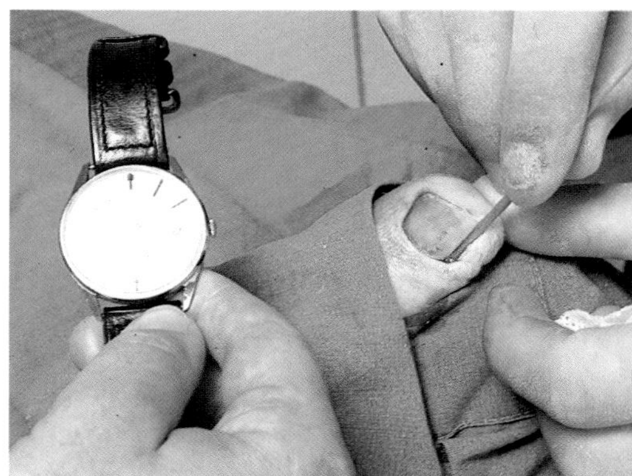

Fig. 26.17 The phenol must be applied for a minimum of three minutes *by the clock*.

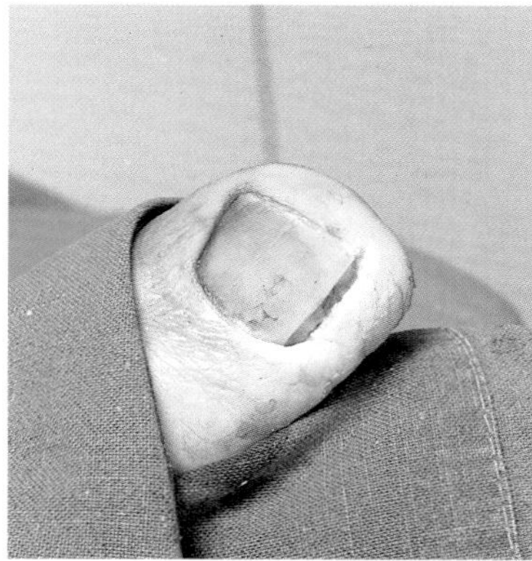

Fig. 26.18 The appearance of the nail bed after applying the phenol.

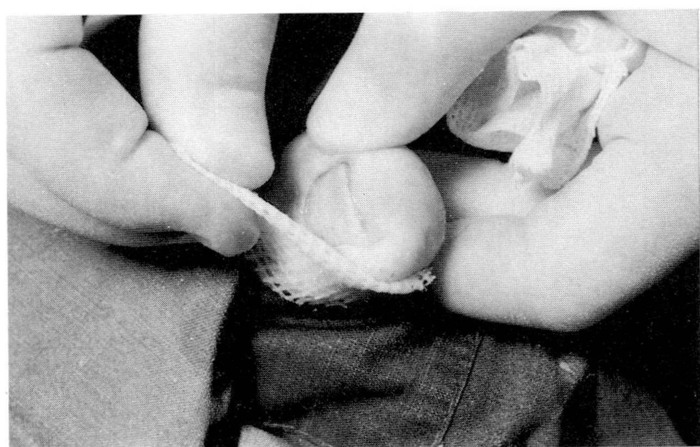

Fig. 26.19 A dressing of Bactigras or fucidin-tulle is now applied.

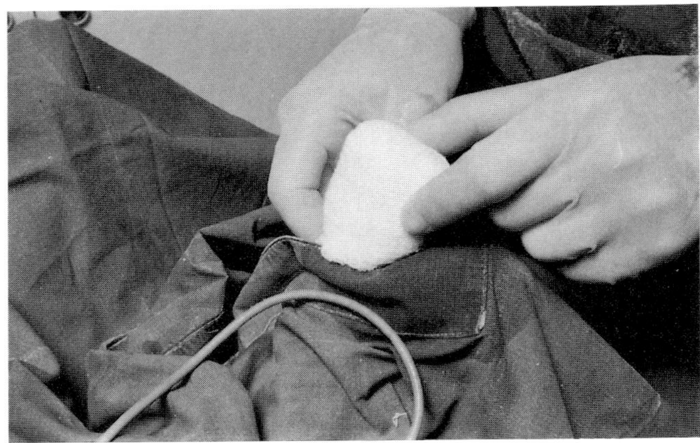

Fig. 26.20 This is now covered with a gauze swab and cotton bandages and left for three days.

A dressing of paraffin tulle impregnated with 5% Chlorhexidine is now applied, covered with one square of sterile absorbent gauze, and the toe bandaged (Figs 26.19 and 26.20).

The tourniquet is released, and the patient allowed home with instructions to rest the foot for 6 hours. Two follow-up dressings are necessary, the first on the 3rd post-operative day, the second, one week later on the 10th day, and this is usually all that is necessary. Frequently on the 10th day dressing the toe is found to be moist and 'messy' – this is thought to be due to a delayed 'phenol reaction', is quite common and needs no special treatment. If discharge or granulations persist, an application of Povidone-iodine spray powder (Disidine) is helpful, covered with a dry dressing.

Incurving, ingrowing nails are treated in an identical manner, removing a narrow strip from either edge of the nail, and phenolizing both sides simultaneously.

TWENTY-SEVEN

Onychogryphosis

'. . . and his nails were like birds' claws'

(Daniel, Chapter 4 verse 33 (RSV))

Onychogryphosis, or irregular thickening of the nail is commonly seen in the elderly; it may follow trauma, or arise secondary to a subungual exostosis, or following chronic hyper-extension of the hallux. Once it has developed, it tends to be permanent, removal of the nail alone is followed by a recurrence many months later; softening and burring of the nail likewise only give temporary relief (Figs 27.1 and 27.2). The only permanent cure, therefore, is removal of the nail and total nail bed ablation.

If the condition is secondary to a subungual exostosis, removal of the nail may predispose to corn formation and further pain; it is therefore important to establish at the outset, the possible aetiology of each case. Where total nail bed ablation is chosen, the method is very similar to that used for ingrowing toe-nails.

Instruments required

(See Chapter 26 plus 1 McDonald's dissector)

27.1 TOTAL NAIL REMOVAL

The preparation, ring block and application of tourniquet are exactly as described for the treatment of the ingrowing toe-nail. To remove the nail, it is first lifted away from the nail bed with a McDonald's dissector or special nail elevator and then split in half using the Thwaites nail nipper. Each half may then be grasped with a strong pair of straight artery forceps and pulled off, using a combination of traction and rotation. If nail nippers are unavailable, the nail may be too thickened to be cut with any other instrument; accordingly it may be removed 'in toto' using a strong pair of artery forceps (Fig. 27.3).

Having removed the nail, the nail bed and germinal epithelium are painted with pure phenol, paying particular attention to the groove containing the nail matrix. As with ingrowing toe-nails, the phenol is left in contact for at least 3 min (Fig. 27.5) then mopped dry, and a paraffin-tulle dressing with 0.5% Chlorhexidine (Bactigras) applied, covered with a sterile gauze swab and bandage.

Follow-up dressings are done on the 3rd and 10th day and thereafter as necessary, any infection is treated with Povidone-iodine powder spray. Healing takes 5–7 weeks, leaving a comfortable and cosmetically acceptable 'toe'.

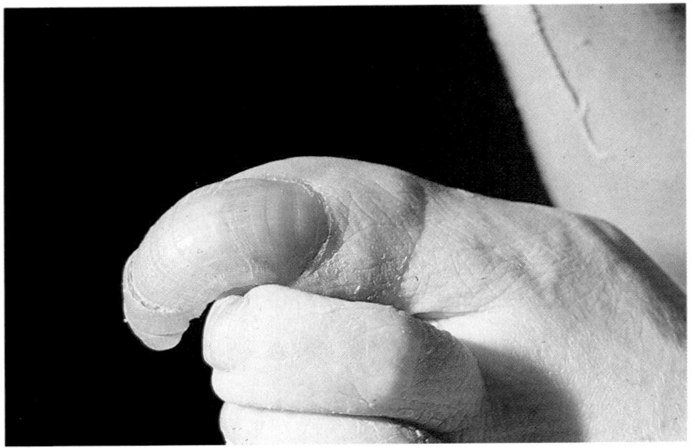

Fig. 27.1 Curved, onychogryphotic nail.

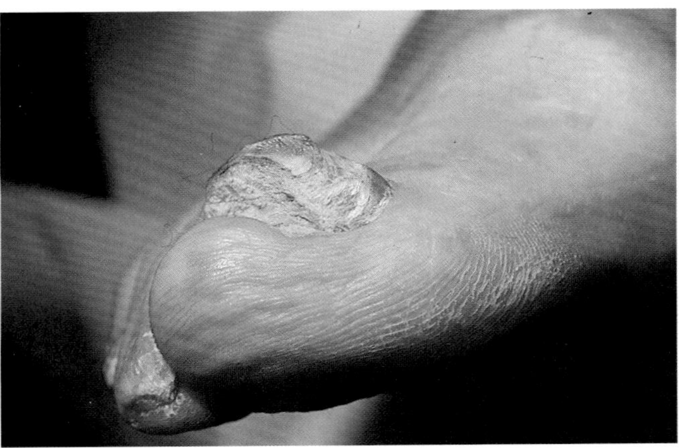

Fig. 27.2 Another onychogryphotic nail.

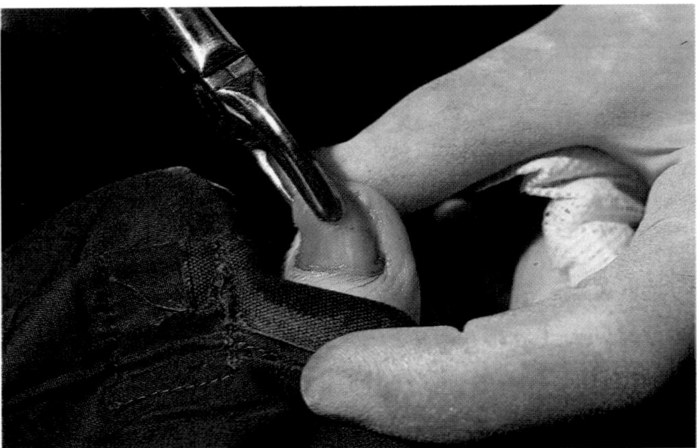

Fig. 27.3 The nail may either be split and removed in two pieces, or whole with a strong pair of forceps.

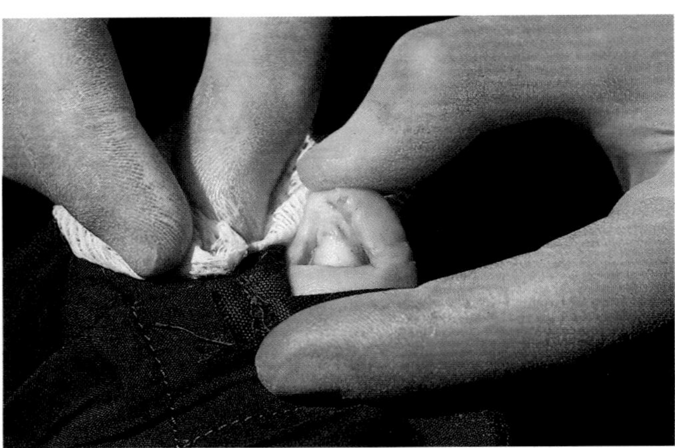

Fig. 27.4 The nail-bed after removal of the onychogryphotic nail.

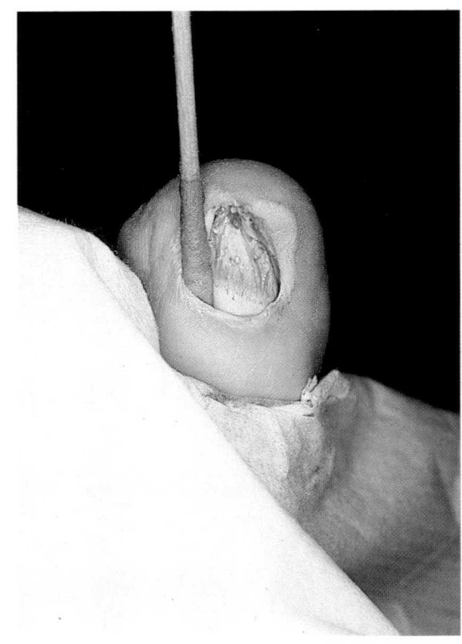

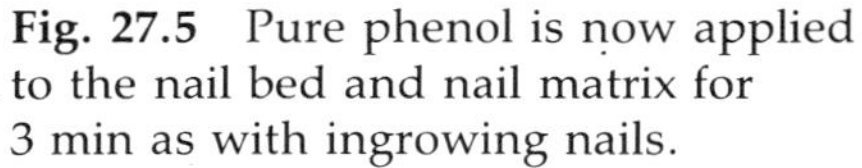

Fig. 27.5 Pure phenol is now applied to the nail bed and nail matrix for 3 min as with ingrowing nails.

TWENTY-EIGHT

Chemical cauterization

'Warts . . . They may be removed also by the knife and the parts from whence they are cut afterwards touched with lunar caustic (silver nitrate) to prevent them from returning. But when this method is practised the operator ought to be certain that he has removed the wart entirely, for where part has been left, the most formidable symptoms have sometimes ensued'

(Encyclopaedia Brittanica, 1797)

The application of caustic chemicals to the tissues can be used to advantage to treat certain lesions; they are cheap, easily obtainable, effective and quick to apply and no special instruments are required. The two disadvantages of using chemicals are difficulty in controlling the exact area treated and the fact that only superficial lesions can be treated. Nevertheless, three substances are used commonly in medical practice, Silver Nitrate, Liquefied Phenol and Monochloro-acetic acid.

28.1 SILVER NITRATE

This has been used for centuries and is well known to most doctors; when applied to moist tissues, it causes them to turn white due to the formation of silver chloride; this then gradually turns black when exposed to light. Unless both patient and operator are particularly careful, accidental touching of the skin with the Silver Nitrate will result in stubborn, unsightly, black stains which are extremely difficult to remove. Similarly if left on plastic work-surfaces in the surgery, Silver Nitrate will cause permanent black staining.

It is produced as a solid pointed stick which may be fixed in a holder, or more recently, individual wooden applicators with a small hard bead at the tip containing 75% Silver Nitrate (see Fig. 32.2). These are disposable, avoid any risks of cross infection, and are easier and cleaner to handle. Finally, Silver Nitrate is made as a solution of any desired strength for topical application.

28.1.1 Granulations

These respond well to the application of Silver Nitrate, often being cured with just one application. Following separation of the umbilical cord in the new-born infant, occasionally messy granulations occur; one or two applications of Silver Nitrate and a dry dressing are all that is required.

28.1.2 Vaginal vault granulations

Vaginal vault granulations following hysterectomy are easily treated with topical Silver Nitrate, rarely needing more than two applications.

28.1.3 Small granuloma pyogenicum

If curette and electrocautery is not available or appropriate, the application of Silver Nitrate may result in a cure.

28.1.4 Epistaxis

Repeated nose-bleeds in children and young adults frequently occur from the small leash of blood vessels in 'Little's Area' which are readily visible. The application of Silver Nitrate directly to this area often results in cure; it is slightly uncomfortable at the time of application and causes reflex watering of the eyes, but is usually acceptable to children (see Chapter 32).

28.1.5 Cervical erosions

Many cervical erosions are asymptomatic and need no treatment; where the patient is experiencing an increased discharge or has symptoms of pain suggesting infection or cervicitis, cauterization of the cervix with Silver Nitrate may be tried. Using the applicator, the whole of the erosion, including the external cervical os is treated with Silver Nitrate; the area so treated becoming white. The patient is warned to expect an increased, watery vaginal discharge for one or two weeks while healing is occurring. Some doctors like the patient to use an antiseptic vaginal cream twice daily during this healing phase.

28.1.6 Ingrowing toe-nails

A Silver Nitrate caustic applicator has been traditionally used for ingrowing toe-nails for years; it is suitable for the treatment of any granulations which occur, but the black staining is a disadvantage, and alternative methods may be more appropriate (see Chapter 26).

28.1.7 Chronic sinus or fistula

Long-standing suppuration and discharge through a skin sinus or fistula may result in the formation of fleshy polypi and/or heaped-up granulations. Both may be helped by the application of Silver Nitrate, often on more than one occasion. Where possible, the underlying cause of the fistula or sinus should be treated.

28.1.8 Chronic conjunctivitis

A weak aqueous solution of Silver Nitrate may be used to treat patients with chronic inflammation of the eye-lids – the so called 'silvering of the eye-lids'. Benoxynate drops are instilled prior to the application of 1% Silver Nitrate, which is then washed out with normal saline.

28.2 PHENOL (CARBOLIC ACID)

Phenol crystals or pure Liquefied Phenol containing 80–90% w/w in water may be used for cauterization, while weaker solutions may be used for injection into hydrocele cavities (Chapter 16) or for the injection of haemorrhoids (see Chapter 36). In each case the treatment relies on the irritant effect of the phenol on the tissues. Used as a 5% solution in glycerine, phenol may also be used for intra-thecal and superficial nerve blocks.

The main use of Liquefied Phenol in general practitioner minor surgery is for ingrowing toe-nails, where it is used to cauterize and destroy the nail matrix (see Chapter 26). In this situation, its threefold action of cauterization, destruction of nerve endings and sterilization makes it an ideal agent.

28.2.1 Granulations

The application of Liquefied Phenol is often an effective treatment for granulation tissue – more than one treatment may be necessary, and a delayed 'phenol reaction' may be seen on the 8th–10th day with increased inflammation and discharge.

28.2.2 Molluscum contagiosum

This condition is caused by a virus infection, and typified by the small, pearly, hard papules with an umbilicated centre. It may be treated with Liquefied Phenol by dipping a sharpened wooden applicator in phenol and then piercing each individual papule, transferring a minute quantity of phenol inside each spot.

28.2.3 Chronic paronychia

Following loss of the nail 'quick' and subsequent infection, often with yeasts, chronic paronychiae may be treated with phenol applied directly with a small wooden applicator sharpened in the shape of a chisel, dipped in phenol. This treatment may be supplemented with topical and occasional systemic antimycotics.

28.2.4 Ear-lobe cysts

Small infected cysts, particularly those occurring in the lobes of the ears may be treated effectively by incision, evacuation of any contents, and the application of pure Liquefied Phenol on a small wooden applicator and cotton wool.

28.2.5 Hydrocele and epididymal cysts (See Chapter 14)

Aspiration alone rarely cures either of these conditions, but aspiration followed by the injection of 2.5% aqueous phenol results in 90–100% cure; the treatment needs to be repeated more than once.

28.2.6 Injection of haemorrhoids

Despite many alternative and more sophisticated treatments for haemorrhoids, 5% oily phenol still remains the treatment of choice for many doctors for their patients with haemorrhoids. The injection is given submucosally in doses of 0.5–5 ml (see Chapter 36).

28.2.7 Nerve blocks

Relief of pain, particularly in terminal malignant disease, may be achieved by selective nerve blocks using 5–10% phenol in glycerine. Similarly, spinal, intrathecal blocks may give relief of pain for many months. The injection is given under full aseptic conditions; after inserting a spinal needle the patient is positioned in such a way that the neurolytic agent is brought into contact with appropriate sensory nerve roots (Fig. 28.1). Small incremental doses of 5% phenol in glycerine are then given until numbness is achieved [27].

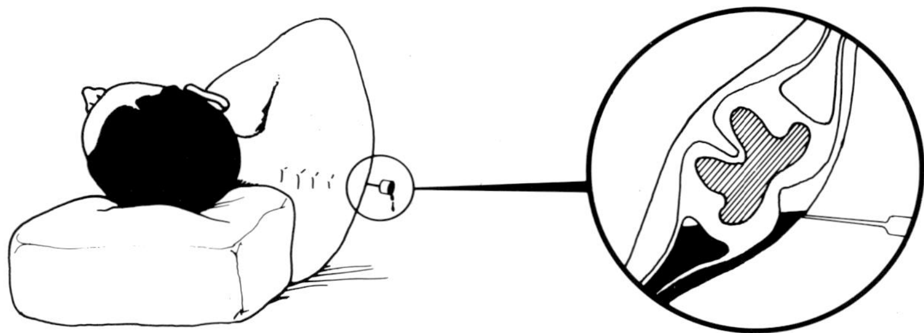

Fig. 28.1 Positioning of the patient to bring the neurolytic agent into contact with the sensory roots.

28.3 MONOCHLORO-ACETIC ACID

This is a simple, effective treatment for small warts, xanthelasmata, and superficial skin lesions.

28.3.1 Warts

Monochloro-acetic acid may be 'pricked' into a wart using a pointed wooden applicator. The concentrated 'saturated' solution should be used. It will be noticed that initially the acid is rapidly absorbed by the wart. More is applied and 'pricked in' until no more is absorbed. Any surplus acid is mopped off the wart which is then left exposed to the air and kept dry. Healing occurs in 8–14 days; and the treatment may be repeated if necessary (see Chapter 16, Fig. 16.2).

28.3.2 Xanthelasma (Xanthoma)

This is a deposit of excess lipids in the skin; commonly found on the medial side of upper and lower eye-lids. Biochemical abnormalities are often not demonstrated and if treatment is requested they may be removed by surgery, electrocautery, cryotherapy or the *very careful* application of monochloro-acetic acid on a small wooden applicator.

28.3.3 Superficial skin lesions

Small naevi, plane warts, superficial keratoses etc. may all be treated by the careful application of monochloro-acetic acid as an alternative to electrocautery, diathermy or cryotherapy.

TWENTY-NINE

The electrocautery

'Put an assortment of olivary cauteries on the fire, large and small, and blow on them until they are well heated. Take one, large or small, apply the cautery to the artery itself after having quickly removed the finger, and keep it there until bleeding is arrested'

(Albucasis, AD 936)

From the earliest times, physicians have used instruments heated to red heat and applied to wounds to control haemorrhage and destroy diseased tissues. The use of an electric current instead of a fire to heat the instrument, enabled much greater control of the cauterization to be achieved, and in practice today most electrocauteries comprise a handle incorporating a switch, and a platinum wire electrode which can be heated to red-heat by the passage of an electric current through it.

Early instruments used a dry battery and rheostat to control the current, and, therefore, the temperature of the wire. These were not entirely satisfactory as the current drain was considerable and the batteries soon became exhausted, often in the middle of a surgical procedure.

With the advent of domestic electricity supplies, lead-acid accumulators were used which could be re-charged at a convenient time and were still portable enough to be taken to a patient's home or doctor's treatment room. Furthermore they could withstand heavy current drain for several hours. As most domestic electricity supplies were direct current, transformers could not be used, and the only means of producing a low voltage and high current necessary for an electrocautery, was by means of a heavy duty variable resistance or rheostat, a method which was wasteful of electricity and not particularly safe for the patient.

The invention of the step-down transformer whereby the domestic electricity supply of 110 V (or subsequently 240 V) alternating current, could be transformed to any chosen voltage now enabled equipment previously run from batteries to be used on domestic supplies, with no worry about unexpected battery failure. In addition, the low-voltage winding of the transformer could be isolated completely from the primary, high-voltage winding, thus ensuring complete electrical safety for the patient and doctor.

Modern cautery transformers still employ this same principle, incorporating a rheostat to vary the output current (Figs 29.1, 29.2, 29.3, 29.4 and 29.6). Unlike many electronic components the electrocautery works equally well on direct current or alternating current; thus there is no necessity to rectify the alternating output from the transformer.

More recently nickel-cadmium rechargeable batteries have been introduced; they have the ability to withstand a heavy current drain, are light in weight, and a completely portable instrument can be produced with no attached wires (Fig. 29.5). However, unless regularly recharged, the batteries can fail suddenly, more so than conventional dry cells, so some form of stand-by is desirable. Also, after several hundred recharges, the

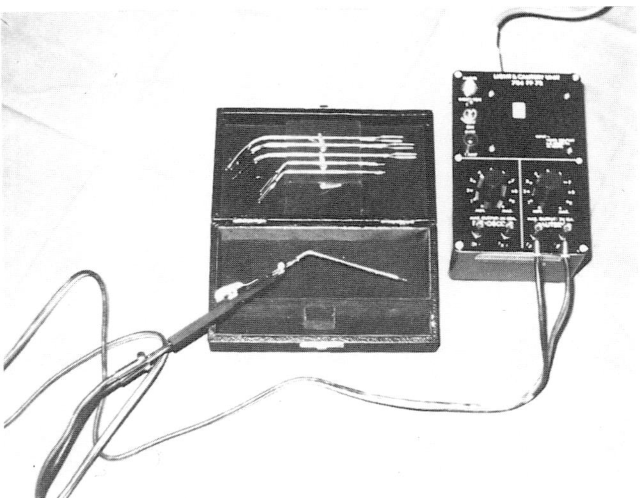

Fig. 29.1 An electrocautery transformer and burners (Rimmer Bros Ltd, London).

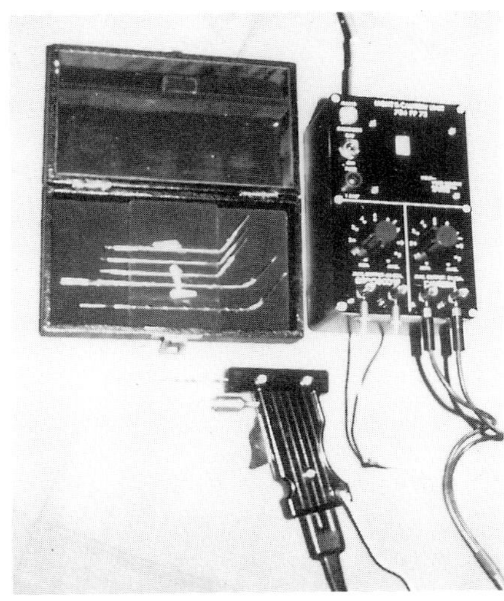

Fig. 29.2 Another electrocautery transformer with pistol grip handle and burners (Rimmer Bros Ltd, London).

Fig. 29.3 A cautery-light transformer with pistol grip and Mark Hovell handles (Down Bros, Mitcham, Surrey).

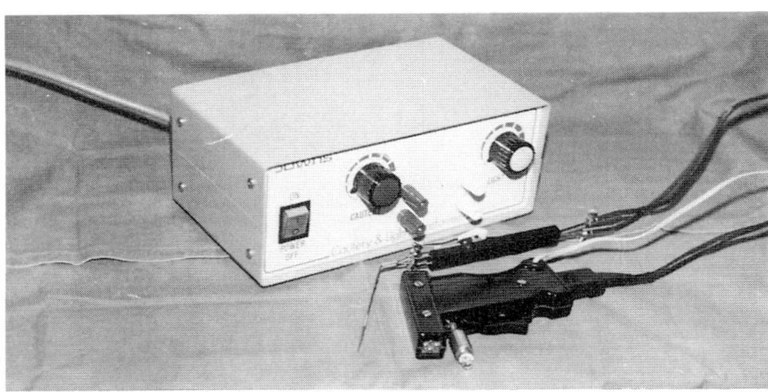

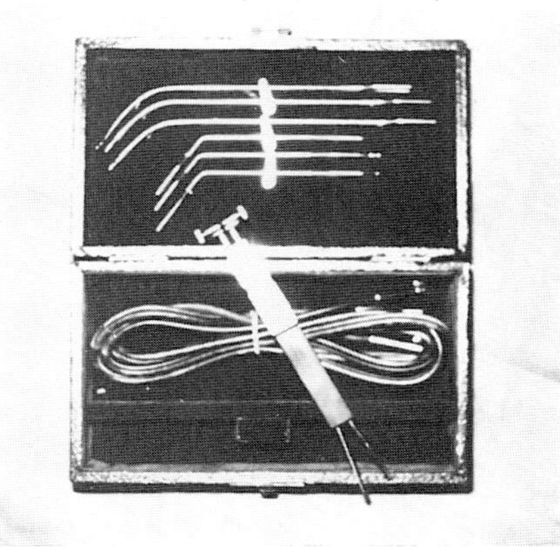

Fig. 29.4 Selection of different shaped burners and Mark Hovell handle.

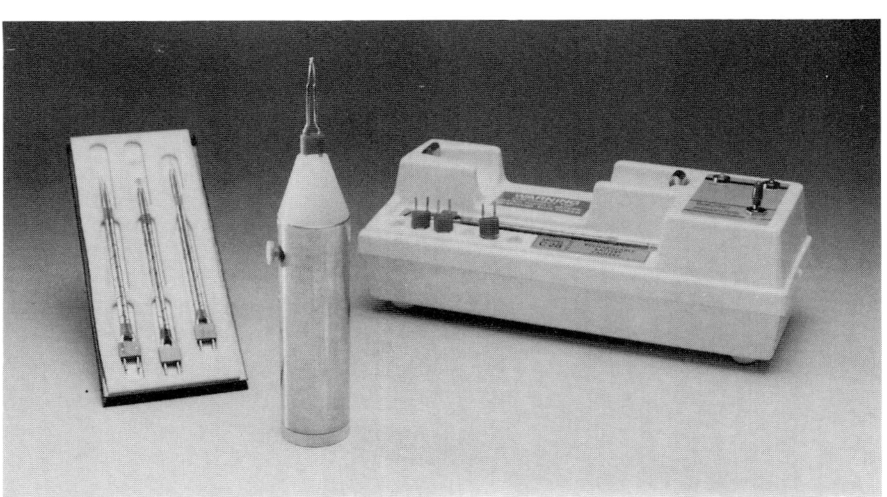

Fig. 29.5 Model C28 cordless rechargeable battery cautery. Quick and simple to use (Warecrest Ltd).

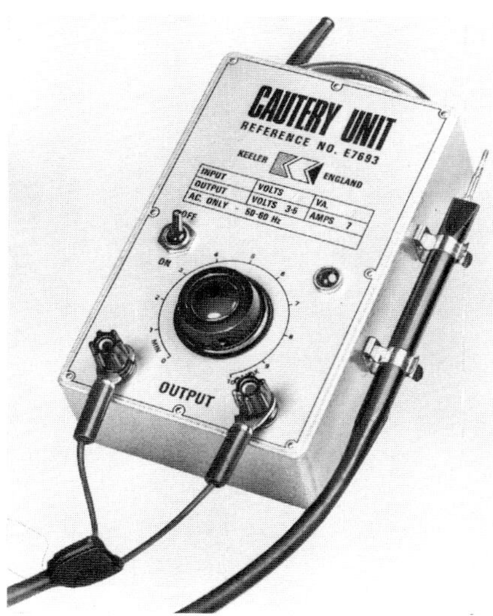

Fig. 29.6 A lightweight electrocautery, designed for ophthalmic use, but very suitable for minor surgical procedures (Keeler Instruments Ltd, London).

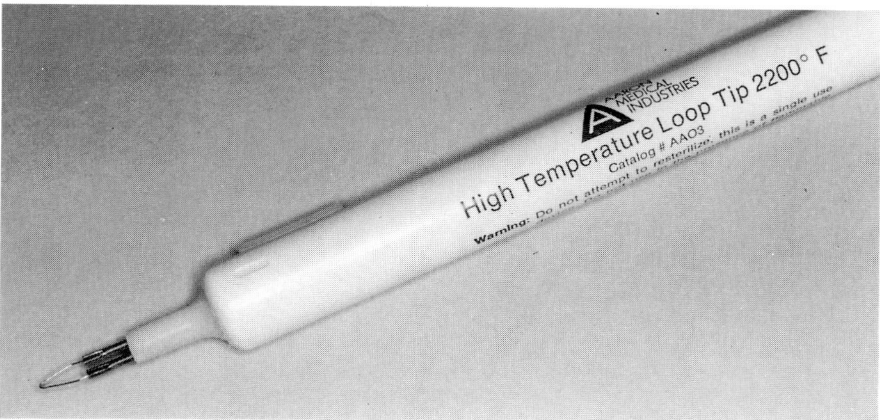

Fig. 29.7 Disposable electrocautery (Aaron Medical Industries USA, Cardiokinetics Ltd UK).

batteries lose their ability to retain a charge, and need to be replaced.

Finally, small, lightweight disposable cauteries have been introduced, incorporating dry-cell, non-rechargeable batteries. These are extremely light, very portable, and most useful for fine cauterization (Fig. 29.7).

The doctor purchasing an electrocautery will be faced with a bewildering array of cautery burners, designed to reach the most inaccessible places, with an equally bewildering variety of shapes and sizes of the actual electrode tip. For the beginner, one simple V-shaped wire electrode is all that is required, preferably with short supporting wires to give greater control of the tip. With increased experience, the doctor may come to prefer a modification of the standard V shape.

29.1 USES OF THE ELECTROCAUTERY

29.1.1 Haemostasis

Small bleeding vessels can be readily sealed by the application of the electrocautery burner. The operator will soon discover the optimum temperature of the wire; generally a dull cherry-red is about right. If not hot enough, the wire will adhere to the tissues – if too hot, it will burn through bleeding vessels without sealing them; an adjustment on the rheostat is all that is required.

29.1.2 Skin tags (see Chapter 18)

These may be picked up with fine-toothed forceps and divided easily with the electrocautery. No pressure is required, a repeated small movement of the red-hot wire will neatly separate the lesion from the base, with no bleeding.

29.1.3 Subungual haematoma (see Chapter 41)

Resting the electrocautery tip against the nail and switching on the current results in a small painless hole in the nail with immediate release of blood.

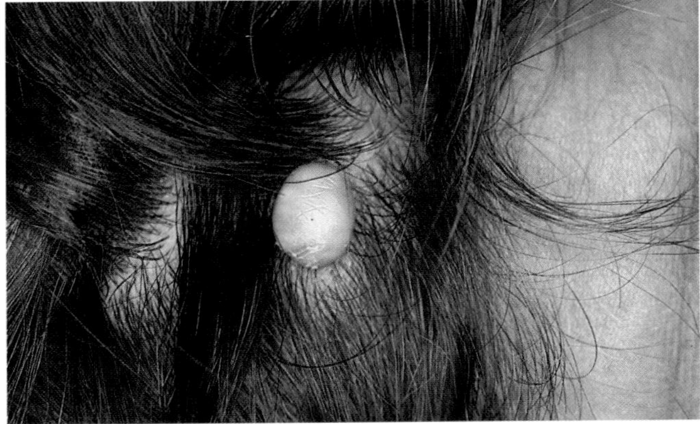

Fig. 29.8 Papilloma on scalp. Base is infiltrated with local anaesthetic.

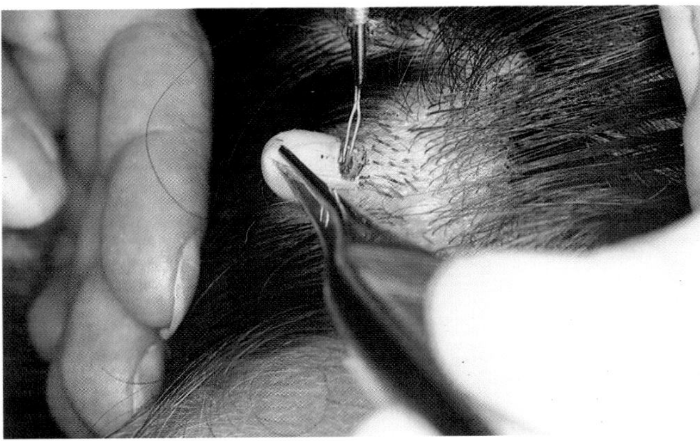

Fig. 29.9 The papilloma is picked up with forceps and separated with the electrocautery.

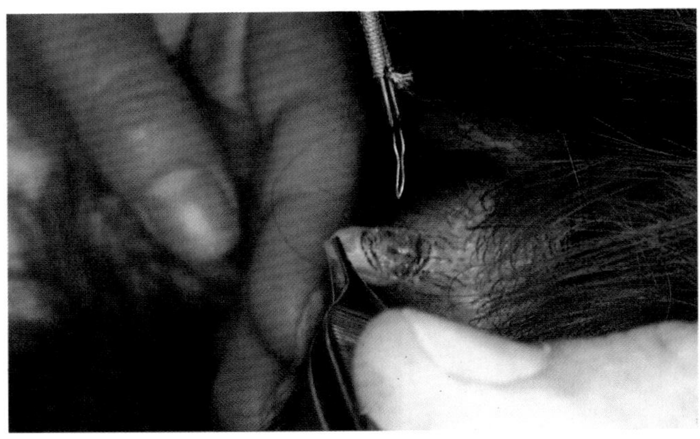

Fig. 29.10 Papilloma nearly separated from its base; notice absence of bleeding.

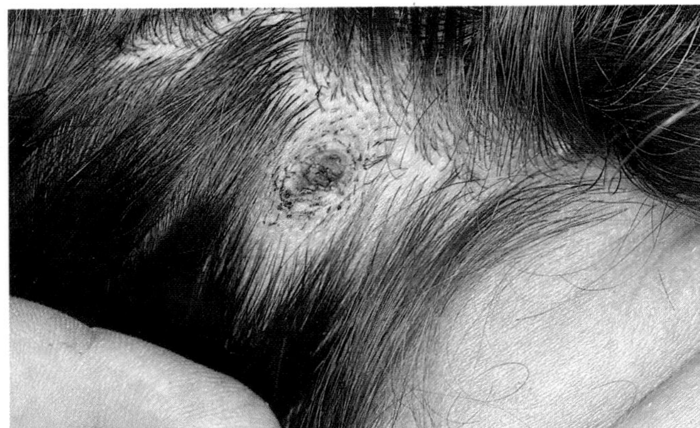

Fig. 29.11 The end-result immediately after removing papilloma. No dressing required.

29.1.4 Accessory digits (see Chapter 41)

Where there is no underlying bony connection, accessory digits may be easily separated at birth using the electrocautery alone.

29.1.5 Basal cell carcinoma (see Chapter 17)

Many small basal celled tumours of the skin may be curetted and the bases extensively cauterized with the electrocautery, with very good results.

29.1.6 Cauterization of the cervix (see Chapter 20)

Cervical erosions are easily treated with the electrocautery; generally no anaesthetic is necessary and the results are good.

29.1.7 Condylomata (see Chapter 16)

Individual condylomata may be destroyed using the electrocautery, small lesions will not require anaesthesia, larger ones can be infiltrated prior to treatment.

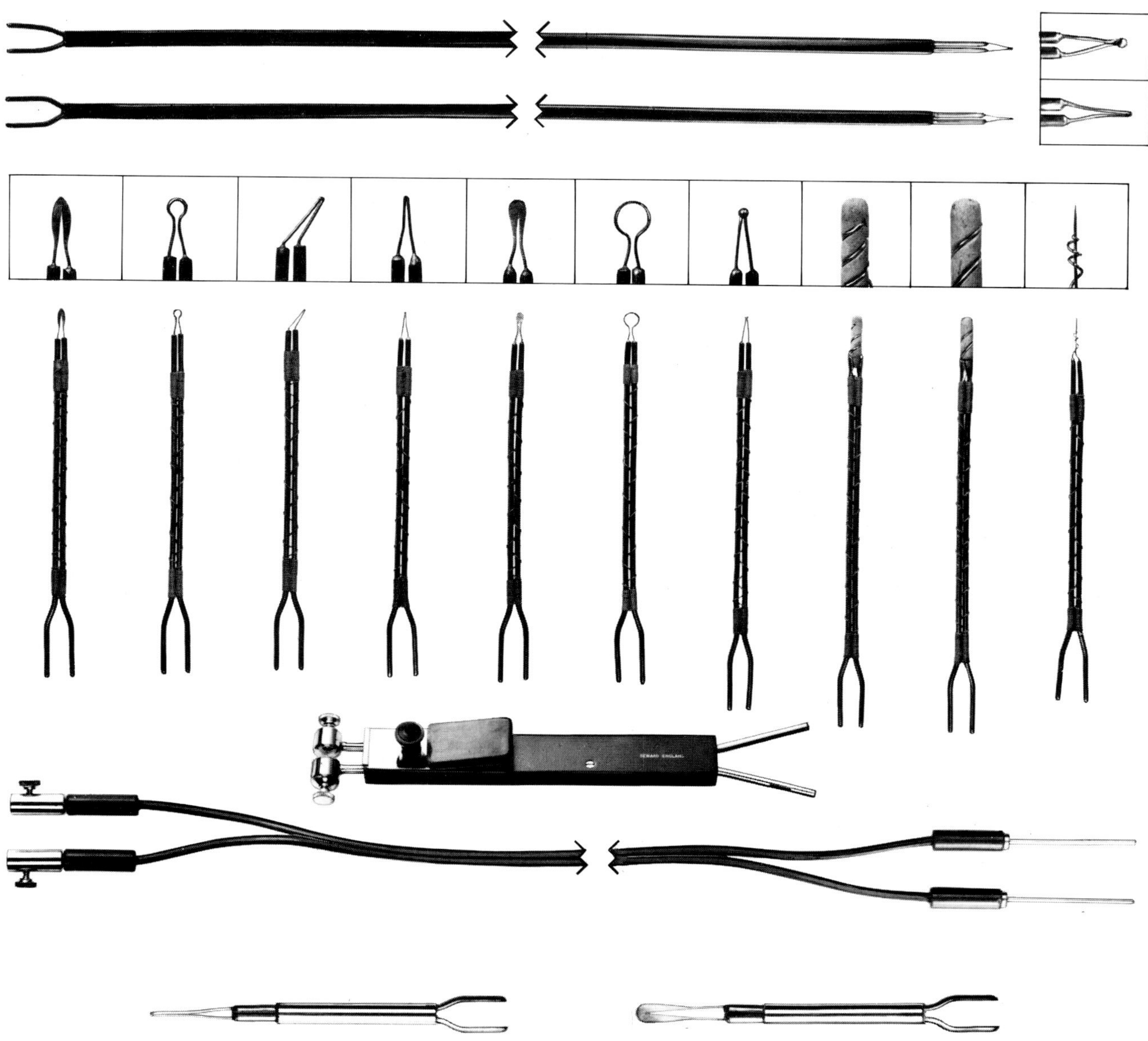

Fig. 29.12 A selection of cautery burners, together with Mark Hovell's cautery handle (Seward Medical).

29.1.8 Entropion (see Chapter 41)

Spot burns with the cautery help to produce fibrosis in the skin/muscle operation for entropion.

29.1.9 Epistaxis (see Chapter 32)

Mild epistaxes are best treated with Silver Nitrate cauterization, but stubborn epistaxes may be treated with electrocautery to Little's area after preliminary topical anaesthesia.

29.1.10 Granuloma pyogenicum (see Chapter 17)

These vascular lesions are ideally treated with curette and electrocautery.

29.1.11 Haemangioma of the lip (see Chapter 41)

After infiltrating with local anaesthetic, a haemangioma on the lip can be treated very effectively by inserting the electrocautery into the centre of the lesion.

29.1.12 Intradermal lesions (see Chapter 17)

Small intradermal lesions may be destroyed by the application of the electrocautery alone; larger lesions may be curetted followed by electrocautery to the base.

29.1.13 Kerato-acanthoma (see Chapter 17)

Curette followed by cauterization of the base is a simple and effective method of treating this rapidly growing tumour.

29.1.14 Molluscum contagiosum (see Chapter 17)

Small lesions are better destroyed with phenol or iodine pricked into each spot, but equally good results may be obtained using the cautery.

29.1.15 Solar keratoses (see Chapter 17)

Most solar keratoses may be removed with a sharp curette and the base cauterized using an electrocautery.

29.1.16 Spider naevi (see Chapter 17)

If the central vessel of a spider naevus is touched with the electrocautery, rapid cure results.

29.1.17 Squamous celled carcinoma (see Chapter 17)

Small squamous celled tumours may be curetted, followed by liberal cauterization of the base.

29.1.18 Warts and verrucae (see Chapter 16)

Almost all warts and verrucae can be removed with a sharp-spoon curette, cauterizing the base afterwards.

29.1.19 Xanthomata (see Chapters 28 and 41)

Used with care, the electrocautery may be a suitable treatment for small xanthelasmata.

THIRTY

The cryoprobe

'Thou shalt make for him cool applications of ice and salt for drawing out the inflammation from the mouth of the wound'

(Edwin Smith, Surgical Papyrus, 3000–2500 BC)

The first recorded use of cold for medical conditions was in the Edwin Smith Surgical Papyrus (3000 BC). Hippocrates described the use of snow and ice for relieving pain and arresting haemorrhage (400 BC) but it is only in the last 100 years that freezing as a recognized treatment has achieved popularity. Liquid air, liquid oxygen and carbon dioxide snow were used at the beginning of the 20th century [28, 29, 30] and in 1950 Dr H. V. Allington described the use of liquid nitrogen as the freezing agent, obtaining excellent results with a variety of skin lesions.

Today closed cryosurgical instruments are in regular use throughout the world; they depend on the Joule-Thompson effect by allowing liquid gas to expand into its gaseous form in a chamber within the cryoprobe, resulting in rapid cooling. Three agents are now used: liquid nitrogen, giving a probe temperature of $-196°$ C; nitrous oxide, giving a probe temperature of $-89.5°$ C and carbon dioxide, giving a probe temperature of $-78.5°$ C (Figs 30.12, 30.2 and 30.1). Tissue destruction occurs if the temperature is reduced to $-25°$ C, and total destruction takes place at $-50°$ C. Modern electronics now enable the doctor to monitor the degree of freezing by the insertion of thermocouples adjacent to the lesion; as experience grows, the thermocouples need not be used.

Whichever cryogen is used, the technique is similar; the area to be frozen is covered with a thin film of K-Y Jelly or glycerine which helps adhesion, and the cryoprobe applied. Immediately the probe has frozen to the skin, it may be gently withdrawn; this has a combined effect of protecting underlying tissues, and reducing the vascularity of the lesion.

A rim of ice will be seen forming in the skin, spreading concentrically from the cryoprobe. Experience will decide how long to leave the probe in contact with the lesion to be treated, but when it is judged to be adequate, the tip is de-frosted, removed, and the lesion allowed to thaw – this generally takes less than 1 min. A second freeze is performed, this appears to give improved results over one single freeze.

The result of freezing is the formation of ice crystals in the intracellular and extracellular fluids, resulting in cell dehydration and shrinkage, an abnormal concentration of electrolytes inside the cell, 'thermal' shock and denaturation of lipid–protein complexes, and cell death. Following cryotherapy, a blister develops, which dries to a scab in about one week and this eventually separates. Occasionally healing takes much longer, but is accompanied by a remarkable absence of pain, and an extremely acceptable cosmetic scar.

Local anaesthetics may be infiltrated below the lesion if necessary, but may alter the freezing response; some throbbing occurs during the first few hours after thawing, but thereafter healing is uncomplicated.

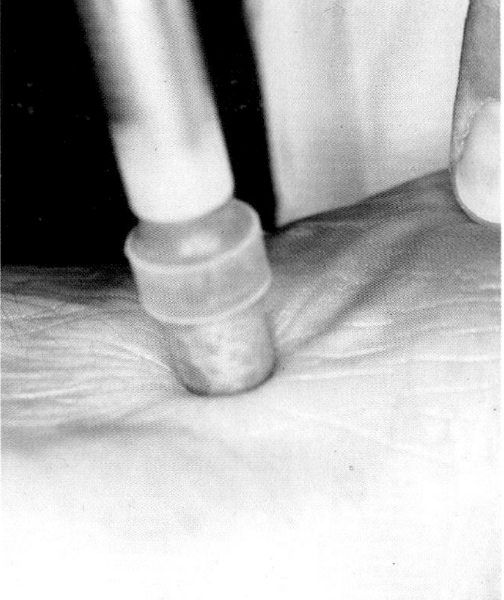

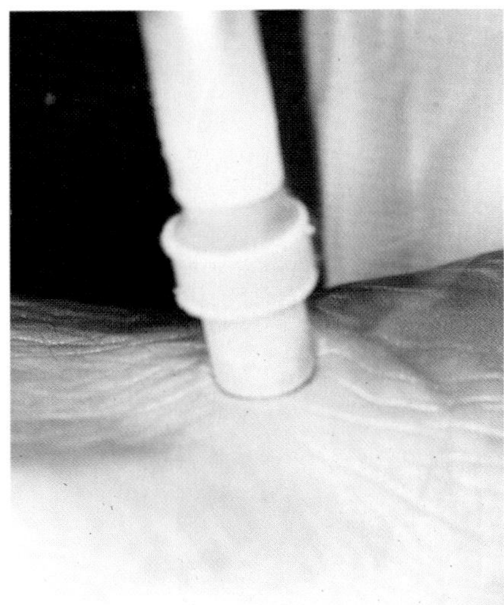

Fig. 30.1 The cryoprobe is applied to the lesion which has been smeared with water-soluble jelly to help adhesion.

Fig. 30.2 Once the probe is adherent to the skin, it may be gently withdrawn as shown.

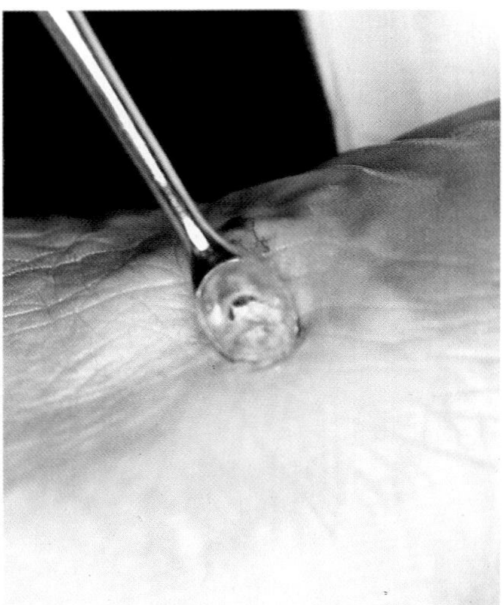

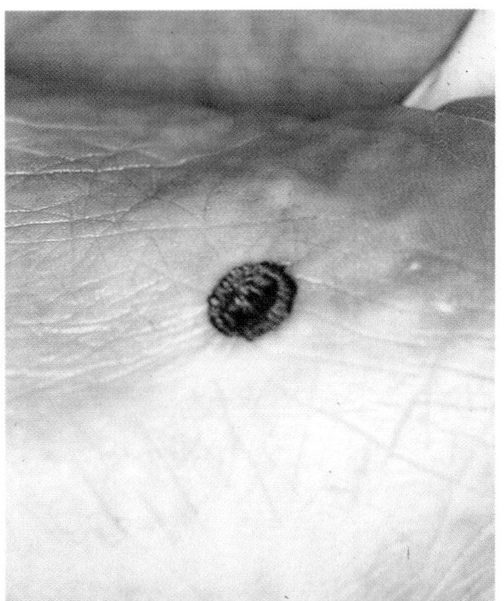

Fig. 30.3 A cryo-biopsy may easily be taken with a sharp-spooned curette.

Fig. 30.4 If necessary the base may be cauterized with the electrocautery as well.

One major advantage of cryotherapy is the ability to take a 'cryo-biopsy' to establish a diagnosis. This is done while the tissues are frozen either with a punch biopsy forceps or curette. A small piece of alginate dressing is placed in the wound to check bleeding as thawing occurs, covered by a dry sterile dressing. Unlike cauterization with heat, freezing does not damage the histology of the cells; the cryobiopsy may therefore be placed directly in 10% formol-saline and sent for routine histology exactly as any other specimen (Fig. 30.3).

Freezing also produces thrombosis in the micro-circulation after 24 hours, so that provided the diameter of the vessels involved is small enough, many vascular lesions can be treated. Intradermal haemangiomata, particularly on the face may be given repeated short freezes every six weeks which will result in a gradual regression and total cure.

Following treatment of any lesion, the area should be kept as dry as possible and if necessary covered with a dry sterile dressing.

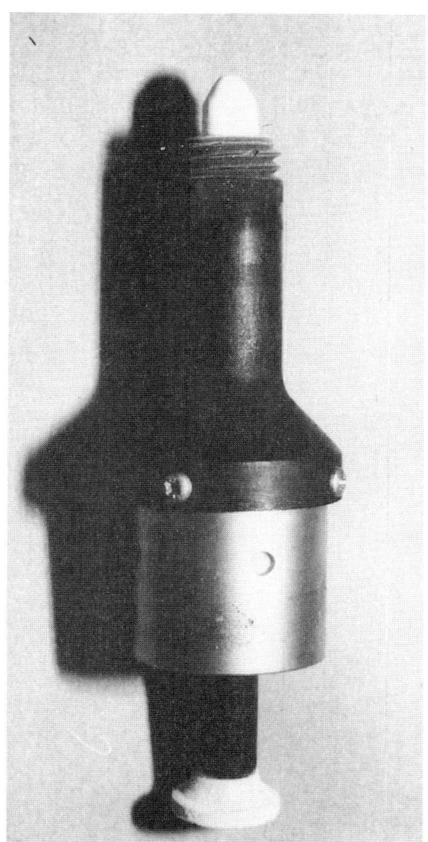

30.1 THE CARBON DIOXIDE SNOW PENCIL (Fig. 30.5)

A small, hand held cryotherapy apparatus is available which utilizes J-size 'Sparklet' carbon dioxide cylinders. The solid carbon dioxide can be compacted to make a pencil, the tip temperature will be about −70° C and is quite suitable for most superficial lesions.

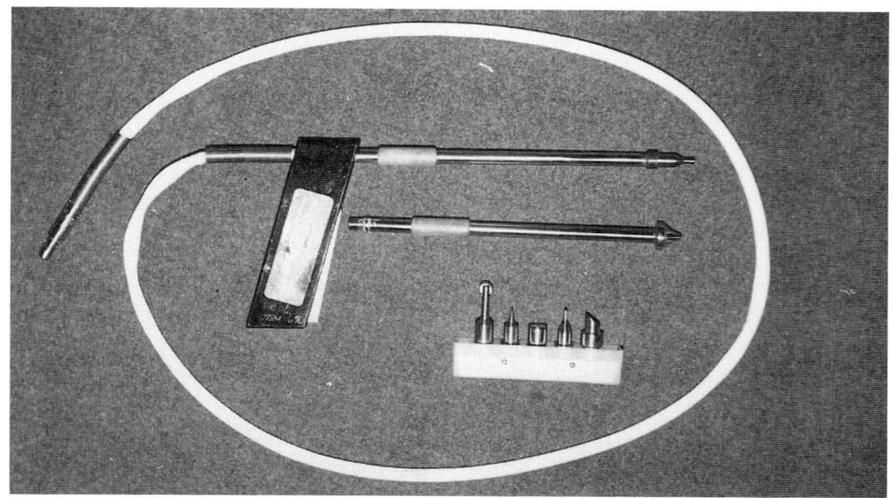

Fig. 30.5 A carbon dioxide pencil which can be made from a J-size CO_2 cylinder.

Fig. 30.6 The nitrous oxide cryoprobe with selection of screw-on probes.

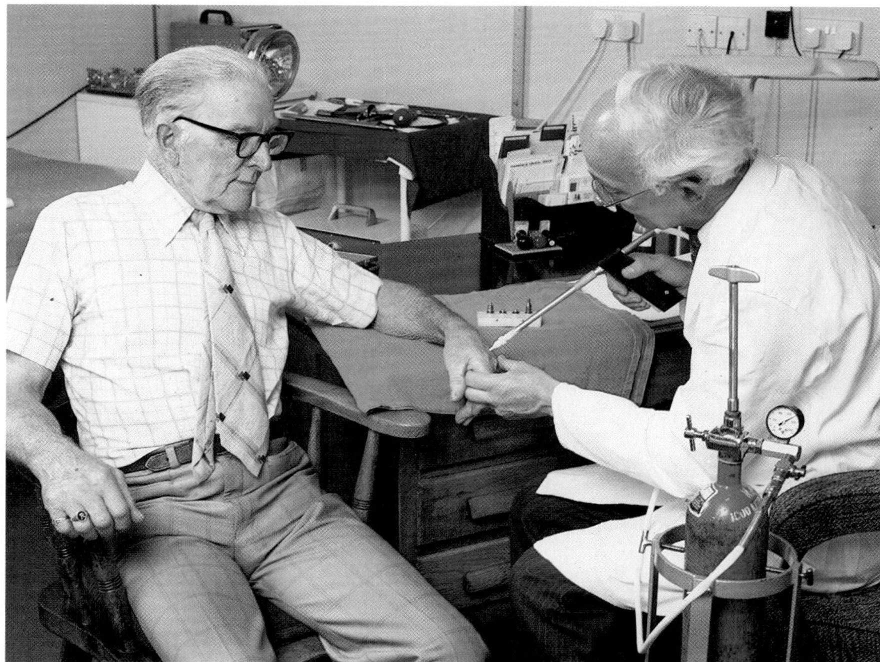

Fig. 30.7 The use of the nitrous oxide cryoprobe in the surgery; treatment is quick and effective.

Fig. 30.8 The nitrous oxide cryoprobe applied to solar keratosis, back of hand.

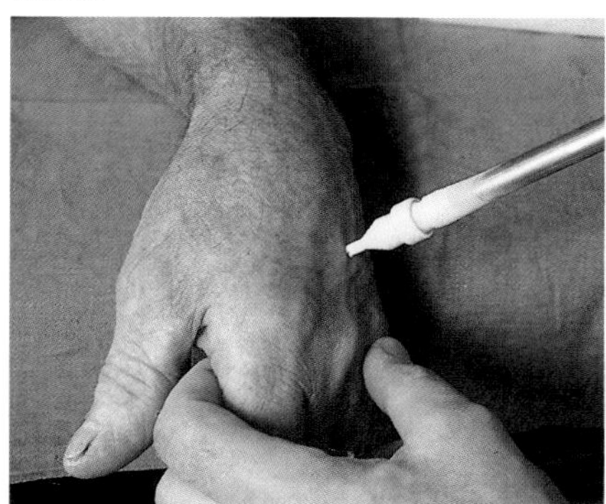

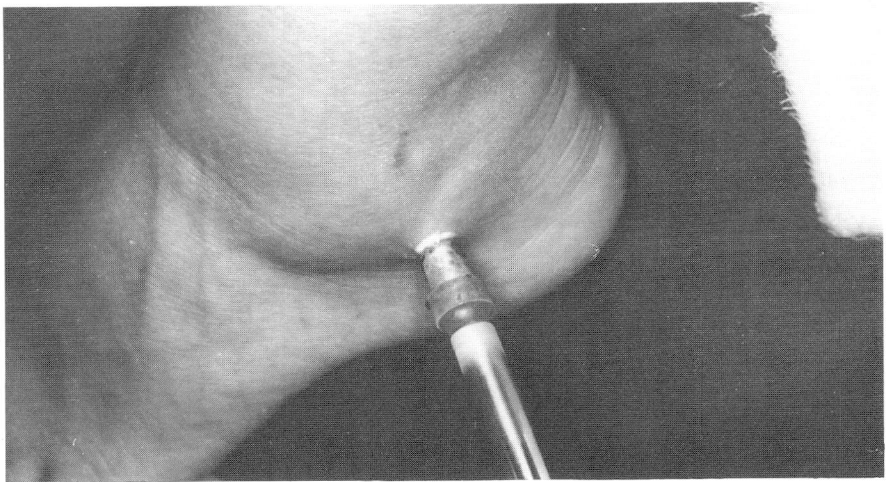

Fig. 30.9 The nitrous oxide cryoprobe applied to a wart on the foot.

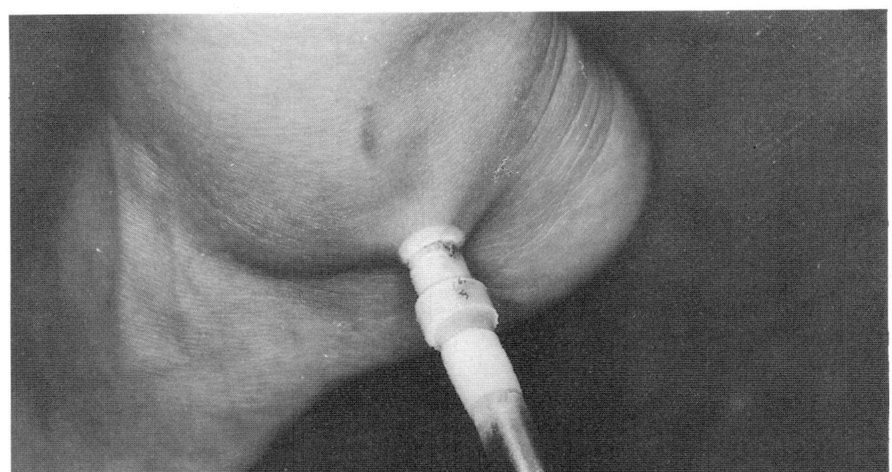

Fig. 30.10 Once the probe is adherent to the wart, gentle traction may be applied.

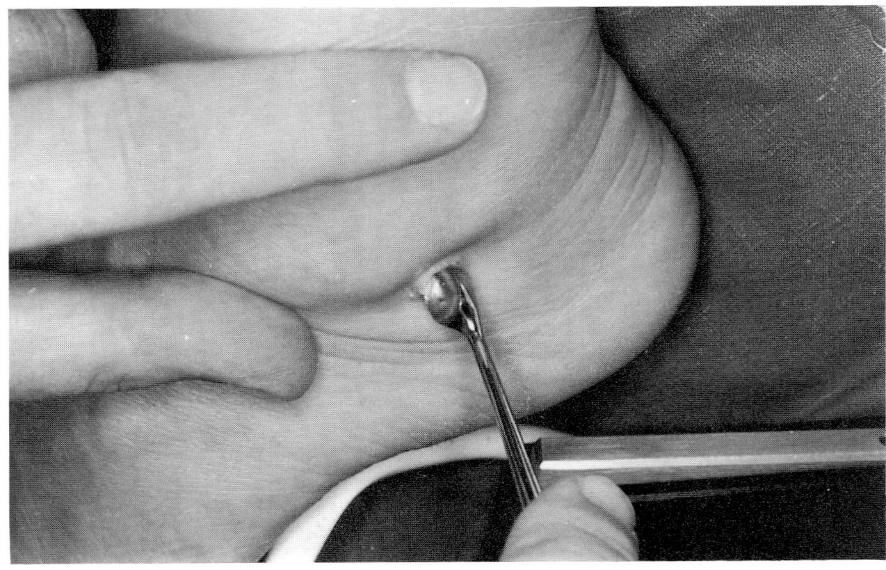

Fig. 30.11 A cryo-biopsy may easily be performed, or the wart removed completely using a sharp-spoon curette.

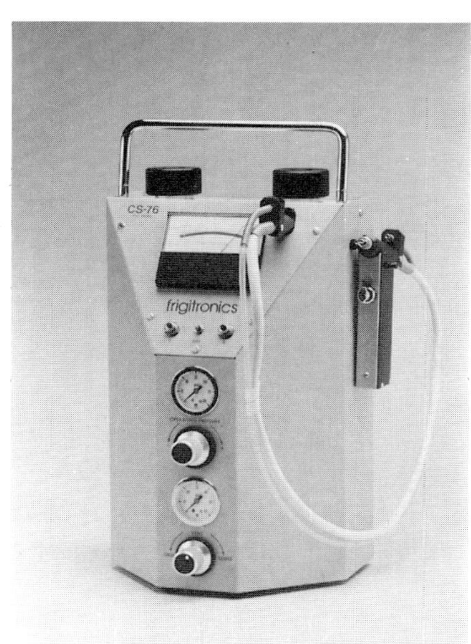

Fig. 30.12 The CS-76 liquid nitrogen cryosurgical unit, which is self pressurizing, portable, and non-electric. It may be used with spray needles and closed-end probes (Frigitronics Ltd, Downs Surgical plc).

30.2 THE NITROUS OXIDE CRYOPROBE [31, 32] (Fig. 30.6)

This is probably the most convenient type of cryoprobe for the general practitioner; although not as effective as the liquid nitrogen instrument, it has the advantage of always being immediately available, whereas a liquid nitrogen instrument depends on regular deliveries of cryogen.

The probes are all of the closed chamber type and can be obtained in a wide variety of different shapes and sizes to suit various lesions. The instrument requires little maintenance, is reliable, and can be sterilized if necessary. Operating pressure is 700–800 lbf/in^2 (2825–5700 kN/m^2) and cylinders generally need to be replaced when the pressure falls below 600 lbf/in^2 (4140 kN/m^2).

Pressures will vary according to the cylinder temperature, being much lower if cold and conversely higher if warm. This fact needs to be remembered if a replacement cylinder has been kept in a cold store-room.

30.3 LIQUID NITROGEN CRYOTHERAPY [33, 34] (Fig. 30.12)

This undoubtedly gives the best results, with probe temperatures as low as −196° C. It may, therefore, be confidently used for malignant skin tumours where cryobiopsy and total destruction is possible. The systems may be closed, or open 'spray' cones. The closed system is similar to the nitrous oxide apparatus, except that the probe tends not to adhere so firmly to tissues during freezing and may be more readily removed. The open 'spray cones' enable a jet of liquid nitrogen to be sprayed over the lesion, under cover of the protective cone.

The main disadvantage of liquid nitrogen is the fact that the doctor has to rely on regular deliveries of liquid nitrogen, and will thus have to collect a 'list' of patients at selected intervals.

THIRTY-ONE

The unipolar diathermy

'An ailment I will treat . . . with the fire-drill'

(Edwin Smith, Surgical Papyrus, 3000–2500 BC)

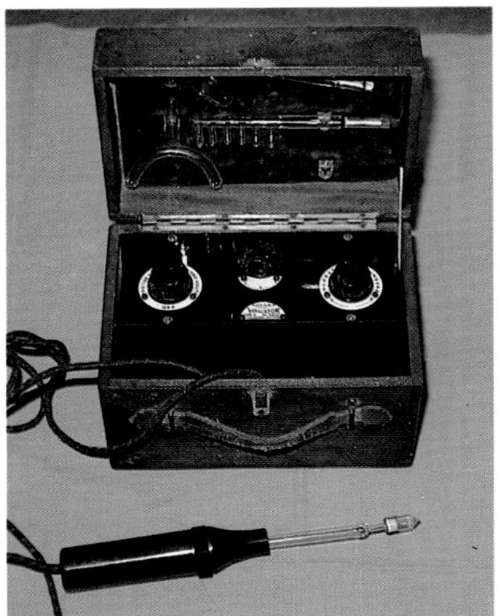

Fig. 31.1 A domestic 'high-frequency machine' belonging to the author's grandfather; 1910 approx. This produced similar currents to the modern 'hyfrecator'.

High-frequency electric currents have been used for minor surgical procedures for 200 years. Early machines used rotating mica discs to generate static electricity which was stored in large Leyden jar condensers, connected to a spark gap and electrodes which were applied to the patient [35]. By the beginning of the 20th century, portable machines were in production which used batteries or domestic electricity supplies; the spark gap was still utilized and is still used in some machines today, being superseded by solid-state electronic circuitry.

The bipolar diathermy machine is a standard item of equipment in almost every operating theatre in the world. A low current at very high frequency and high voltage is passed through the patient. Two electrodes are needed to complete the circuit – one is large in area and is usually strapped to the patient's thigh, the other is usually connected to diathermy forceps or an electrode. If this latter electrode is placed in contact with the patient, a current sufficient to heat the tissues is generated. By varying the waveform and intensity of the current, tissues may be coagulated or cut.

The unipolar diathermy utilizes a similar principle – it generates a very high voltage, at very high frequency but relatively low current, but unlike the bipolar diathermy does not require a large second electrode to be connected to the patient. This makes it more suitable for use in minor surgery where large currents are not needed. A high-frequency current may be used in one of three ways, viz: desiccation, fulguration and coagulation.

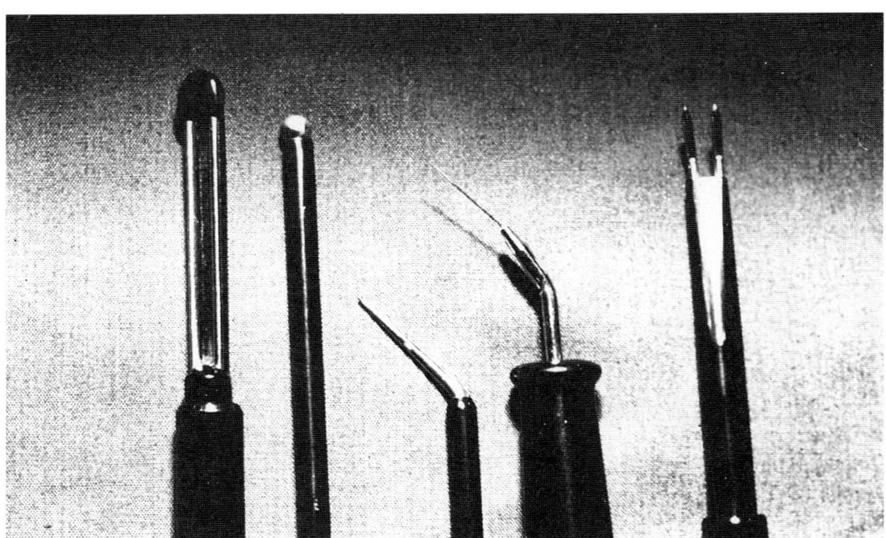

Fig. 31.2 Selection of unipolar diathermy electrodes.

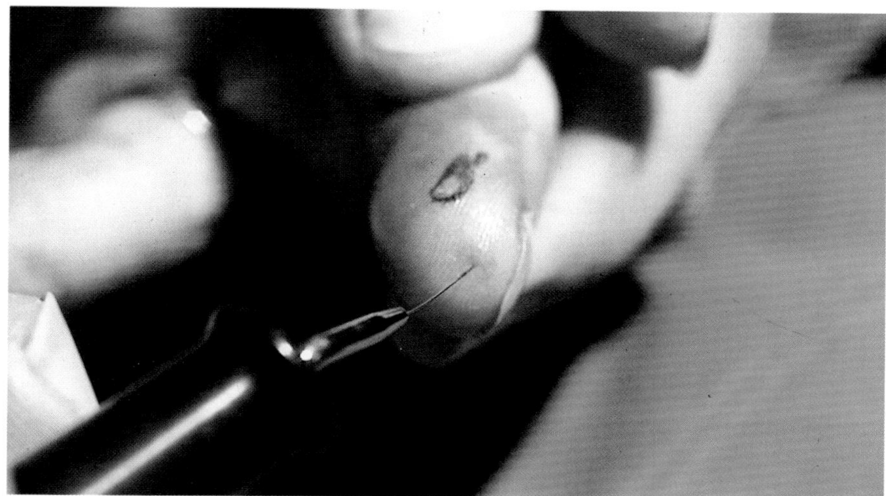

Fig. 31.3 Showing the needle electrode of the unipolar diathermy being used to treat a wart on the finger-tip.

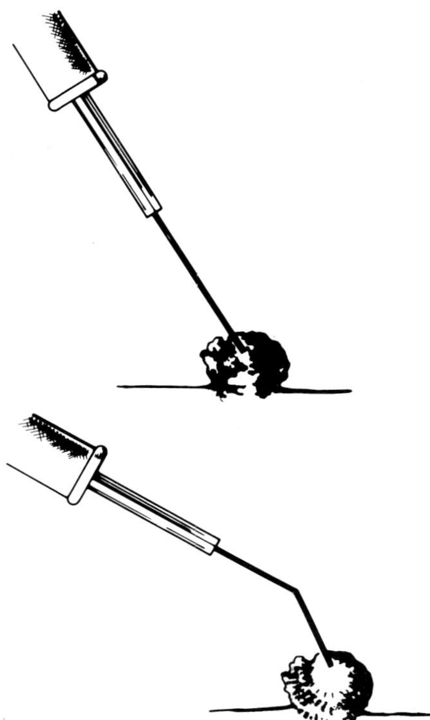

Fig. 31.4 Desiccation of a wart by inserting a needle electrode into the lesion and passing a current through it. This generates heat within the wart and destroys it.

In desiccation the electrode is inserted into the lesion to be treated to the depth at which the tissue is to be destroyed. The heat generated in the electrode dries out, and thus destroys the tissue which separates in a few days (Figs 31.3 and 31.4).

Fulguration is achieved by holding the electrode just above the surface to be treated and drawing a stream of sparks from the electrode to the point of treatment. The tissues are charred and destroyed, being rejected in a few days (Fig. 31.5).

In coagulation a bipolar electrode is used which is connected to a separate winding on the transformer. It is placed on the surface to be treated and an electric current flows between the two poles of the electrode, generating heat and thus destroying the tissues (Fig. 31.6).

As individual machines vary, the doctor who has not used a hyfrecator before can experiment using a piece of raw meat held in the hand, and applying different electrodes, desiccation, fulguration and coagulation. The depth and extent of treatment can then be assessed by cutting through the meat and examining the lesions produced.

Small cutaneous lesions and those affecting the cervix, vagina and bowel can be treated without the need for a local anaesthetic. For the majority of other lesions, however, it is more comfortable to infiltrate with local anaesthetic prior to treatment.

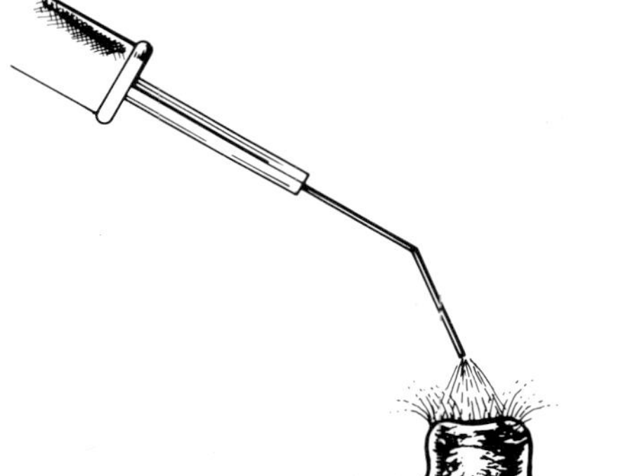

Fig. 31.5 Fulguration of a wart by holding the electrode just above the lesion and allowing a stream of sparks to pass from the electrode to the wart, thus generating heat and destroying it.

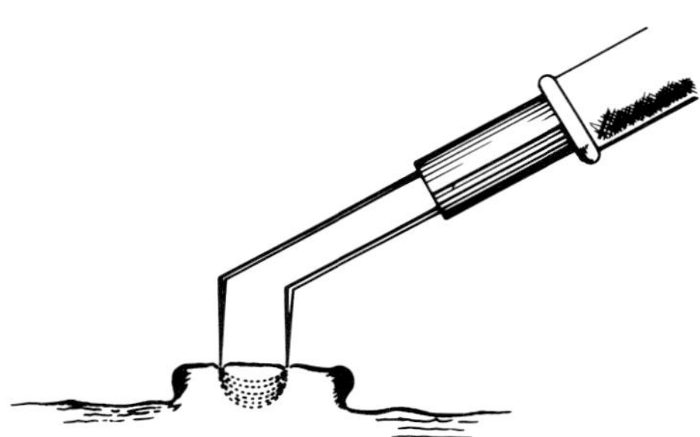

Fig. 31.6 Coagulation using a bi-polar electrode pressed against the skin. Tissue destruction is confined to the area between the electrodes.

31.1 ADVANTAGES OF HIGH-FREQUENCY CURRENTS

1. Quick, effective destruction of lesions with no blood loss.
2. Accuracy – most lesions can be destroyed with minimal damage to adjacent tissues.
3. The treated area is left sterile.
4. Good cosmetic results with little post-operative pain.
5. Excellent for vascular lesions.

31.2 DISADVANTAGE

As with the electrocautery the lesion is destroyed, and cannot be examined histologically except by taking a preliminary biopsy.

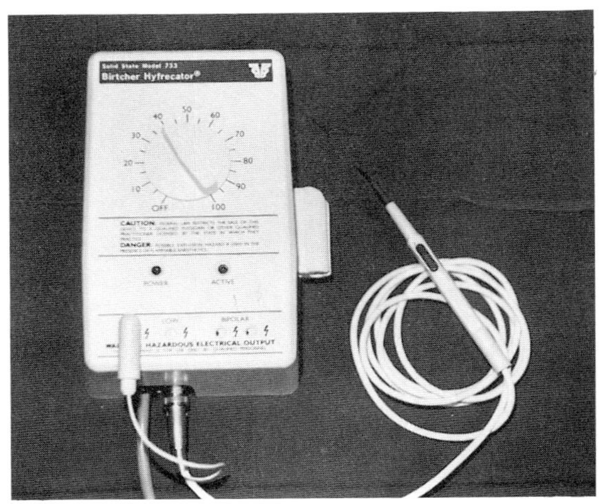

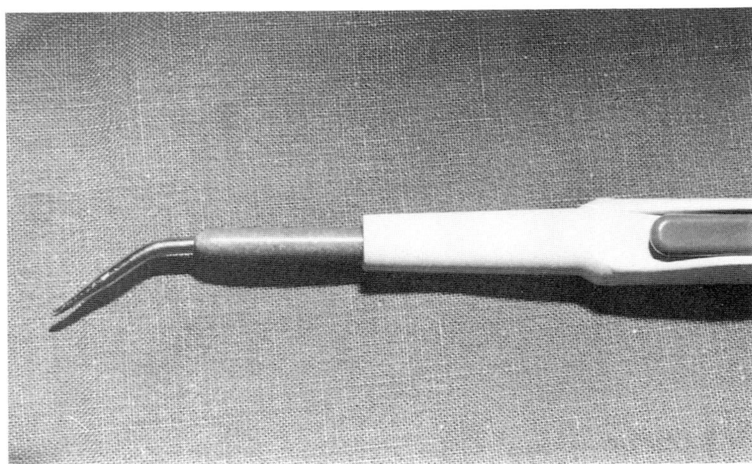

Fig. 31.7 The Birtcher Hyfrecator.

31.3 SOME APPLICATIONS OF HIGH-FREQUENCY TREATMENT

31.3.1 Warts

Infiltrate the base of the wart with local anaesthetic and desiccate it with a fine needle electrode inserted to base of wart.

31.3.2 Verrucae

The technique is similar to that for warts.

31.3.3 Haemangiomata

As with warts use a method of desiccation. Haemangiomata may require more than one treatment depending on their size.

31.3.4 Large haemangiomata

Infiltrate the base with local anaesthetic and then use bi-polar coagulation. The treatment may need to be repeated.

31.3.5 Spider naevus

Local anaesthesia is not used. The needle electrode should be inserted into the main blood vessel, usually in the centre.

31.3.6 Xanthelasma

The treatment is light fulguration with or without local anaesthesia.

31.3.7 Solar keratosis

Infiltrate with local anaesthetic; then curette followed by fulguration to the base.

31.3.8 Cervical erosions

These may be treated with fulguration without local anaesthesia.

31.3.9 Papillomata

Small papillomata may be desiccated or fulgurized without anaesthesia. Larger lesions should have the base anaesthetized first.

31.3.10 Naevi

Large naevi may be better excised, but small naevi can be easily destroyed by desiccation. If pigmented, the area desiccated should include a narrow area of healthy adjacent skin.

As can be seen, almost any skin lesion can be effectively treated with a high-frequency current; as the tissue immediately following treatment is sterile, healing may be promoted by the application of a sterile dry dressing, and advising the patient to keep the area dry until healing is complete.

THIRTY-TWO

Epistaxis

'Clean out for him the interior of both nostrils with two swabs of linen until every worm of blood which coagulates in the inside of his nostrils comes forth. Now afterwards thou shouldst place two plugs of linen saturated with grease and put into his nostrils'

(Edwin Smith, Surgical Papyrus, 3000–2500 BC)

Most nose bleeds, particularly in children, are self-limiting; recurrent epistaxes often arise from a small collection of blood vessels in 'Little's area' just inside the nose on either side of the nasal septum. These can be successfully sealed by a variety of treatments, including the following.

32.1 SILVER NITRATE CAUTERIZATION

This is probably the simplest method. With the patient facing the doctor, and good illumination, Little's area is inspected on either side. Silver Nitrate is now applied, using a disposable Silver Nitrate wooden applicator or using a pointed Silver Nitrate pencil stick held in an applicator (Fig. 32.2). The treated area immediately turns white; some reflex watering of the patient's eyes always occurs. The patient is requested not to blow their nose for several hours, and normally only one treatment is necessary. No anaesthetic is required.

32.2 ELECTROCAUTERIZATION OF LITTLE'S AREA

More stubborn recurrent epistaxes may be treated with the electrocautery; but the nose must be anaesthetized. This is achieved by spraying the inside of the nose with Xylocaine pressurized spray (Lignocaine metered dose

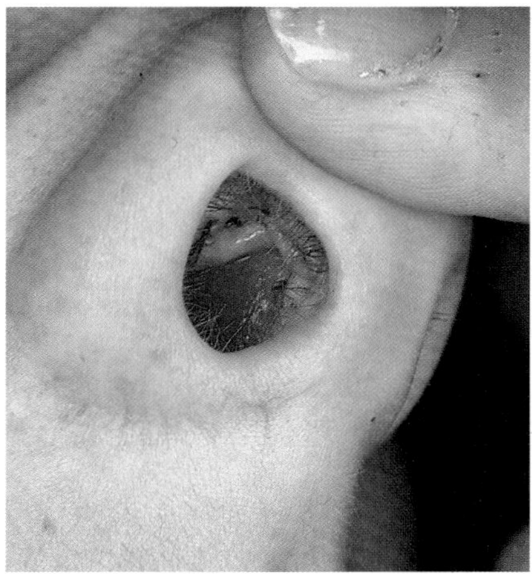

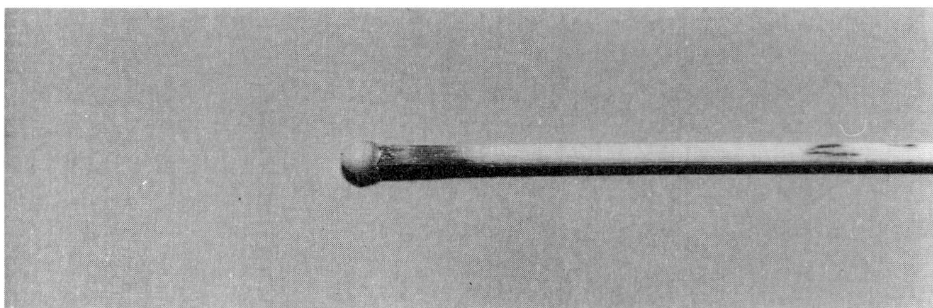

Fig. 32.1 The majority of nose-bleeds occur from 'Little's area' just inside the nostril as shown.

Fig. 32.2 Single-use Silver Nitrate applicators are ideal for cauterizing 'Little's area'.

aerosol 100 μg per dose) or by the application of pledgelets of cotton wool soaked in 4% Lignocaine or similar topical anaesthetic.

With good illumination, the offending blood vessels are cauterized with the electrocautery. Only dull-red heat is used, and sparingly. Over enthusiastic electrocauterization can lead to perforation of the nasal septum, and only one side should be cauterized at a time.

32.3 DIATHERMY OF LITTLE'S AREA

This may be achieved using the unipolar diathermy or hyfrecator. As with electrocautery, the preliminary application of local anaesthesia is necessary. The area to be treated may be fulgurized by holding the needle electrode a very short distance away from the tissues and allowing a stream of sparks to play over the area. The current is turned down to minimum to avoid damage to the nasal septum.

32.4 CRYOTHERAPY TO LITTLE'S AREA

Effective control may be achieved by freezing; the use of local anaesthesia is desirable but not always necessary. It is important to check that the probe will just cover the area to be frozen without accidentally touching any other part of the nose, otherwise this may become adherent to the probe and result in an additional 'frost-burn'.

32.5 PHOTOCOAGULATION OF LITTLE'S AREA

An infra-red photocoagulator with narrow applicator may be used to control recurrent epistaxes. The topical application of local anaesthetic is necessary but the technique is simple and gives good results.

32.6 THE ACUTE BLEED

None of the aforementioned treatments is applicable during an acute nosebleed, which must be controlled either by digital pressure or packing the nose with ribbon gauze soaked in 1:1000 adrenalin (plus 4% Lignocaine if necessary). Should either of these fail, and particularly if the patient is elderly, where the source of bleeding is unlikely to be from Little's area, they should be referred to hospital.

THIRTY-THREE

The use of the proctoscope

'The discharge of blood from the rectum is a disease chiefly confined to those advanced in life. It is occasioned by full living, abuse of purgatives, violent passions or habitual melancholy. To this effect, leeches and warm fomentations applied to the anus are the most efficacious remedies'

(Encyclopaedia Brittanica, 1817)

Examination of the anal canal in all patients with rectal symptoms is mandatory, but patients are still seen with inoperable cancers who missed having an early rectal examination.

Rectal bleeding is an extremely common symptom, fortunately in the majority it arises from haemorrhoids which can be visualized easily with a proctoscope. Instruments may be disposable or non-disposable, each having their own advantages and disadvantages.

33.1 DISPOSABLE PROCTOSCOPES

These consist of a plastic tube with central obturator; they may be pre-sterilized in individual packs, and if sterilizing facilities are available (see Chapter 5) they can be used on more than one occasion. External illumination is necessary for the majority of instruments, although some have provision for internal illumination.

33.2 NON-DISPOSABLE PROCTOSCOPES

These are generally made of stainless steel and consist of an outer tube and handle, together with a central obturator. Illumination can be from an external source, from in-built illumination in the form of a tungsten-filament or quartz bulbs, or from an external fibre-optic light source. They can be sterilized by autoclaving, dry heat oven or immersion (see Chapter 5).

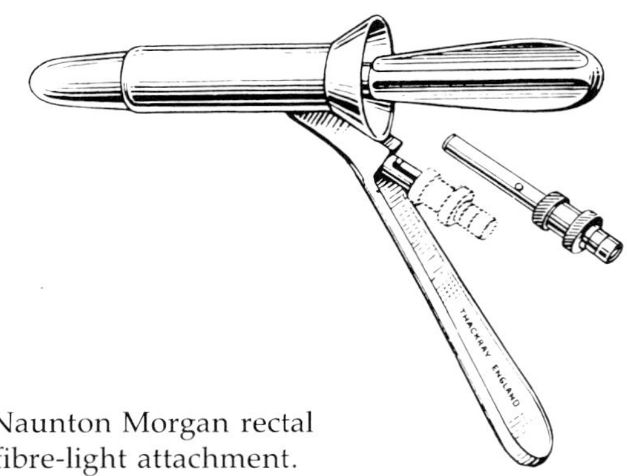

Fig. 33.1 The Naunton Morgan rectal speculum with fibre-light attachment.

33.2.1 Technique

If the patient is lying in the left lateral position, with knees drawn up, the direction of the anal canal is upwards and forwards. A digital rectal examination is performed, and any abnormality in the rectum noted. The muscle tone of the anal sphincter is noted, as is the degree of discomfort caused by the examination. This may give a clue to the diagnosis of anal fissure, typified by pain and spasm. The examining finger is withdrawn, and the glove examined for any signs of blood. Next, the proctoscope is lubricated and very gently inserted into the anal canal; as soon as the instrument is felt to have passed through the sphincter, its direction is changed slightly posteriorly to take account of the direction of the rectum. The instrument is inserted fully to the flange, and the obturator withdrawn and the illumination switched on. The normal mucous membrane is pale, but capillaries and tributaries of the superior haemorrhoidal vein are visible. Any pathology is noted, and the proctoscope slowly withdrawn, during which the mucous membrane begins to close in. Prolapsing internal haemorrhoids become easily visible at this stage, and their positions may be noted for future reference. As the proctoscope is further withdrawn, lesions of the anal canal may be seen such as proctitis, or fissure.

Where the patient gives a history of bleeding on defaecation, it is worth re-introducing the proctoscope and asking the patient to strain down as the instrument is slowly withdrawn. In this way, a bleeding haemorrhoid or fissure can be identified. If suspected haemorrhoids are revealed on proctoscopy, it is often convenient to treat them at the time of the initial examination (see Chapter 36).

THIRTY-FOUR

Sigmoidoscopy

'Signs, forsooth, of ulceration are these: the patient cannot abstain from going to the privy because of aching, and he passes a stinking discharge mixed with watery blood. Ignorant leeches will assure the patient that he has dysentery, when truly it is not. I never saw, nor heard of any man that was cured of cancer of the rectum, but I have known many that died of the aforesaid sickness'

(John of Arderne, 1306–1390)

Sigmoidoscopy is considerably easier to perform than is generally realized [36, 37]. It is not a difficult technique to learn, and with regular use the practitioner will quickly learn to recognize both the normal and abnormal appearances. It can be one of the most valuable instruments in general practice; combined with a pair of biopsy forceps, rapid diagnosis of carcinoma of the rectum, ulcerative colitis, rectal polypi, proctitis and haemorrhoids can be made.

The first sigmoidoscope was invented by Bodenhamer in 1863 and consisted of a flexible tube of reflecting mirrors; unfortunately it was found to be impractical and it was not until 1895 that Kelly described a sigmoidoscope, very similar to those found today. His instrument had the light bulb placed distally, which had the disadvantage of soiling by faeces and bulb failure. In 1912 Yeomans designed an instrument with proximal illumination and air insufflation, and apart from slight modifications today's instruments are very similar.

Improvements in illumination using fibre-optic light sources and cables have enabled better visualization to be obtained, and most recently, flexible, fibre-optic sigmoidoscopes have been introduced which will examine more of the rectum and sigmoid colon than the conventional rigid instrument.

34.1 INDICATIONS FOR USE

Sigmoidoscopy forms an integral part of the routine investigation of all patients presenting with rectal bleeding, change in bowel habit, prolonged diarrhoea, and of the follow-up of patients who have had rectal surgery.

The standard adult stainless-steel Lloyd-Davies sigmoidoscope with proximal illumination gives good visualization, is easy to use, is well constructed and virtually indestructable (Fig. 34.1). A smaller diameter instrument is also available but for the majority of examinations, the adult

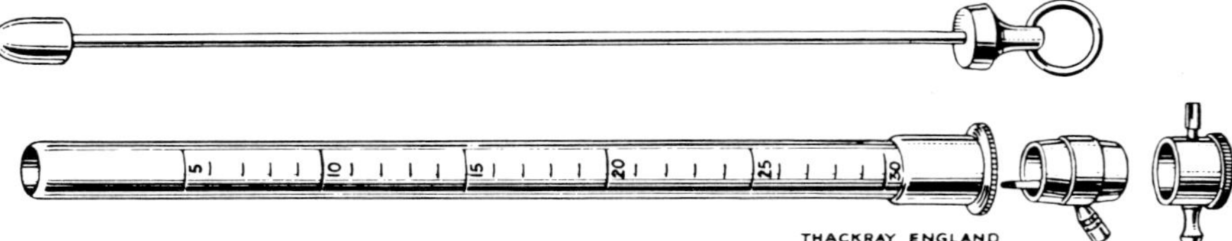

Fig. 34.1 The Lloyd Davies stainless steel adult sigmoidoscope fitted with proximal fibre-light chamber.

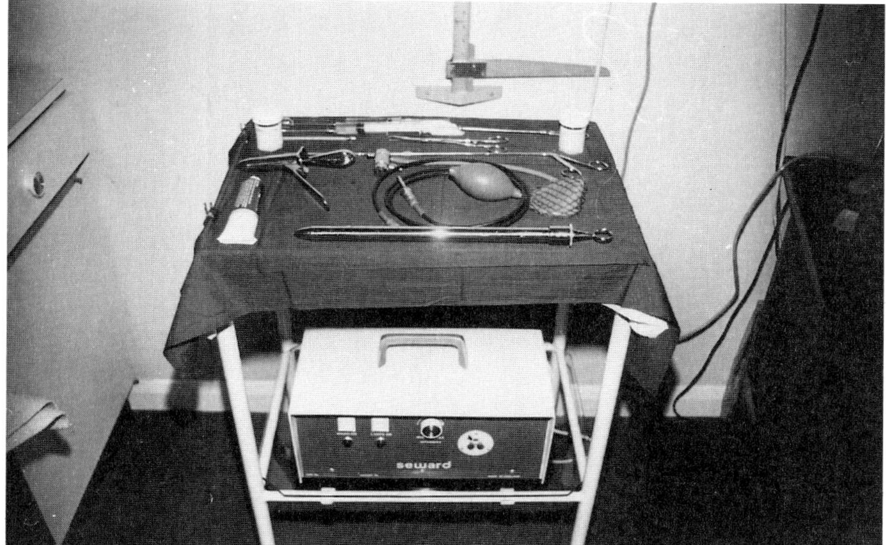

Fig. 34.2 It is a good idea to keep all instruments and accessories for sigmoidoscopy on one trolley for immediate use.

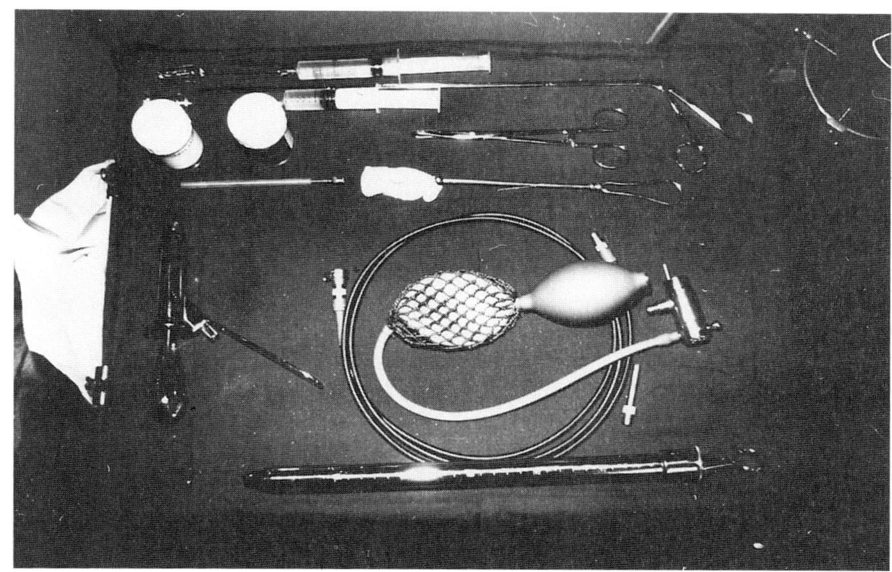

Fig. 34.3 Instruments ready for sigmoidoscopy.

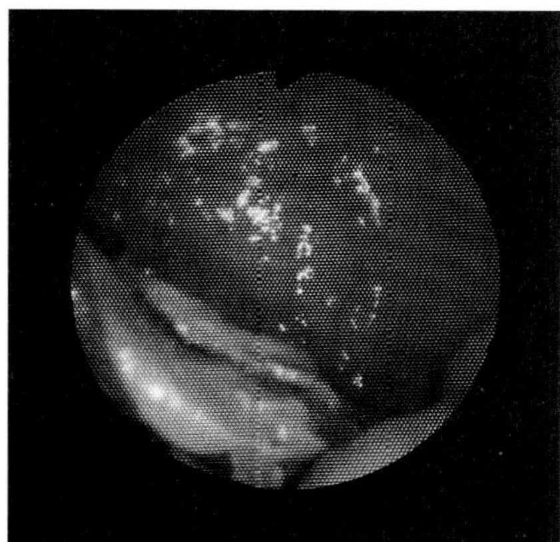

Fig. 34.4 View through sigmoidoscope on entering rectum. Small quantity faeces which are negotiable.

size will be found to be more than adequate. Tungsten filament or quartz halogen bulbs give good illumination, but if a fibre-optic light source can be obtained this is even better and more reliable.

Reasonably priced disposable sigmoidoscopes are also available; these have the advantage of not requiring repeated sterilization and cleaning, but will work out more expensive in the long run compared with the stainless steel models.

A telescope attachment with magnification is a valuable accessory giving much improved views of the mucosa. Having assembled all the necessary instruments for sigmoidoscopy it is better to keep them all on a separate 'rectal trolley' ready for immediate use; this may then be taken from one consulting room to another at a moment's notice (Fig. 34.2). Biopsy forceps, although expensive, are invaluable, and enable the doctor to take an immediate biopsy of any suspicious lesions. In order to take a biopsy,

Fig. 34.5 Paterson biopsy forceps.

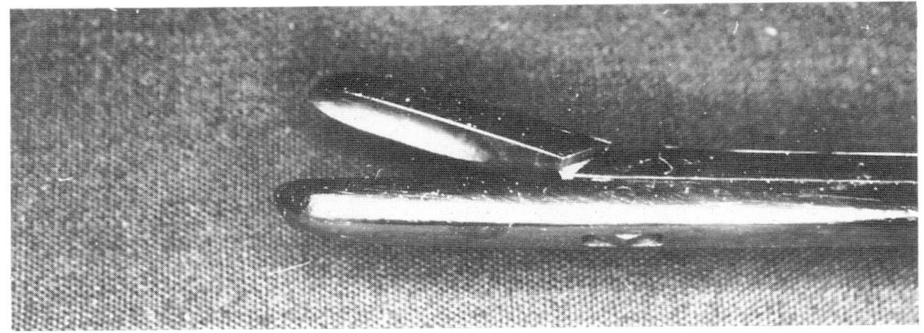

the window or telescope attachment at the operator's end of the sigmoidoscope needs to be removed in order to introduce the forceps, and this occasionally causes slight problems with loss of insufflated air, prolapse of mucosa, or poor visibility. Paterson's biopsy forceps, Chevalier Jackson's biopsy forceps, or Yeoman's rectal biopsy forceps are all suitable for the taking of biopsies. Other instruments which may be kept on a 'rectal trolley' include a proctoscope, haemorrhoid injection syringe and needles, ampoules of 5% oily phenol, specimen containers with 10% formol-saline for histology, K-Y Jelly, swabs, haemorrhoid ligator, grasping forceps and neoprene bands, plus swab holder and swabs.

34.2 PREPARATION OF THE PATIENT

Normally no preliminary bowel preparation is necessary, nor desirable, as the instrument can usually be manoeuvred past any faeces. Enemas or bowel wash-outs, as well as inflaming the mucosa, will wash away tell-tale blood-streaks or secretions. If the bowel is completely occluded with faeces, it is better to abandon the examination and attempt it on another occasion after defaecation.

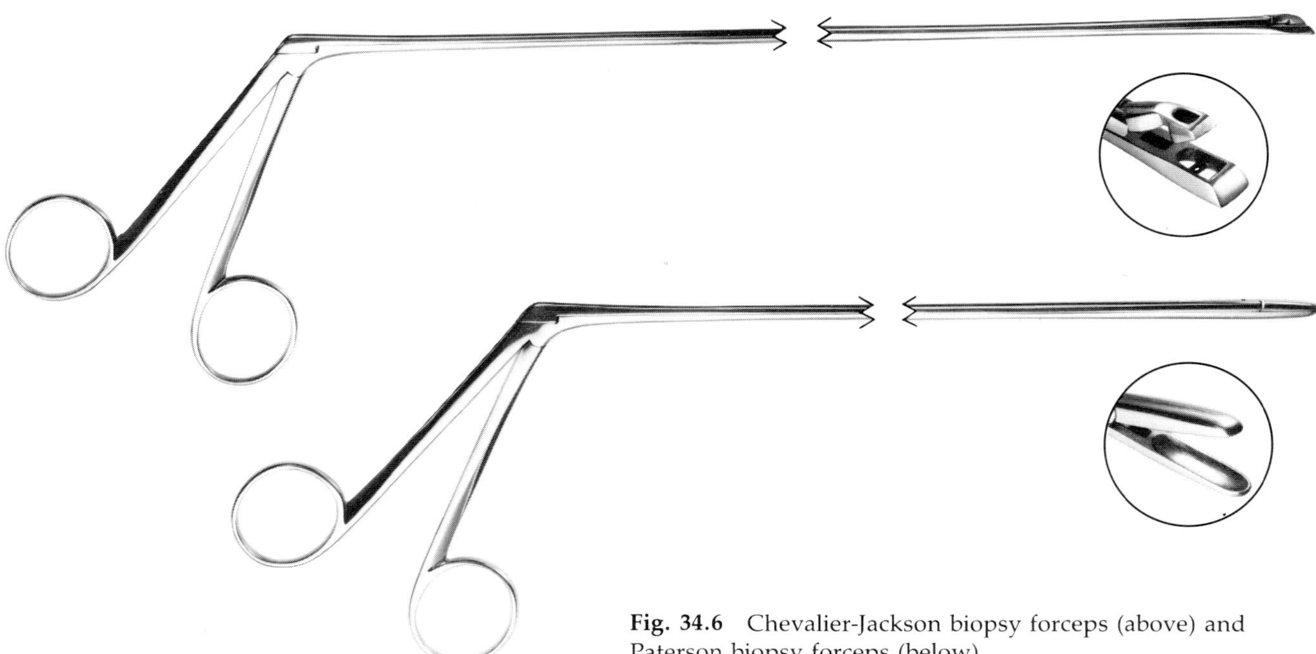

Fig. 34.6 Chevalier-Jackson biopsy forceps (above) and Paterson biopsy forceps (below).

34.3 TECHNIQUE OF SIGMOIDOSCOPY

The actual sigmoidoscopic examination only takes a few minutes, thus, if the instruments are always ready assembled for immediate use, it may be included in the initial consultation. The left lateral position is both comfortable and adequate for most sigmoidoscopies. The patient should be positioned with the buttocks at the edge of the couch, and knees and feet at the opposite edge, curled up.

A careful explanation of what will be done should always be given to the patient, in particular they may feel embarrassed in case they lose faeces or blood and soil the examination couch; reassurance that the patient, and doctor, are protected by a glass window will allay much anxiety.

The sigmoidoscope is assembled, the light checked, and the distal end lubricated with water-soluble K-Y jelly. Specimen containers and biopsy forceps are placed in an accessible position for the operator, and a digital rectal examination performed. This will reveal any low-lying masses, as well as lubricating the anal canal.

Holding the sigmoidoscope, and with the palm of the hand covering the obturator to prevent it being extruded, the instrument is *gently* inserted into the anal canal, in the direction of the umbilicus. It helps at this stage to ask the patient to quietly breathe in and out of his or her mouth. As soon as the sigmoidoscope has entered the rectum, the obturator is removed, and the inspection window or telescope attached, together with the bellows; a little air is introduced, from now on the instrument is advanced under direct vision. The lower valve of Houston is seen on the left, then the middle valve on the right. The apex of the rectum often appears to be a blind end, but by gently withdrawing the sigmoidoscope and pointing it towards the left and slightly forwards, the entrance to the sigmoid can be seen. This is usually the most difficult part of the examination, but with gentleness and patience, it can usually be negotiated. The instrument may now be passed to 20–25 cm provided the patient does not complain of pain. Any lesions or blood stained discharges are noticed, and the sigmoidoscope gradually withdrawn.

A better examination of the rectum is obtained as the instrument is being withdrawn than when it is being introduced. Any suspicious lesions can be biopsied and their exact distance from the anus measured on the scale printed on the side of the sigmoidoscope.

If blood or a blood-stained discharge is seen coming from further inside the bowel, a colonoscopy and/or barium enema should be arranged. Similarly if any infective lesion is suspected, rectal swabs can be taken for culture.

During the examination, air should be gently blown in with the bellows to keep the bowel lumen opened out, forcible air distention should be avoided as it may cause pain and spasm.

An analysis of sigmoidoscopies performed in general practice showed that the presenting symptom of bleeding occurred in 49%, and of those, 14% were found to have rectal cancer; 70% of these could not be felt on digital examination but could all be seen with the sigmoidoscope. Thus although the commonest cause of rectal bleeding is still haemorrhoids, nevertheless 1 in 7 (14%) were found to have a carcinoma [38].

THIRTY-FIVE

Thrombosed external haemorrhoids

'But wit thou, . . . that an abscess breeding near the anus should not be left to burst by itself . . . be it boldly opened with a very sharp lancette so that . . . the corrupt blood may go out'

(John of Arderne, 1306–1390)

More correctly described as peri-anal haematoma, the 'thrombosed external haemorrhoid' is a common condition, occurring spontaneously in young adults, sometimes associated with straining at defaecation, but often not. They are painful and can vary in size from a small pea to a large walnut; left untreated, they gradually absorb, leaving a small skin tag (Fig. 35.1). Surgical treatment offers a quick, effective cure, takes only a few minutes, and gives immediate relief of symptoms.

Instruments required

- 1 2 ml syringe
- 1 25 SWG × $\frac{5}{8}$" (0.5 mm × 16 mm) needle
- 1% Lignocaine with adrenalin 1:200 000
- 1 pair toothed dissecting forceps 5" (12.7 cm)
- 1 pair iris scissors, straight $4\frac{1}{2}$" (11.4 cm)

With the patient lying on his or her left side, and knees drawn up, the base of the haematoma is infiltrated with local anaesthetic. If an assistant is available, they should be asked to pull the upper buttock upwards to expose the thrombosed haemorrhoid – if an assistant is not available, the patient may do this themselves. An ellipse of skin is cut out using the iris scissors and dissecting forceps; this immediately reveals the typical black blood-clot inside the haemorrhoid which may either be expressed by pressure or lifted out with the forceps. The wound is checked to make sure there is only one haematoma – occasionally two or three loculated clots are found and each should be removed. Generally there is only a little bleeding, which can be controlled by the application of a sterile gamgee dressing (Fig. 35.2). The patient is advised to have twice-daily salt baths until healing is complete.

Small peri-anal haematoma may conveniently be left to absorb spontaneously, but if surgery is contemplated, just a radial incision and expression of the clot may suffice.

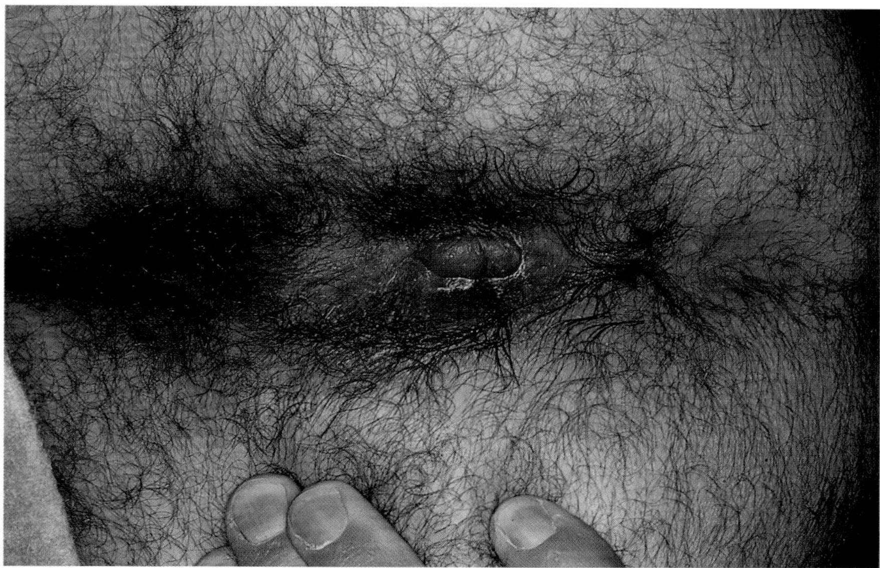

Fig. 35.1 Typical thrombosed external haemorrhoid.

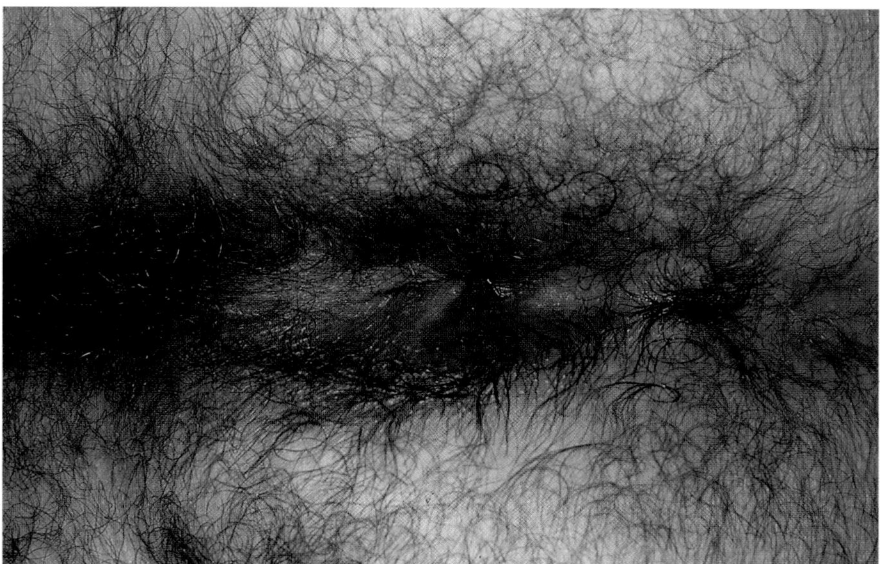

Fig. 35.2 Immediately after excising thrombosed external haemorrhoid; no stitch needed – the skin edges contract together. Bleeding is generally only slight.

THIRTY-SIX

The treatment of internal haemorrhoids

'When there are chronic haemorrhoids in the anus, sear the patient with three cauterisations over the lower dorsal vertebra'

(Albucasis, 11th Century)

It is a wise rule to suspect all haemorrhoids as being due to carcinoma of the rectum until proved otherwise. For this reason it is essential to examine every patient complaining of rectal bleeding with the proctoscope, and if possible the sigmoidoscope as well.

Three types of internal haemorrhoids can be recognized.

36.1 TYPES OF HAEMORRHOIDS

36.1.1 First degree

The haemorrhoids are small, bleed freely, especially after defaecation and though not palpable with the examining finger, are visible when examined through the proctoscope. This type is eminently suitable for treatment in general practice by injection, photo-coagulation or cryotherapy.

36.1.2 Second degree

These haemorrhoids are larger, and tend to protrude after defaecation, but will generally reduce themselves. Bleeding may be less marked because fibrosis is developing in the pile. Treatment by injection, photo-coagulation and cryotherapy is still possible, as is neoprene-band ligation, but the results are not consistently as good as first degree haemorrhoids.

36.1.3 Third degree or prolapsing haemorrhoids

In this type, prolapse is severe, requiring digital replacement by the patient or doctor; strangulation is a common complication. Such haemorrhoids are not generally suitable for general practitioner treatment and should be referred to a general surgeon. Most uncomplicated haemorrhoids are painless; the presence of pain indicates inflammation, strangulation, thrombosis, or anal fissure.

36.2 TREATMENT OF FIRST DEGREE AND SECOND DEGREE INTERNAL HAEMORRHOIDS BY INJECTION OF SCLEROSING FLUID

This is still the method favoured by the majority of surgeons in the UK; the solutions used, and the technique employed have changed little over the last 100 years and still give excellent results [39, 40].

Instruments required

1 proctoscope with illumination
1 sigmoidoscope with illumination
1 haemorrhoid injection syringe and needle
5 ml ampoules of 5% Oily Phenol BPC

With the patient lying in the left lateral position a digital rectal examination is performed to exclude any low-lying tumours, followed by a sigmoidoscopy. If there is any suspicion of blood coming from higher in the large bowel, either from the history or examination, colonoscopy and/or barium enema examination should be arranged.

A well lubricated proctoscope is now inserted to its full length and the obturator removed. By gently withdrawing the instrument, any haemorrhoids will become easily visible; these are commonly situated at three o'clock, seven o'clock and eleven o'clock positions corresponding with the termination of the branches of the superior haemorrhoidal artery.

It may be necessary at this stage to gently re-insert the proctoscope so that the base of each haemorrhoid can be seen. A submucosal injection of 5% phenol in almond oil is now given. This must be done at the upper end of the haemorrhoid and above the ano–rectal ring. Injections given below the ano–rectal ring are extremely painful. The bevel of the needle should be directed towards the mucosa rather than the lumen of the rectum, and the phenol injected slowly, until blanching is seen; the amount injected varies from 1 ml to 5 ml or occasionally even more if the mucosa is very lax.

All three primary haemorrhoids may be treated simultaneously, or if one is larger (commonly the right anterior) this may be given two injections, followed by subsequent treatments at a later visit.

The patient is given advice about avoiding constipation, put on a high roughage diet, and allowed home. Follow-up examinations and injections can be at the discretion and preference of the doctor – weekly if other injections are anticipated, or after six weeks if routine follow-up is desired.

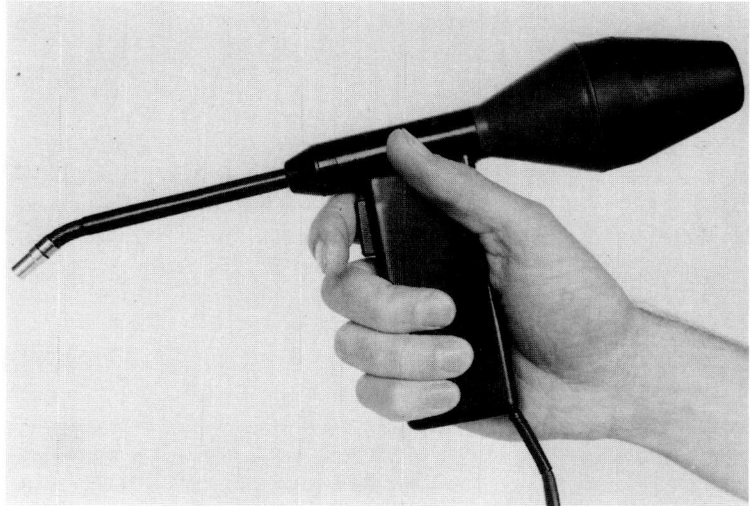

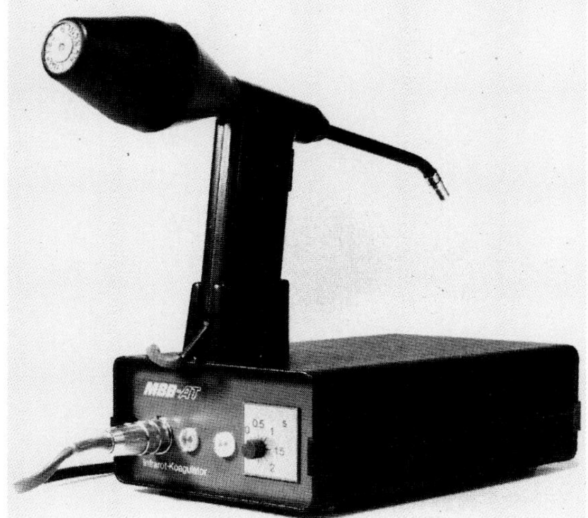

Fig. 36.1 The infra-red coagulator; very quick and simple to use; three burns required at the base of each haemorrhoid (Chilworth Medicals Ltd).

36.3 CRYOTHERAPY TREATMENT OF INTERNAL HAEMORRHOIDS

Where a cryoprobe is available, satisfactory treatment of first and second degree haemorrhoids can be obtained, and if the patient is judged to be unfit for haemorrhoidectomy, even third degree haemorrhoids can be treated [41]. The cryoprobe is applied to the haemorrhoid itself and a two minute freeze given.

The nitrous oxide cryoprobe has the added advantage that it adheres to the tissue, so that gentle traction may be applied to prevent freezing of deeper tissues. The probe must then be re-warmed before it can be separated from the haemorrhoid. Treatment is well tolerated, some patients experience a dull ache during and immediately after freezing. The patient should be warned to expect a profuse watery, blood-stained discharge for many weeks following treatment.

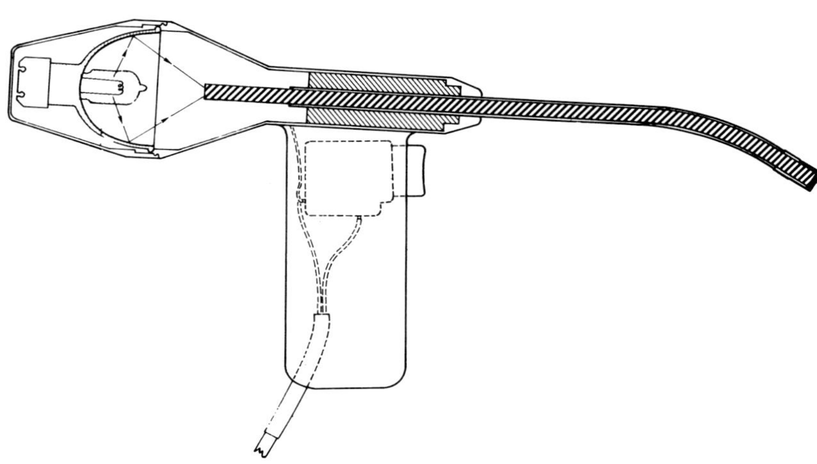

Fig. 36.2 How the photo-coagulator works (Chilworth Medicals Ltd).

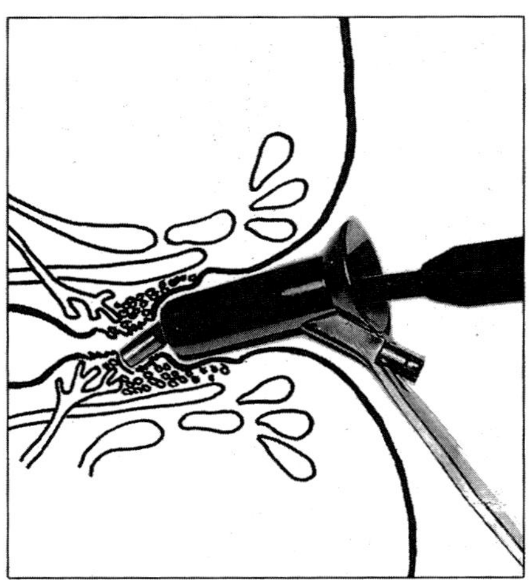

Fig. 36.3 Showing placement of photo-coagulator within proctoscope (Chilworth Medicals)

36.4 INFRA-RED PHOTO-COAGULATION OF INTERNAL HAEMORRHOIDS

A relatively new, and simple instrument for the treatment of internal haemorrhoids is the infra-red photo-coagulator. This consists of a low-voltage quartz–halogen bulb with gold plated reflector and a solid quartz rod which transmits infra-red radiation to a teflon coated tip (Figs 36.1, 36.2 and 36.3). A 1.5 s pulse of infra-red radiation produces an accurately defined necrosis 3 mm deep and 3 mm in diameter. The probe may be used through the proctoscope in the same way as injection therapy, and is applied at exactly the same sites, i.e. above the base of each haemorrhoid. Three separate areas of coagulation are required at the base of each haemorrhoid for optimum results. Of all treatments currently available for internal haemorrhoids, photo-coagulation is one of the simplest, safest, and quickest, and can be rapidly learned by any doctor [42].

36.5 NEOPRENE BAND LIGATION OF INTERNAL HAEMORRHOIDS

Rubber-band ligation has been used successfully for the treatment of haemorrhoids, but the technique requires more skill and practice than injection or photo-coagulation [43, 44, 45]. It is suitable only for haemorrhoids whose base is more than 2 cm above the ano–rectal ring; if bands are applied below this level, severe pain is caused, and the removal of any constricting band is extremely difficult! An assistant is required to hold the proctoscope; the haemorrhoids are visualized, and the rubber-band ligator, loaded with one band is passed through the proctoscope. Using a pair of haemorrhoid grasping forceps, the haemorrhoid is pulled through the ring of the applicator, and the band slipped over the base by pressing the handle on the instrument (Figs 36.4 and 36.5). Secondary haemorrhage occurs in 1% of patients and can be severe.

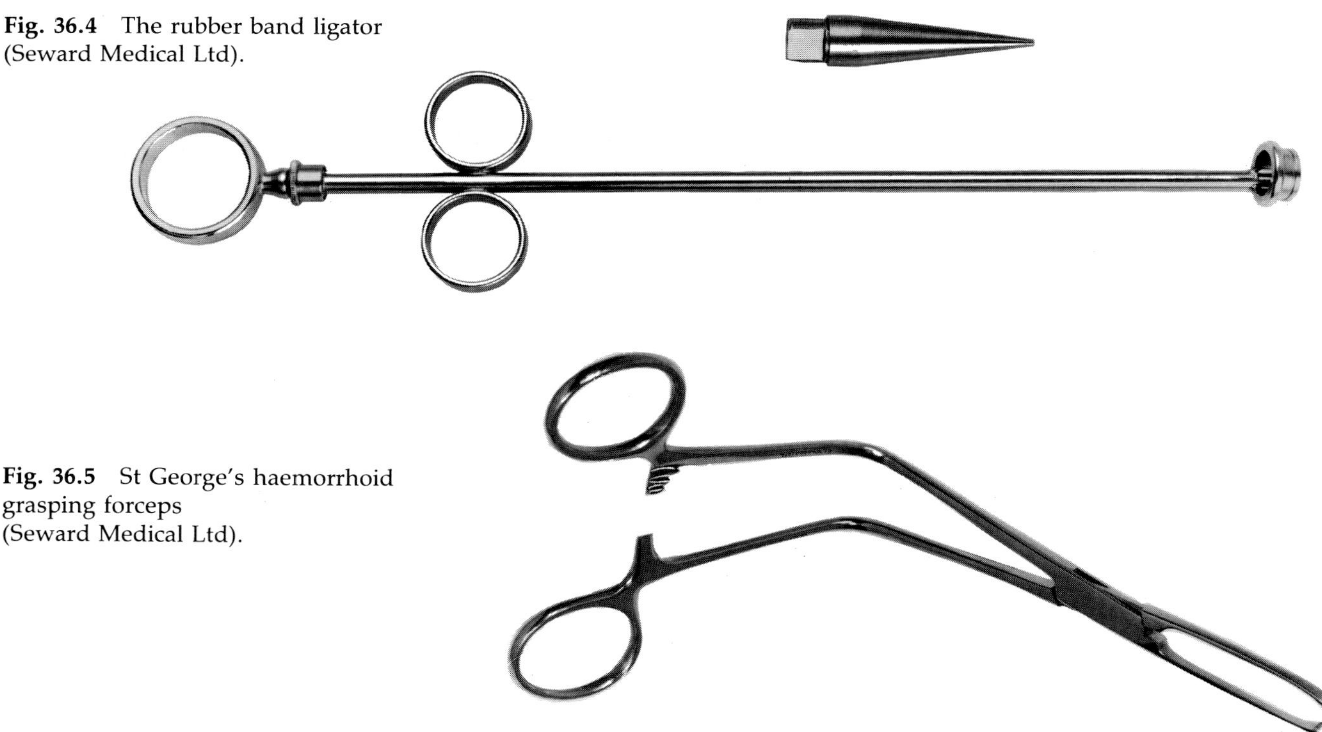

Fig. 36.4 The rubber band ligator (Seward Medical Ltd).

Fig. 36.5 St George's haemorrhoid grasping forceps (Seward Medical Ltd).

36.6 MANUAL DILATION OF THE ANUS

This treatment for haemorrhoids was known in ancient Greece, practiced in the Middle Ages, and recently revived by Peter Lord [46]. Normally done under a general anaesthetic, nevertheless it can be performed under local infiltration or caudal anaesthesia. Young patients with much anal spasm, and haemorrhoids associated with anal fissure seem to achieve most relief from this procedure; contra-indicated are the elderly and those with a lax anal canal, who fare particularly badly, with a risk of permanent incontinence of faeces.

THIRTY-SEVEN

Vasectomy

'But amongst other causes of barreness in men, this also is one that maketh them barren . . . the incision, or cutting of their veins behind their ears'

(De Morbis Foemineis, 1686)

Vasectomy as a method of contraception has become increasingly popular in the last decade; it is an operation which can be performed by the general-practitioner surgeon under local anaesthesia, but because of the medico–legal implications, extra attention must be given to counselling, record-keeping, technique, histology and follow-up. It involves resecting a small portion of the vas deferens on either side of the scrotum. Although the operation should be considered irreversible, due to increasing divorce rates, patients change their minds, so a technique of vasectomy which will allow reversal should be performed if possible.

37.1 PRE-OPERATIVE COUNSELLING

Husband and wife should be seen together and the details of the operation explained to them. A cervical smear and gynaecological examination should be offered to the patient's wife to exclude the possibility of her needing a hysterectomy.

A consent form needs to be signed by both partners, and for the doctor's protection should include the sentence 'I understand that in extremely rare circumstances, a pregnancy can occur despite the operation'. If either partner has any reservations about vasectomy it is wiser not to undertake the operation until these are resolved.

Instruments required

Warm, aqueous Povidone-iodine (Betadine solution).
1 2 ml syringe
2 25 SWG × $\frac{5}{8}$″ (0.5 mm × 16 mm) needles
1 scalpel handle size 3
1 scalpel blade size 15
1 pair fine pointed straight iris scissors 4$\frac{1}{2}$″ (11.4 cm)
1 pair toothed dissecting forceps 5″ (12.7 cm)
2 pairs fine, curved, Halstead Mosquito artery forceps
1 pair 'vasectomy' forceps or fine Allis forceps
1 Kilner needle holder
1 Hyfrecator (optional)

Surgical sutures:

1 catgut metric gauge 2 (4/0) curved cutting needle. Ref. Ethicon W 480 (chromic) or W 470 (plain)
1 braided polyester (Mersilene) metric gauge 1.5 (4/0) curved cutting needle. Ref. Ethicon W 316

37.2 TECHNIQUE

All instruments should be sterilized by autoclaving or using a hot-air oven, and an absolutely aseptic technique employed throughout; an infected post-operative scrotal haematoma is disastrous. The patient should shave the scrotal skin on both sides, and follow this with a bath.

A right handed surgeon should stand on the left of the patient; this allows gentle traction to be applied to each vas with the left hand.

Each vas is identified by careful palpation and the presence of any abnormality such as a varicocele excluded.

The skin is painted with warmed Povidone-iodine aqueous solution (Betadine), the vas identified, and isolated to the lateral side of the cord. A small intradermal weal of Lignocaine is raised and a 1 cm incision made in the skin, down to the outer sheath of the vas, which is then further anaesthetized with a second injection of Lignocaine into the sheath surrounding the vas. Using special vasectomy forceps or fine Allis forceps, the vas in its sheath is picked up, and the sheath separated using fine-pointed iris scissors. The vasectomy forceps are now re-applied, this time around the vas inside the sheath, and a short section of vas freed from its sheath posteriorly. The sheath is mobilized from the front of the vas distally for about 1 cm to prepare a pocket for burying the vas later. It is now possible to apply a pair of fine Halstead mosquito artery forceps at either end of the isolated portion of vas and excise the middle piece which is sent for histology. A 1 cm portion of 'mesentery' is separated from the proximal portion of vas, and then ligated with 4/0 (metric gauge 2) catgut, as is the vas itself.

The distal end of the vas is ligated with non-absorbable braided polyester 4/0 (metric gauge 1.5). Each end of the divided vas is now coagulated with the unipolar diathermy (Hyfrecator). To prevent any chances of re-anastamosis, the proximal and distal ends of the vas are enclosed in different fascial planes as follows: the lower end is buried in the pocket of the sheath previously prepared, while the upper end of the vas is secured outside the sheath.

Skin closure is achieved by inserting one blade of a small pair of Allis forceps inside the incision deep to the dartos muscle, the other in the skin and suturing through both with 4/0 (metric gauge 2) plain catgut. The same procedure is then performed on the opposite side and both skin incisions painted with Whitehead's varnish, nobecutane or collodion.

A scrotal support or close fitting pants are applied and the patient allowed to return home after 15 minutes rest.

It is essential to warn the patient that he will continue to produce viable spermatozoa for three months or more following vasectomy, and thus must continue with alternative forms of contraception until two consecutive sperm tests are returned showing no motile spermatazoa in fresh (less than 2 hours old) specimens. Failure to take notice of this advice has resulted in more than one unplanned pregnancy.

For medico–legal reasons, it is important to record the following in writing:

1. That the patient and his wife have had the operation carefully explained to them.

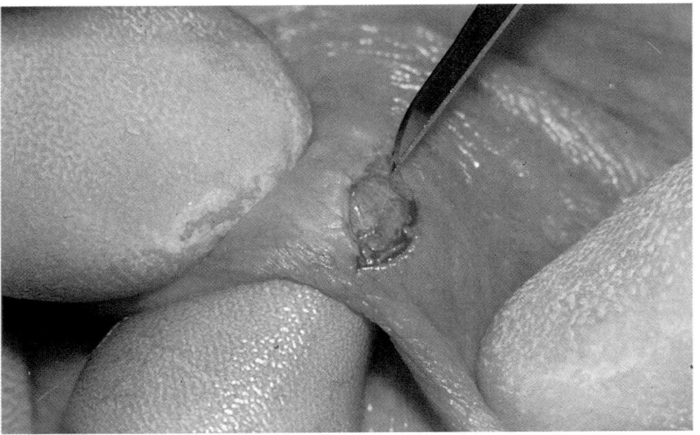

Fig. 37.1 The vas is isolated always lateral to the cord, and held between the finger and the thumb of the left hand. After raising a small intradermal weal with the Lignocaine, a 1 cm incision is made through it down to the outer surface of the sheath of the vas.
(Figures 39.1–39.20 by kind permission of Mr W. Keith Yeates.)

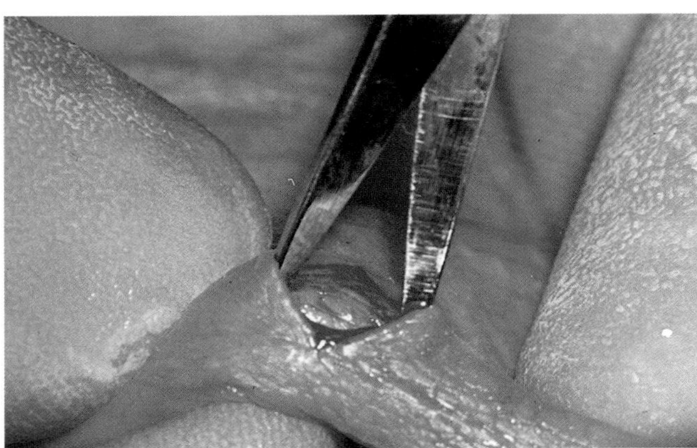

Fig. 37.2 After another very small amount of Lignocaine has been injected on each side of the vas and into its sheath, the sheath is delineated by introducing and opening the blades of fine pointed scissors.

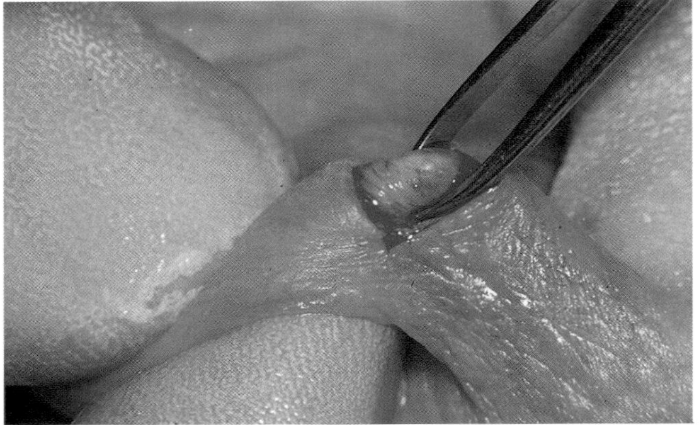

Fig. 37.3 The vas in its sheath is then picked up with a fine pair of Allis forceps.

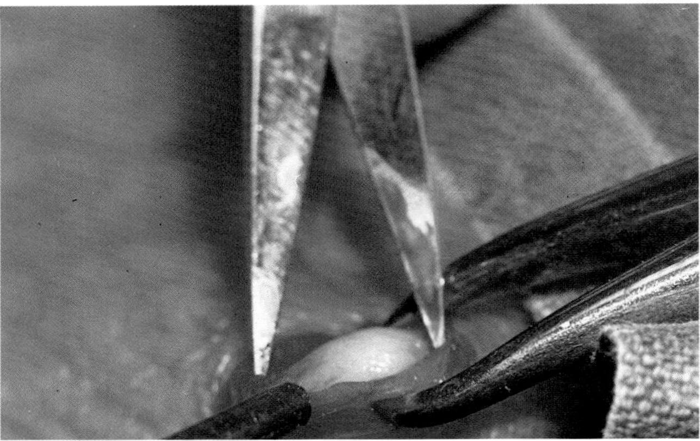

Fig. 37.4 A blunted towel clip is applied round the vas in its sheath; the latter is then opened with the fine pointed scissors exposing the bare vas.

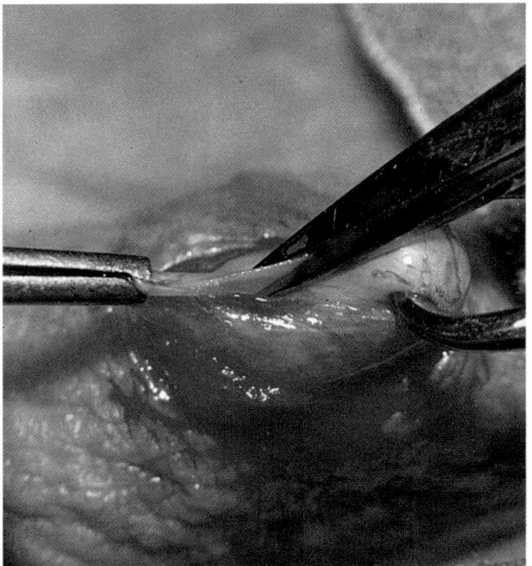

Fig. 37.5 The towel clip is opened and re-applied inside the sheath, under the vas itself. The lower part of the sheath of the vas is then picked up with small toothed dissecting forceps, and the fine adhesions between it and the vas divided with the scissors.

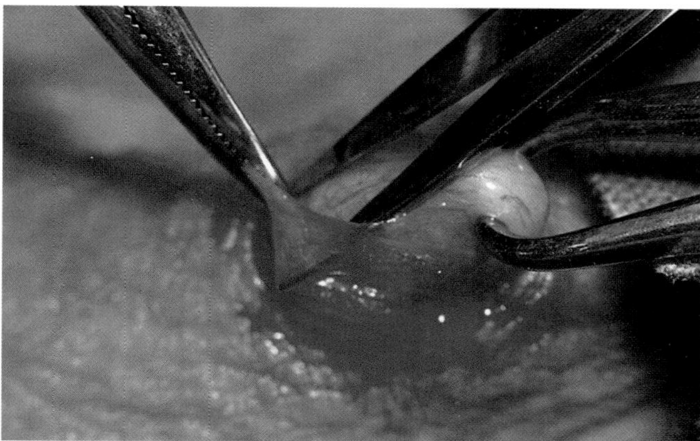

Fig. 37.6 The lower edge of the pocket created is held with haemostatic forceps, which are then left on.

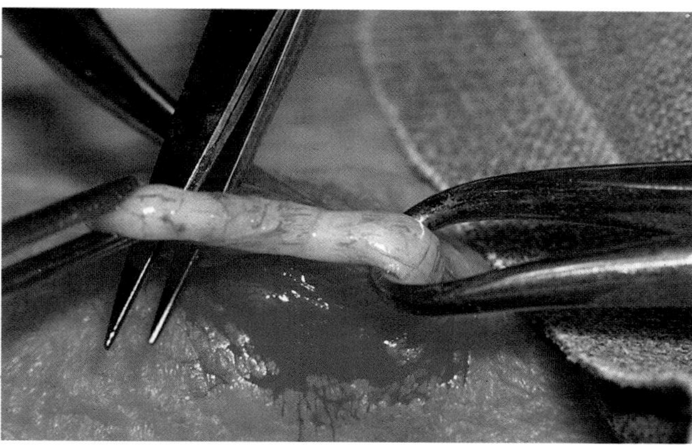

Fig. 37.7 A short section of vas is picked up with the toothed dissecting forceps, and isolated from the posterior part of its sheath.

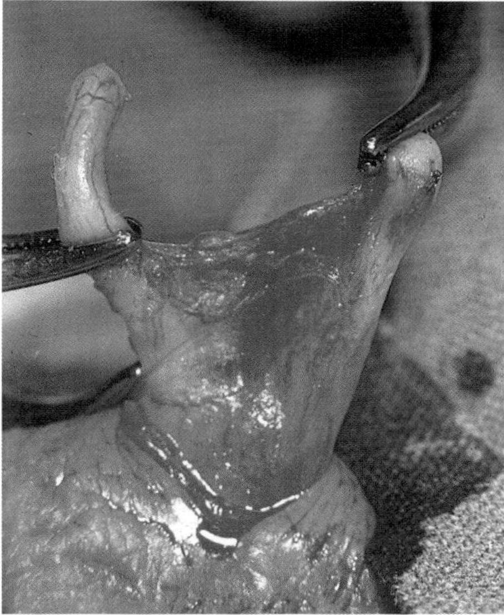

Fig. 37.8 A pair of haemostatic forceps is applied at each end of the isolated section of the vas, which is then excised for histological examination.

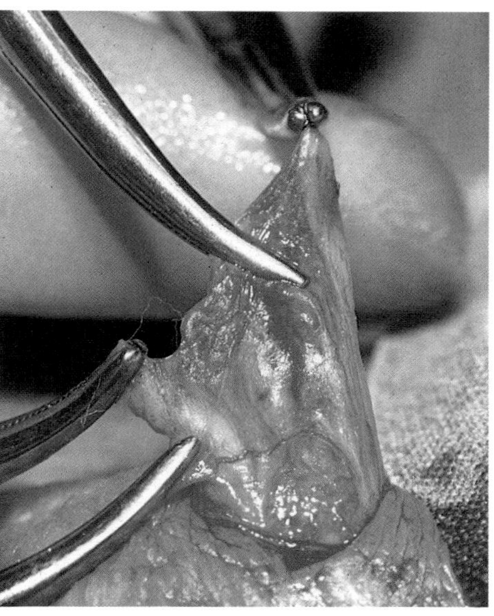

Fig. 37.9 The 'mesentery' attached to the upper end of the vas is then held with haemostatic forceps, which are used to strip off the mesentery from the upper end for about 1 cm.

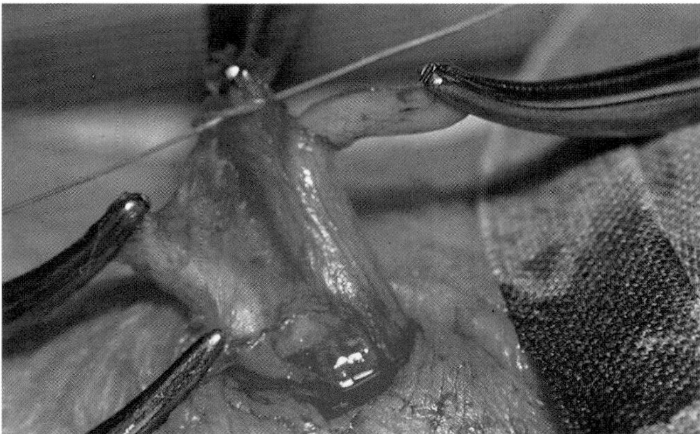

Fig. 37.10 The mesentery is ligated with 4/0 catgut.

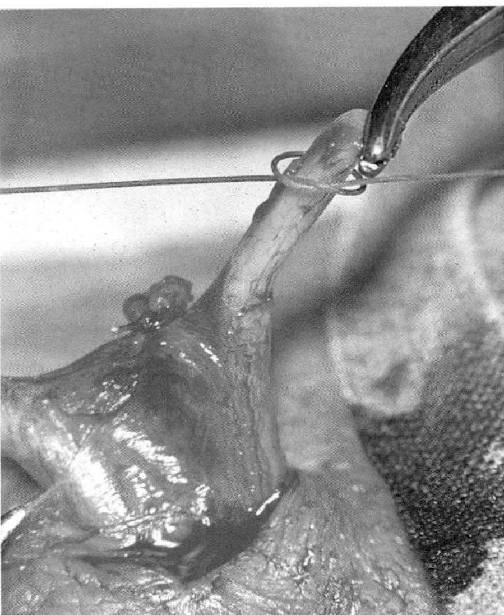

Fig. 37.11 The upper end of the vas is ligated with 4/0 catgut.

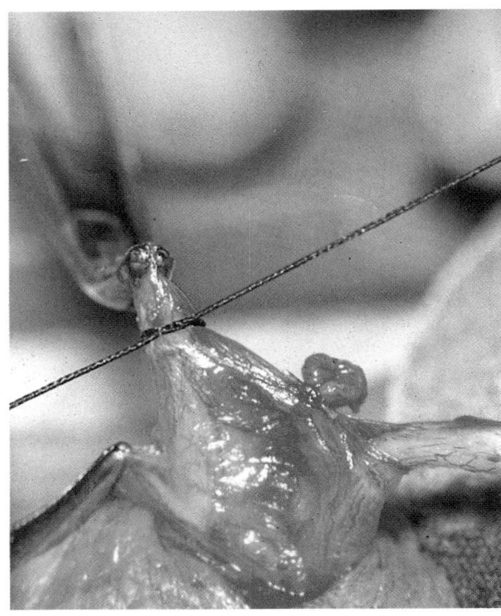

Fig. 37.12 The lower end is ligated with non-absorbable material (silk or braided nylon).

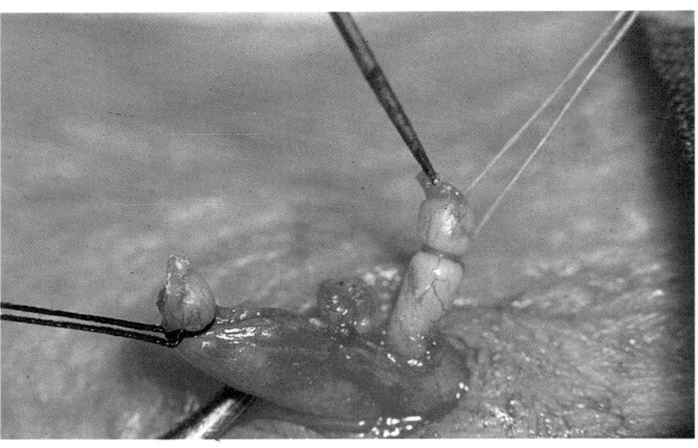

Fig. 37.13 The ligatures round each end of the vas are left long and held in haemostatic forceps, which keeps the field on full view throughout the procedure. Diathermy is applied to both cut ends.

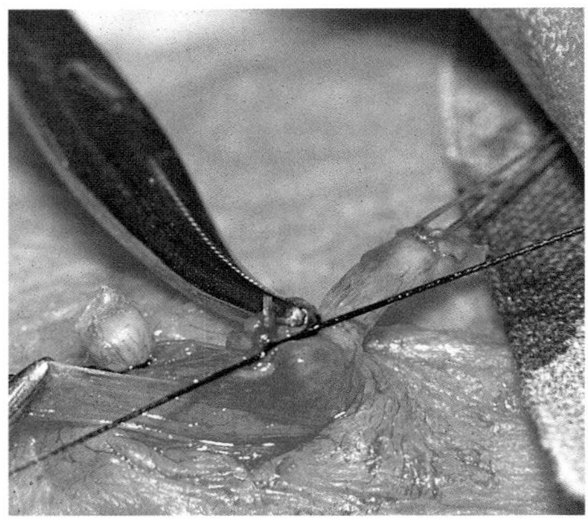

Fig. 37.14 The lower end is then buried in the pocket in the sheath previously prepared. The closing suture of non-absorbable material is first tied round a haemostat, which picks up the site of the ligation of the mesentery.

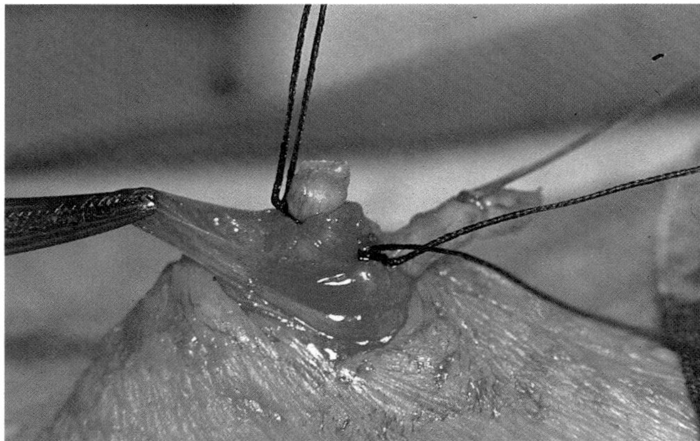

Fig. 37.15 The lower edge of the pocket is opened by traction on the haemostat previously applied.

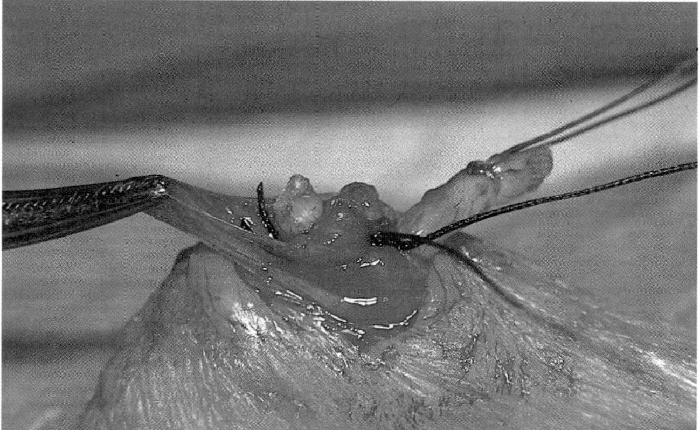

Fig. 37.16 The ligature round the lower end of the sectioned vas is cut.

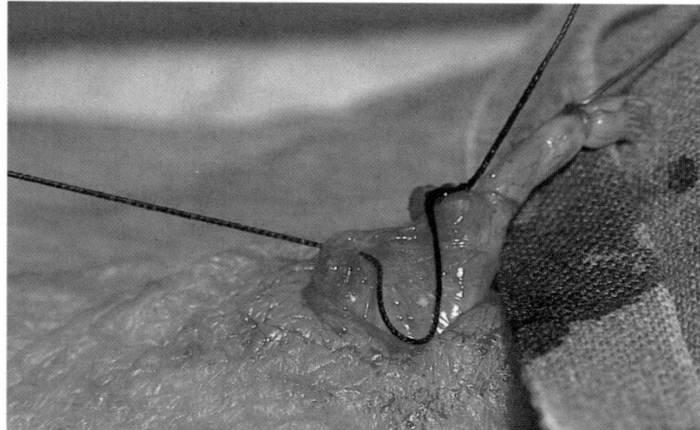

Fig. 37.17 The suture is passed through the margins of the sheath.

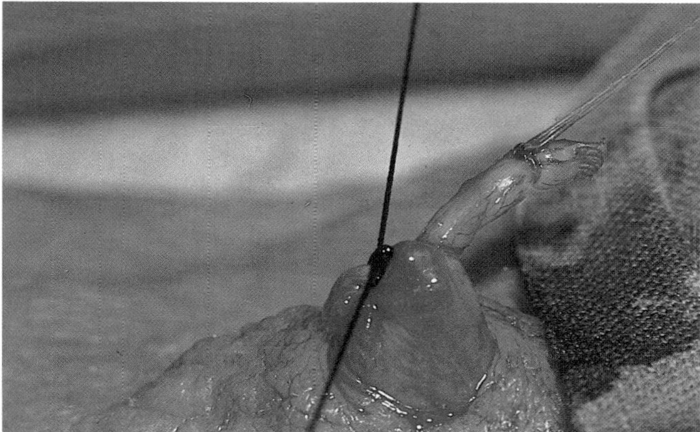

Fig. 37.18 The sheath is then closed over the lower end of the vas.

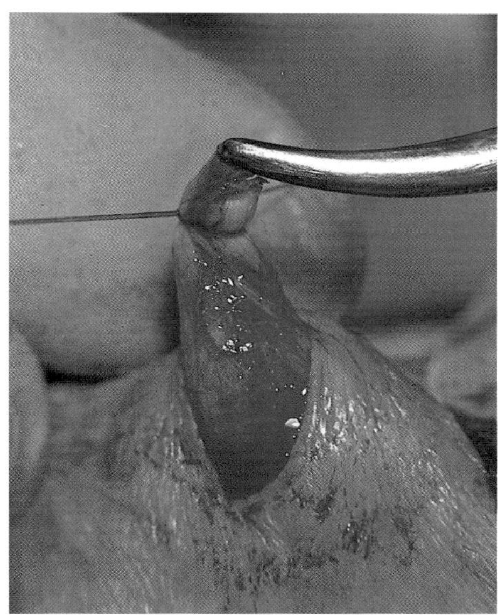

Fig. 37.19 The ends of the catgut ligature round the upper end of the vas are tied round a tented-up piece of loose fascia outside the sheath and then cut short.

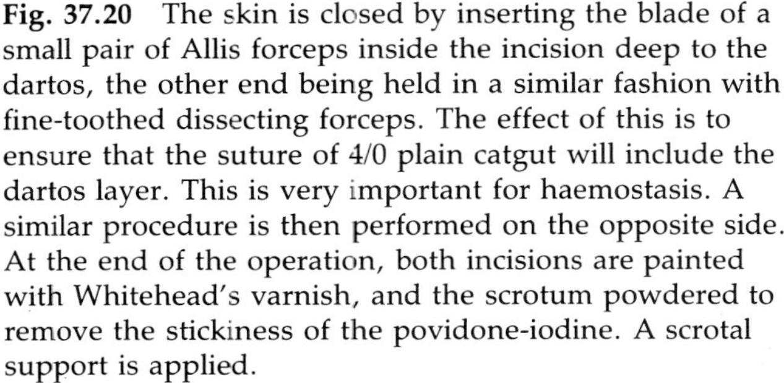

Fig. 37.20 The skin is closed by inserting the blade of a small pair of Allis forceps inside the incision deep to the dartos, the other end being held in a similar fashion with fine-toothed dissecting forceps. The effect of this is to ensure that the suture of 4/0 plain catgut will include the dartos layer. This is very important for haemostasis. A similar procedure is then performed on the opposite side. At the end of the operation, both incisions are painted with Whitehead's varnish, and the scrotum powdered to remove the stickiness of the povidone-iodine. A scrotal support is applied.

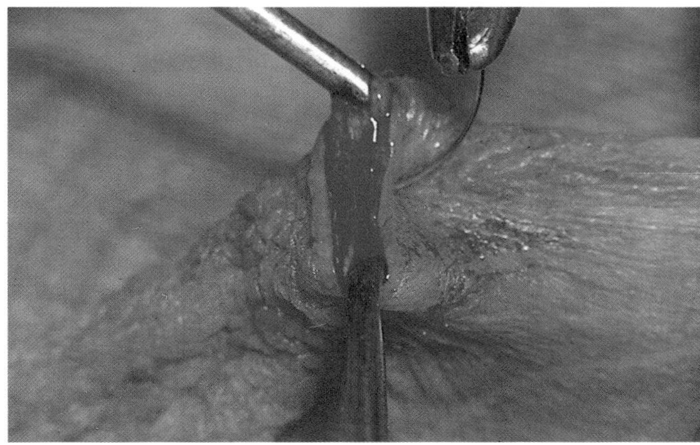

2. That the exceptionally rare possibility of failure has been explained and is understood.
3. A histology report confirming that a portion of vas has been excised on either side.
4. Two negative sperm tests following operation.

Photocopies of duplicate forms of each should be given to the patient, with the originals being kept permanently by the doctor.

37.3 POST-OPERATIVE CARE

The patient may experience discomfort, but not usually pain, which can be controlled with mild analgesics. He should be advised to keep the skin dry for four days; no restrictions need be imposed on intercourse, provided contraception is practised until azoospermia is achieved. Mild bruising is common and of no significance; very rarely, a large haematoma occurs, which can look alarming, but which normally settles on conservative treatment alone. Given careful selection, adequate counselling and the doctor's personal knowledge of the patient, vasectomy is an excellent method of contraception once a couple feel their family is complete.

THIRTY-EIGHT

Excision of ganglion

'They are most frequently met with over the tendons upon the back of the wrist: the most certain method of treatment is to make a small puncture into the sac, and to draw a cord through it, or after the puncture is made, to press out the contents and then inject some gently stimulating fluid, as port wine and water heated blood warm'

(Encyclopaedia Brittanica, 1797)

Ganglia are extremely common; they are cystic swellings surrounded by a fibrous tissue wall, occurring in the vicinity of joint capsules and tendon sheaths. Most have crystal clear gelatinous contents, apart from some in which bleeding has occurred. The cause is not fully understood, but may be a degenerative process in the mesoblastic tissues surrounding the joint. The commonest site is the dorsum of the wrist (Fig. 38.1) (60–80%) followed by the flexor aspect of the wrist adjacent to the radial artery (15–20%). Smaller ganglia occur in the flexor sheaths of the fingers, dorsum of foot, ankle and head of fibula.

Untreated, many ganglia disappear spontaneously; many others appear not to trouble the patient and may be left alone. Treatment is indicated if the patient is complaining of unacceptable symptoms, usually pain or limitation of function. Many treatments have been advocated – all carry a recurrence rate, and the patient should be advised of this accordingly. Simple rupture of the cyst by pressure occasionally succeeds, as does incision with a tenotomy knife, aspiration and injection of sclerosants [48], but most surgeons recommend excision as offering the best chance of cure.

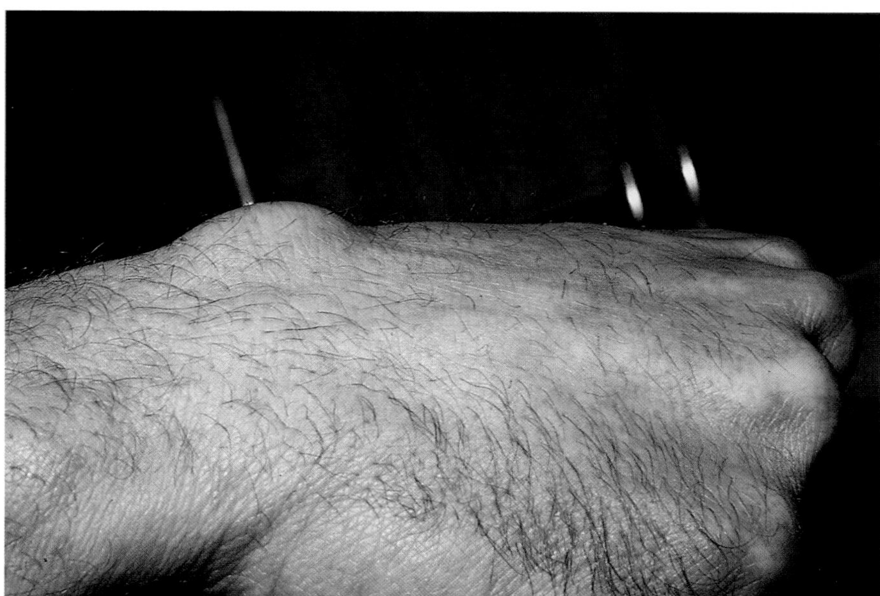

Fig. 38.1 Typical ganglion on dorsum of wrist.

It is essential to have a bloodless operating field, secured by a pneumatic tourniquet, as the dissection can be quite difficult, and the ganglion extend deeper than anticipated. Thus a general anaesthetic or intravenous regional block is required; the latter being the method chosen for the average general practitioner (see Chapter 7).

Many patients will assume that excision of a ganglion will be no different from a small sebaceous cyst; it is therefore important to let them know that it is quite a complicated procedure, that they should not drive a car immediately following operation and that, despite a meticulous dissection, recurrence is still possible.

Instruments required

Povidone-iodine in spirit (Betadine alcoholic solution)
1 scalpel handle size 3
1 scalpel blade size 15
1 pair McIndoe's scissors, curved, 7″ (17.8 cm)
1 Kilner needle holder 5″ (12.7 cm)
1 pair Adson's fine-toothed dissecting forceps, 4¾″ (12 cm)
2 Kilner double-ended retractors (Cat's paw retractors)
1 self-retaining retractor (Kocher's thyroid or similar)
surgical suture sterile polyamide 6
monofilament gauge 2 (3/0) with curved cutting reverse needle. Ref. Ethicon W 320
skin closure strips 3M Code GP41 6 mm × 75 mm

Items required for intravenous regional block:

1 orthopaedic pneumatic tourniquet
1 sphygmomanometer + cuff
1 4″ (10 cm) Kling bandage
1 3″ (7.6 cm) Esmarch rubber bandage
1 intravenous cannula 18 SWG, 0.9 mm (Abbocath – T or equivalent)
2 20 ml syringes
1 1 ml syringe
1 5 ml syringe
1 vial 50 ml 0.5% Prilocaine (Citanest)
1 ampoule Diazepam 10 mg
1 ampoule pethidine 50 mg

38.1 TECHNIQUE OF INTRAVENOUS REGIONAL BLOCK (SUMMARY)

For full details and precautions, the reader is recommended to read Chapter 7.)

1. Remove any rings from fingers on affected hand.
2. Explain procedure in detail to patient.
3. Give intravenous 'pre-medication' injection of pethidine (Demerol) and Diazepam in opposite arm.
4. Apply pneumatic tourniquet over cotton wool to upper arm, and second 'sphygmomanometer' cuff distal to first cuff.

5. Cover both with non-stretch cotton bandage to prevent ballooning of either cuff.
6. Inflate 1 cuff to just below arterial pressure to distend veins at wrist.
7. Insert intravenous cannula in suitable vein (avoiding the ganglion).
8. Deflate cuff and attach 1 ml syringe prefilled with 0.5% Prilocaine to i/v cannula.
9. Raise arm and apply Esmarch bandage from fingers to proximal cuff.
10. Inflate orthopaedic tourniquet (proximal cuff) to 300 mm Hg.
11. Unwind Esmarch bandage.
12. Ask assistant to watch pressure in pneumatic tourniquet from now until end of operation **without fail!**
13. Inject 30 ml 0.5% Prilocaine (Citanest) through intravenous cannula.
14. Leave cannula and 1 ml syringe in place (gives access to circulation if needed should the cuff fail).
15. Now inflate second cuff (distal) to 300 mm Hg.

38.2 THE OPERATION [49]

The overlying skin is liberally painted with Povidone-iodine in spirit (Betadine alcoholic solution); a sterile drape is applied over the area, and full aseptic precautions observed. (A surgical gown, mask and gloves should be worn.)

The incision should follow a skin crease, normally transverse (Fig. 38.2), about 4 cm long, and any underlying nerves dissected free. The extensor retinaculum overlying the ganglion is incised, and a self-retaining retractor inserted. The bulk of the ganglion is seen superficial to the tendons, but when these are retracted, the deeper part of the ganglion may be seen (Figs 38.3 and 38.4) extending to the wrist joint or intercarpal joint. Gradually the main part of the ganglion is dissected free using a scalpel, applying traction with toothed dissecting forceps. Usually at this stage, the capsule is incised, liberating the typical clear jelly. This is often an advantage and makes the remaining dissection easier. The ganglion is now detached (Fig. 38.6) excising part of the joint capsule as well. It is quite in order to leave adjacent tendons without a synovial covering.

Closure is by one subcuticular monofilament Polyamide suture, strengthened by skin closure strips (Figs 38.7, 38.8, 38.9 and 38.10). A sterile dry gauze dressing is applied covered with cotton wool and an elastocrepe bandage. The assistant now applies direct pressure over the site of the incision, and the doctor releases both tourniquets.

If all is well, the dressings are left undisturbed until the 10th post-operative day, when the suture is removed, leaving the Steri-strips in position. A light sterile dressing is reapplied over these for four more days and then removed.

38.3 EXCISION OF RHEUMATOID SYNOVIOMA
(Figs 38.11 and 38.12)

This is performed using an identical approach to the excision of ganglion.

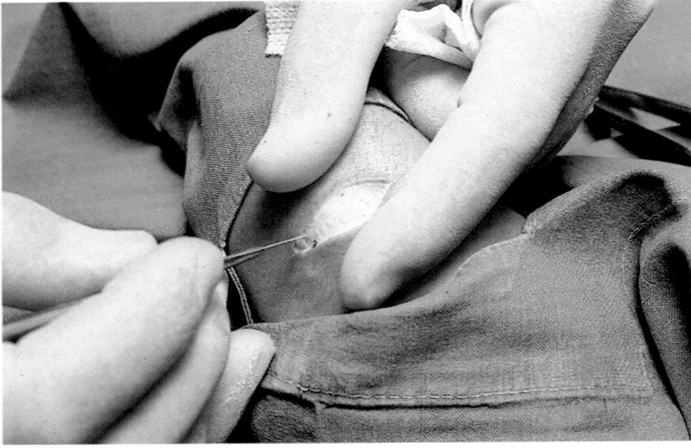

Fig. 38.2 A transverse incision is made over the ganglion in the line of a skin crease.

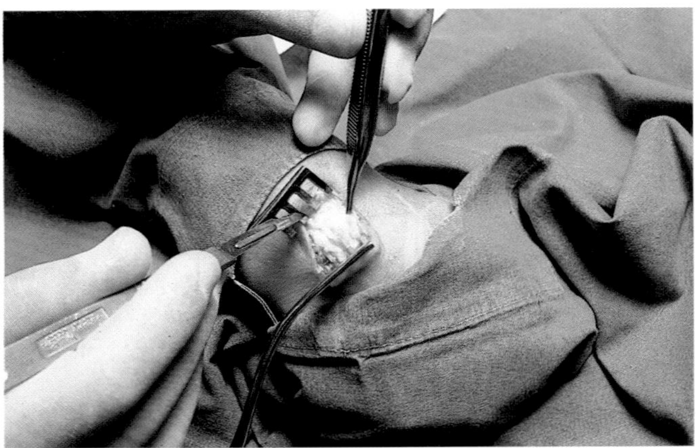

Fig. 38.3 A self-retaining rectractor is inserted.

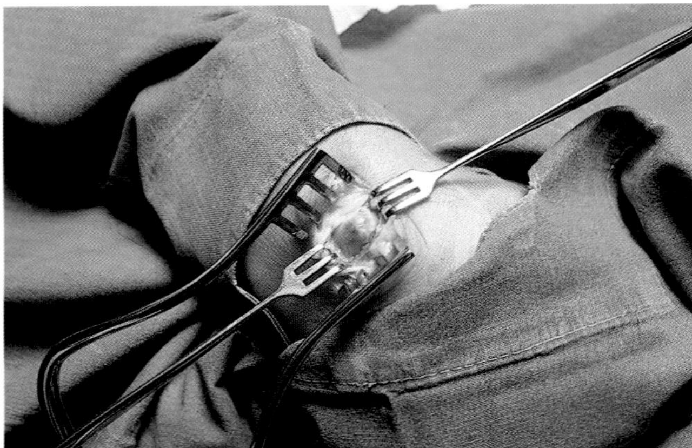

Fig. 38.4 If necessary, two cat's paw retractors may be used as well to improve access.

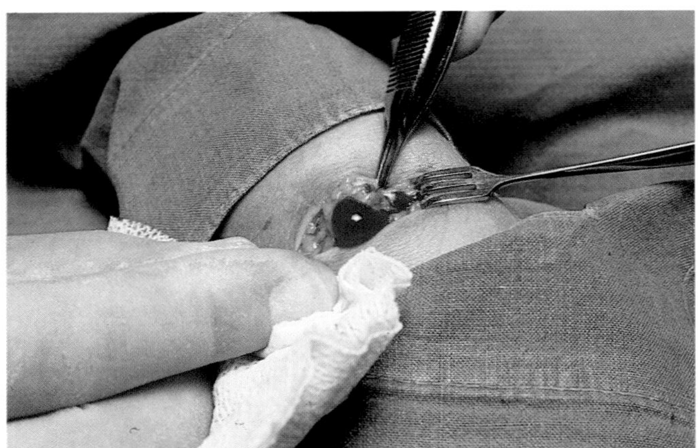

Fig. 38.5 The ganglion has been opened; blood-stained jelly is seen; this indicates possible previous trauma. Normally, the jelly is clear.

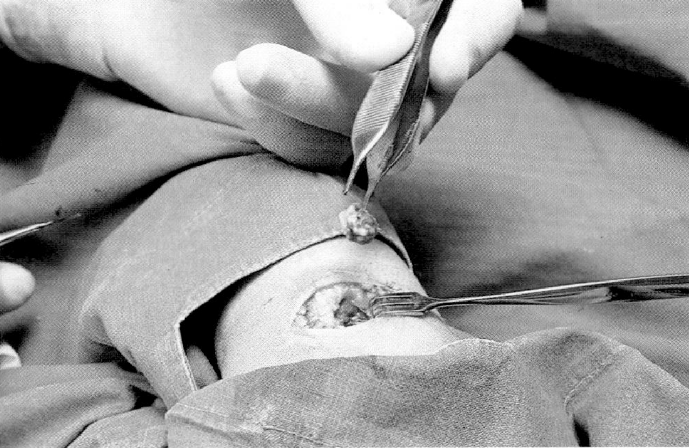

Fig. 38.6 The capsule of the ganglion has been excised.

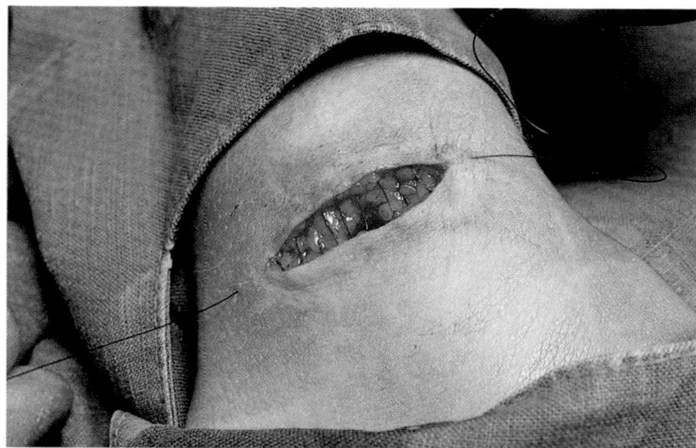

Fig. 38.7 A sub-cuticular monofilament nylon suture gives a neat scar.

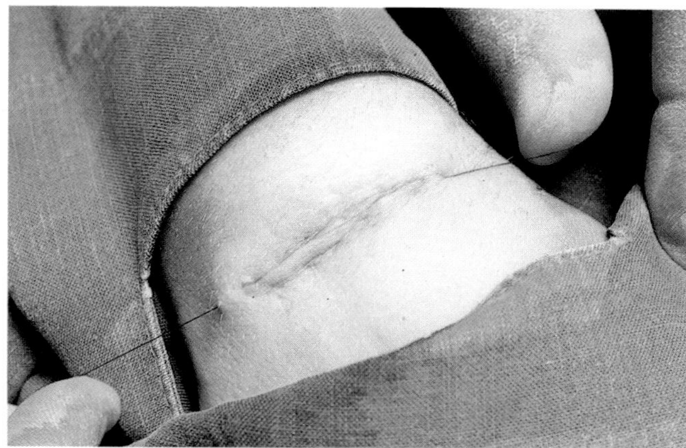

Fig. 38.8 Skin edges approximated with the subcuticular nylon stitch.

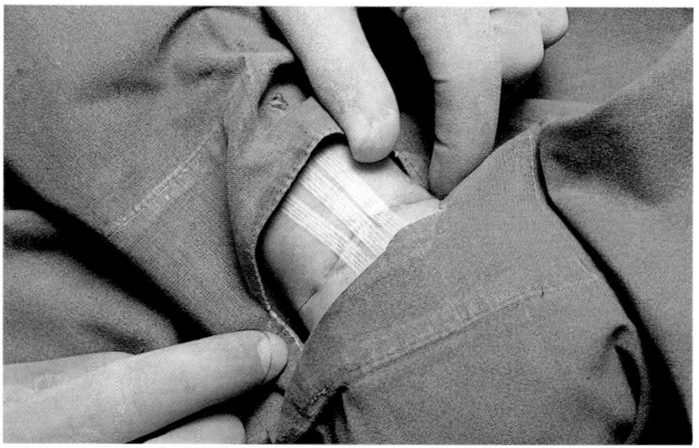

Fig. 38.9 Additional support may be given by the application of skin closure strips.

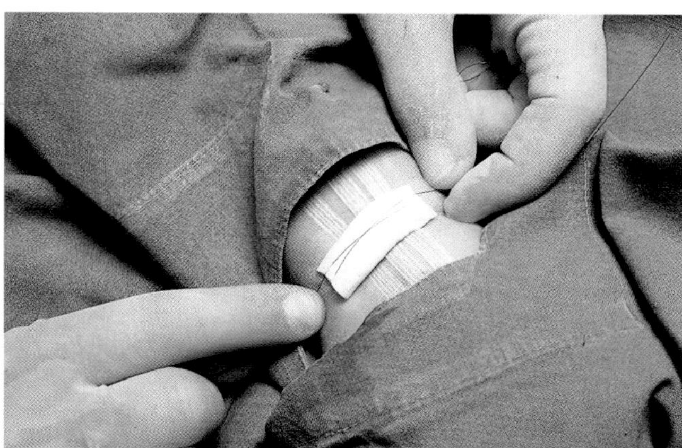

Fig. 38.10 The ends of the nylon suture are folded over a cotton wool roll, and taped in position.

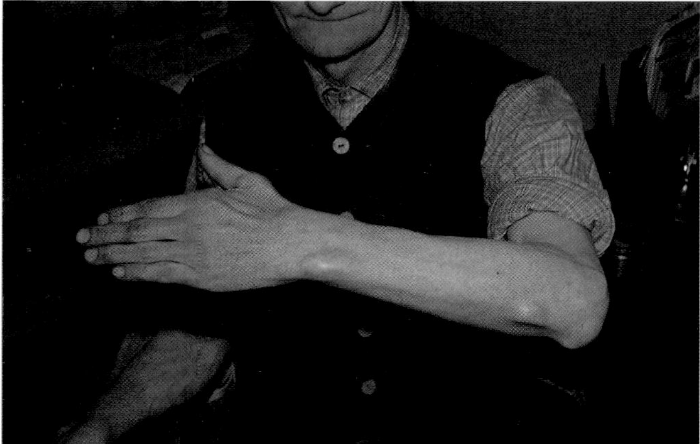

Fig. 38.11 Rheumatoid 'nodule' may be excised as for ganglion.

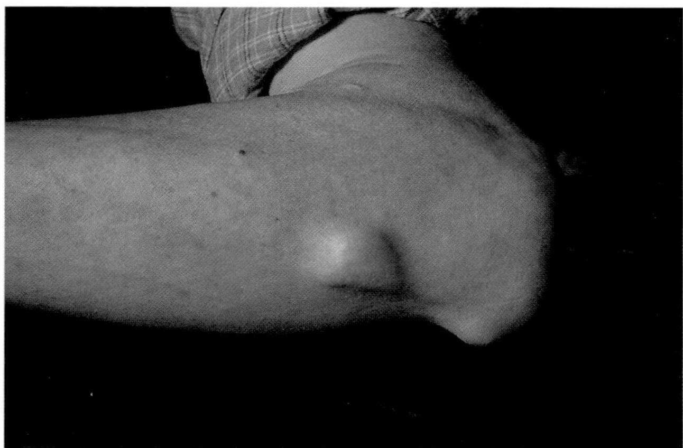

Fig. 38.12 Rheumatoid 'nodule'.

THIRTY-NINE

Decompression of the carpal tunnel

'She is woke up nightly by pains in the fingers, hands, and up the fore-arms. The hands seem to become stiff and useless, and when she gets up look, she says, as if they were dead. The pain is severe and prevents sleep.

She connects her complaint with the use of water for scrubbing floors; she gave up her place as servant on this account and her hands improved afterwards'

(J. A. Ormerod, On a peculiar numbness and paresis of the Hands, 1883)

Decompression of the median nerve in the carpal tunnel is now one of the commonest operations on the hand; yet the first recorded carpal tunnel decompression was only done in 1941 [50]. The presenting symptoms are paraesthesia affecting the middle three fingers, with pain radiating up the forearm; the patient is commonly a woman, and the right hand is affected more than the left; typically the pain and 'pins and needles' wake the patient at night, and relief is sometimes obtained by shaking the arm and hanging it out of bed.

Confirmation of the diagnosis may be obtained by applying pressure over the carpal tunnel to reproduce the symptoms, by tapping the carpal tunnel (Tinel's Sign) or by acutely flexing the wrist and fingers. If early warning symptoms are ignored, wasting of the thenar muscles occurs, and even if the nerve is subsequently decompressed, recovery of wasted muscle seldom occurs. It should also be remembered that cervical nerve root entrapment at C7 level will give pain in the hand and numbness of the middle finger, so it is important to check the neck at the time of the initial examination.

Non-surgical treatment is worth trying; this consists of splinting, diuretics, and steroid injection (Chapter 6). If a steroid injection relieves the symptoms, only to recur, at least the doctor knows decompression will work and can thus confidently recommend it.

Surgical decompression is a much simpler operation than is generally realized. A bloodless operating field is essential therefore a general anaesthetic or intravenous regional block with pneumatic tourniquet is necessary. Likewise, complete aseptic operation conditions are mandatory; this means CSSD packs or autoclaving, gowns, masks, and surgical gloves.

Instruments required

- Povidone-iodine in spirit (Betadine alcoholic solution)
- 1 scalpel handle size 3
- 1 scalpel blade size 15
- 1 self retaining retractor (Kocher's Thyroid or similar)
- 2 Kilner double-ended retractors (Cat's paw retractors)
- 1 McDonald's dissector (double-ended)
- 1 stitch scissors 5″ (12.7 cm)

1 Kilner needle holder $5\frac{1}{4}''$ (13.3 cm)
1 pair fine toothed Adsons dissecting forceps $4\frac{3}{4}''$ (12 cm)
surgical suture sterile polyamide 6
monofilament metric gauge 2 (3/0) 26 mm curved reverse cutting needle Ref. Ethicon W320
skin closure strips 3M Ref. GP 41 6 mm × 75 mm

Items required for intravenous regional block

1 orthopaedic pneumatic tourniquet
1 sphygmomanometer + cuff
1 4″ (10 cm) Kling cotton bandage
1 3″ (7.6 cm) Esmarch bandage
1 intravenous cannula size 18 SWG (0.9 mm) (Abbocath-T or equivalent)
2 20 ml syringes
1 5 ml syringe
1 1 ml syringe
1 vial 50 ml 0.5% Prilocaine (Citanest)
1 ampoule Diazepam 10 mg
1 ampoule Pethidine 50 mg

39.1 TECHNIQUE OF INTRAVENOUS REGIONAL BLOCK (SUMMARY)

(For full details and precautions see Chapter 7.)

1. Remove any rings from fingers on affected hand.
2. Explain procedure in detail to patient.
3. Give intravenous 'pre-medication' injection of Pethidine (Demerol) and Diazepam in opposite arm.
4. Apply pneumatic tourniquet over cotton wool to upper arm, and second 'sphygmomanometer' cuff distal to first cuff.
5. Cover both with non-stretch cotton bandage to prevent ballooning of either cuff.
6. Inflate 1 cuff to just below arterial pressure to distend veins at wrist.
7. Insert intravenous cannula in suitable vein.
8. Deflate cuff and attach 1 ml syringe prefilled with 0.5% Prilocaine to i/v cannula.
9. Raise arm and apply Esmarch bandage from fingers to proximal cuff.
10. Inflate orthopaedic tourniquet (proximal cuff) to 300 mm Hg.
11. Unwind Esmarch bandage.
12. Ask assistant to watch pressure in pneumatic tourniquet from now until end of operation **without fail!**
13. Inject 30 ml 0.5% Prilocaine (Citanest) through intravenous cannula.
14. Leave cannula and 1 ml syringe in place (gives access to circulation if needed should the cuff fail).
15. Now inflate second cuff (distal) to 300 mm Hg.

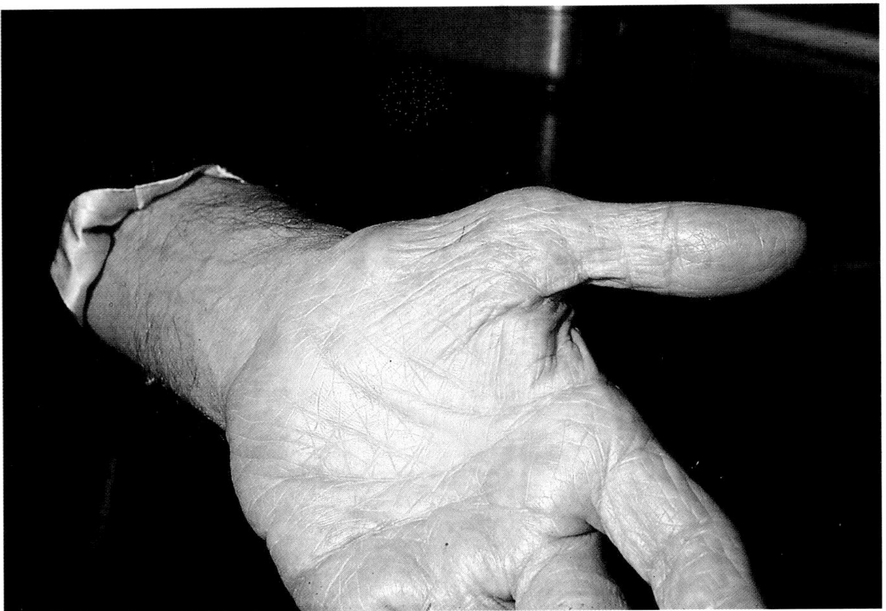

Fig. 39.1 Untreated, compression of the median nerve may result in severe wasting of the thenar muscles.

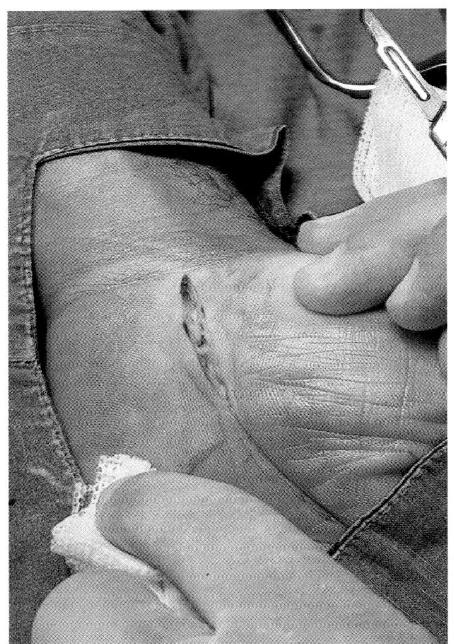

Fig. 39.2 The incision is made in the proximal palmar crease as shown.

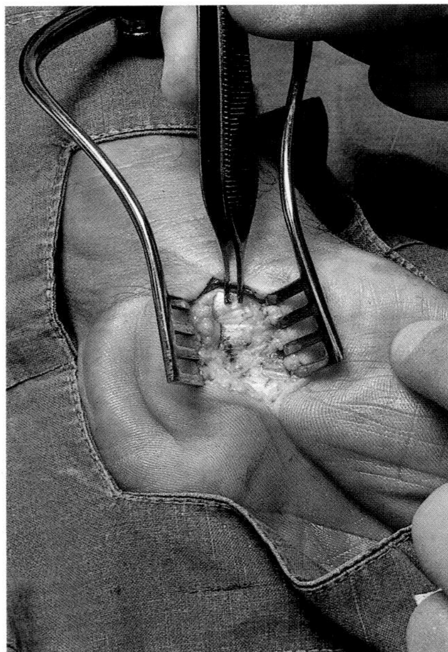

Fig. 39.3. A self-retaining retractor makes the operation much easier.

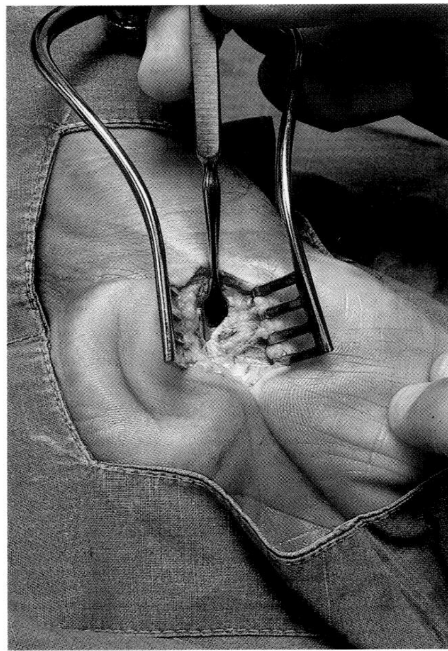

Fig. 39.4 The McDonald's dissector is slipped under the retinaculum, in front of the nerve.

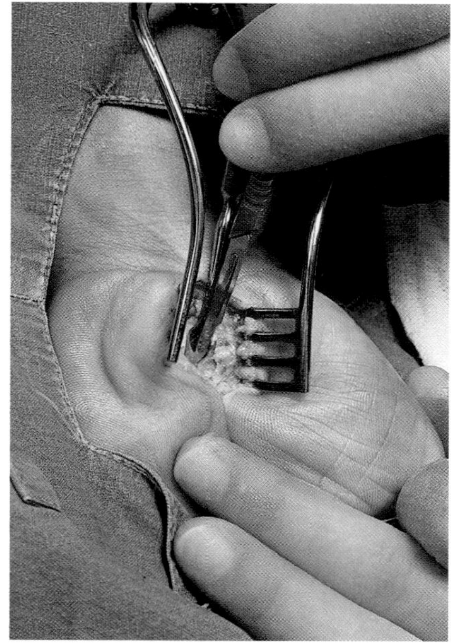

Fig. 39.5 With the McDonald's dissector protecting the nerve, the retinaculum is split with a small scalpel blade.

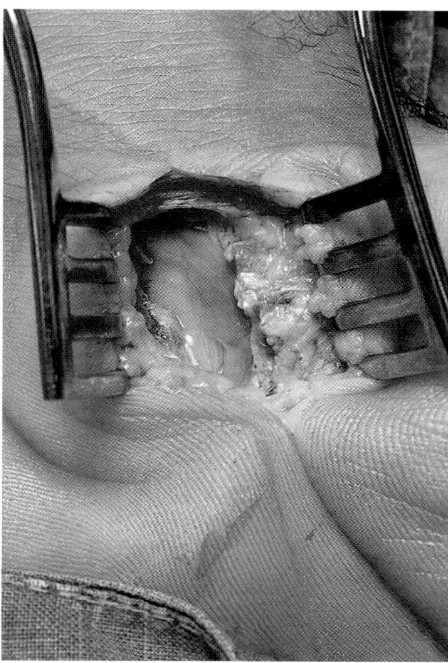

Fig. 39.6 The median nerve is now exposed. (Note what a large structure it is.)

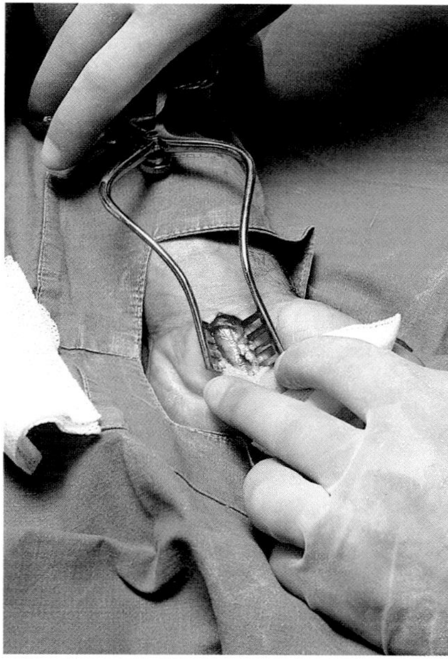

Fig. 39.7 The retractor may now be removed.

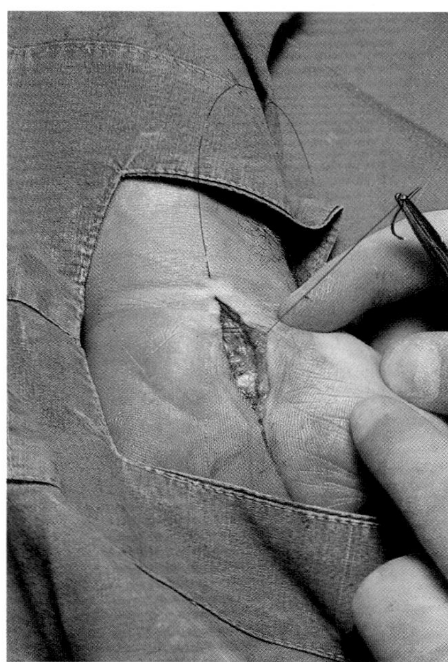

Fig. 39.8 Skin closure is with a subcuticular monofilament nylon suture alone.

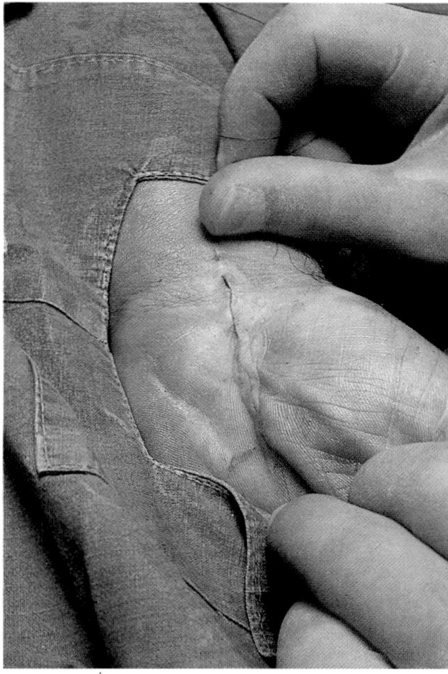

Fig. 39.9 A subcuticular stitch gives a neat scar, and it is quick to insert and is easy to remove.

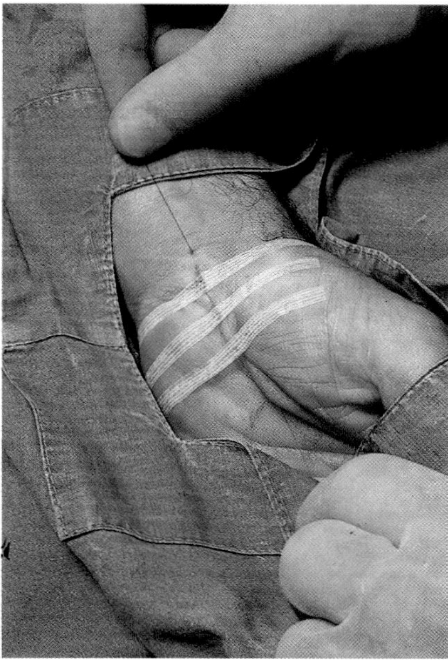

Fig. 39.10 Additional support may be given by the application of skin-closure strips.

39.2 THE OPERATION [51, 52]

The overlying skin is liberally painted with Povidone-iodine in spirit (Betadine alcoholic solution) and a sterile drape placed over the area. As with excision of ganglion and release of trigger finger, full aseptic technique is employed – this means wearing sterile surgical gown, mask and gloves.

A skin incision is made in the thenar crease as shown (Fig. 39.2), correctly placed it will be exactly between the thenar and hypothenar muscles, exactly over the median nerve. Self retaining or individual hand-held retractors are now placed in the wound and opened, to expose the underlying fatty tissues and dense fibrous transverse ligament (Fig. 39.3). The incision is cautiously deepened until the glistening median nerve is seen. At this stage, the McDonald's dissector (Fig. 39.4) is gently introduced below the transverse ligament and in front of the median nerve, and the ligament divided by cutting down on the blade of the dissector which is protecting the nerve. The median nerve may now be freed both proximally and distally with the aid of the McDonald's dissector, and particular note made of any branches to the thenar muscles or skin, which should be preserved (Fig. 39.6).

When the operator is satisfied that the median nerve is no longer compressed within the carpal tunnel, the retractors may be removed and the wound closed. Just the skin is sutured; either with interrupted braided silk 3/0 (metric gauge 2) or a neater scar may be obtained by using a subcuticular monofilament polyamide 6 3/0 (metric gauge 2) suture, strengthened with adhesive skin closure strips Ref. 3M GP41 6 mm × 75 mm (Figs 39.8, 39.9 and 39.10). Sterile gauze swabs are now folded in half and taped in position over the incision to act as a mild pressure dressing – these are then covered with cotton wool and a firm elasto-crepe bandage. When applying the cotton wool, it is important to place it between all the fingers.

The arm is now elevated, and the assistant applies pressure over the incision while the doctor releases both tourniquets. Pressure is maintained for at least five minutes; following this the arm is placed in a triangular sling with the palm of the operated hand on the opposite shoulder.

Assuming all is well, the dressing is left undisturbed until the 10th post-operative day when the sutures are removed, leaving the Steri-strips. A sterile dry dressing is reapplied over the strips and lightly bandaged and left in place for a further four days, by which time healing is complete.

The patient usually obtains immediate relief of all symptoms – occasionally it may take several months to recover, and frequently there is a tender area underneath the scar which arises from the exposed nerve – this likewise recovers gradually over several months; however, if any significant degree of muscle wasting has occurred, this does not usually recover.

Carpal tunnel syndrome, diagnosed before irreversible damage to the nerve has occurred is one of the most satisfactory conditions to treat surgically.

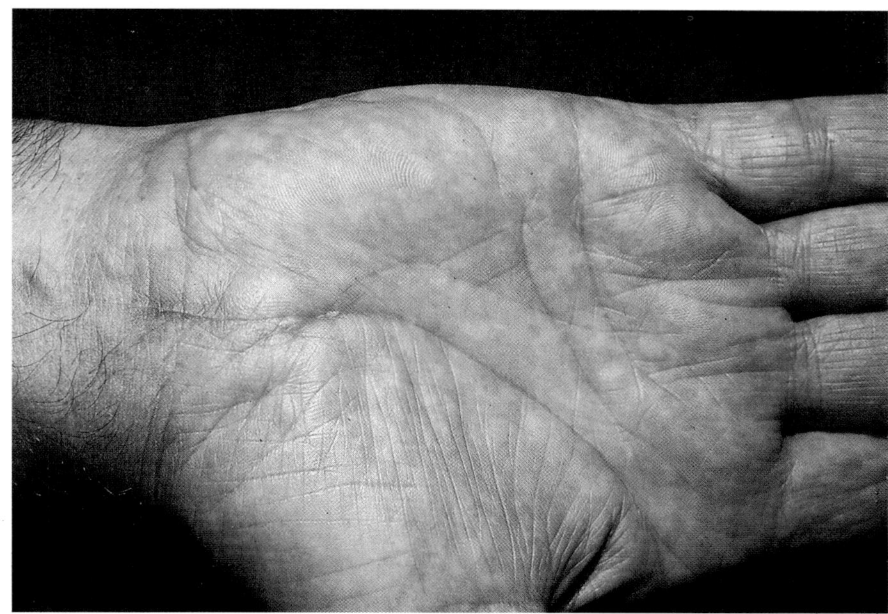

Fig. 39.11 The scar, six weeks later.

FORTY

Release of trigger finger
(Tenovaginitis stenosans and De Quervain's syndrome)

'It seemed most likely that it was a thickening of the tendon sheath at a specific point. On March 7th 1894 I excised the common tunnel of extensor pollicis brevis over a length of one centimetre'

(Fritz de Quervain, Concerning a Form of Chronic Tenovaginitis, 1868–1940)

Trigger finger and trigger thumb are caused by a constriction of the flexor tendon sheath combined with a secondary localized thickening of the tendon. This results in difficulty extending the joint, which often straightens suddenly with a palpable 'click'. Commonly the constriction occurs in front of the metacarpo-phalangeal joint under the annular ligament. Relief may be obtained by injecting corticosteroid (Methylprednisolone acetate) into the sheath, but if the condition recurs, surgery is indicated.

Instruments required

- Povidone-iodine in spirit (Betadine alcoholic solution)
- 1 scalpel handle size 3
- 1 scalpel blade size 15
- 1 McDonald's double-ended dissector
- 2 pairs Halsteads mosquito artery forceps curved 5″ (12.7 cm)
- 1 Kilner needle holder $5\frac{1}{4}$″ (13.3 cm)
- 1 pair McIndoe's scissors, curved 7″ (17.8 cm)
- 1 pair Kilner double-ended retractors (Cat's paws retractors) or small self-retaining retractor
- 1 pair fine toothed Adson dissecting forceps $4\frac{3}{4}$″ (12 cm)
- surgical suture, sterile polyamide 6
- monofilament metric gauge 2 (3/0) with 26 mm curved reverse cutting needle. Ref. Ethicon W 320
- skin closure strips 3M Ref. G.P.41 6 mm × 75 mm

Items required for intravenous regional block

- 1 orthopaedic pneumatic tourniquet
- 1 sphygmomanometer + cuff
- 1 4″ (10 cm) Kling bandage
- 1 3″ (7.6 cm) Esmarch rubber bandage
- 1 intravenous cannula 18 SWG 0.9 mm (Abbocath – T or equivalent)
- 2 20 ml syringes
- 1 1 ml syringe
- 1 5 ml syringe
- 1 vial 50 ml 0.5% Prilocaine (Citanest)
- 1 ampoule Diazepam 10 mg
- 1 ampoule Pethidine 50 mg

40.1 TECHNIQUE OF INTRAVENOUS REGIONAL BLOCK (SUMMARY)

(For full details and precautions, the reader is recommended to read Chapter 7.)

1. Remove any rings from fingers on affected hand.
2. Explain procedure in detail to patient.
3. Give intravenous 'pre-medication' injection of Pethidine (Demerol) and Diazepam in opposite arm.
4. Apply pneumatic tourniquet over cotton wool to upper arm, and second 'sphygmomanometer' cuff distal to first cuff.
5. Cover both with non-stretch cotton bandage to prevent ballooning of either cuff.
6. Inflate one cuff to just below arterial pressure to distend veins at wrist.
7. Insert intravenous cannula in suitable vein.
8. Deflate cuff and attach 1 ml syringe prefilled with 0.5% Prilocaine to i/v cannula.
9. Raise arm and apply Esmarch bandage from fingers to proximal cuff.
10. Inflate orthopaedic tourniquet (proximal cuff) to 300 mm Hg.
11. Unwind Esmarch bandage.
12. Ask assistant to watch pressure in pneumatic tourniquet from now until end of operation **without fail!**
13. Inject 30 ml 0.5% Prilocaine (Citanest) through intravenous cannula.
14. Leave cannula and 1 ml syringe in place (gives access to circulation if needed should the cuff fail).
15. Now inflate second cuff (distal) to 300 mm Hg.

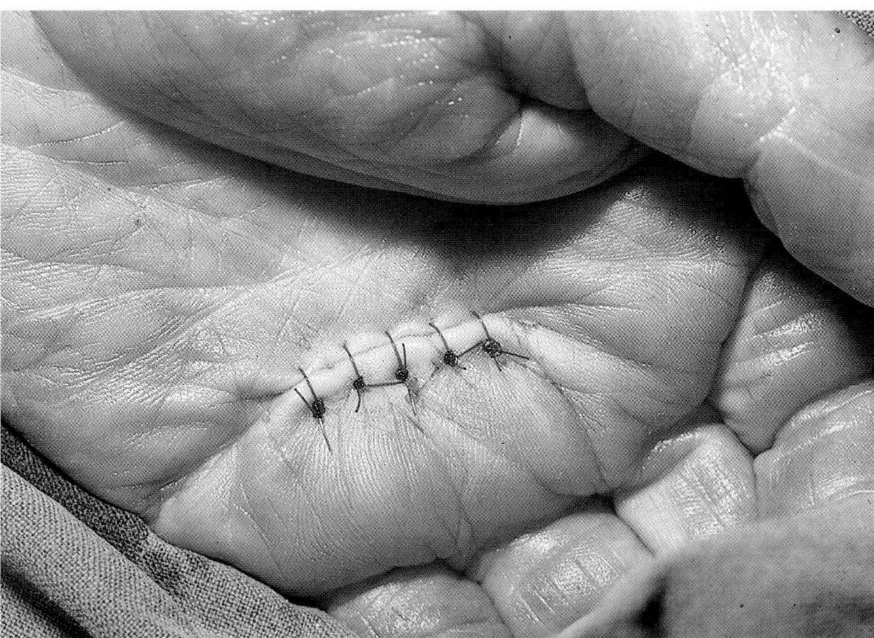

Fig. 40.1 Showing the site for incision for release of fourth trigger finger.

40.2 THE OPERATION [53]

The overlying skin is liberally painted with Povidone-iodine in spirit (Betadine alcoholic solution), a sterile drape is placed over the area, and full aseptic precautions observed. A surgical gown, mask and gloves should be worn.

A small transverse incision is made in the distal palmar crease for trigger fingers, and the proximal thumb crease for trigger thumb (Fig. 40.1).

The incision is deepened until the flexor sheath is exposed, taking care to avoid the digital nerves and blood vessels on either side. For this stage of the operation it is easier and safer to use curved fine artery forceps for dissection rather than scissors or scalpel.

The proximal part of the annular ligament and tendon sheath is divided, and the patient asked to move the fingers, to demonstrate that any triggering has been released. It is preferable to leave the distal portion of the annular ligament, as troublesome bowing of the tendon can occur if this is divided. It is not necessary, nor desirable, to remove any thickening of the tendon itself for fear of subsequent weakening and spontaneous rupture.

Closure is by one subcuticular monofilament suture, supplemented by skin closure strips.

A sterile dressing is applied over the incision, covered with cotton wool and an elastocrepe bandage, and the arm placed in a triangular sling with the affected hand on the opposite shoulder.

The dressing is left completely undisturbed until the suture is removed on the 10th post-operative day. The skin closure strips are left in place, and the hand lightly bandaged for two more days, after which no restrictions need be imposed, and the patient is encouraged to use the fingers as much as possible.

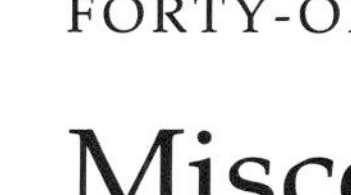

FORTY-ONE

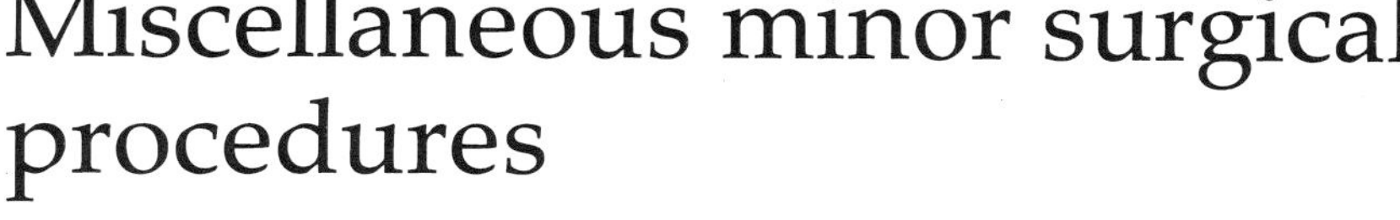

Miscellaneous minor surgical procedures

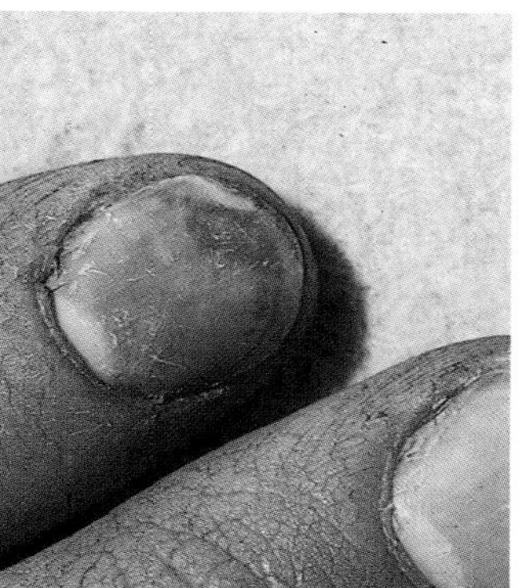

Fig. 41.1 Sub-ungual haematoma.

To draw out splinters
'Incence, Dough, Sea-salt, Wasp's Dung, Fat, Red-lead and Wax. Apply thereto: it draws the matter out'

(Ebers Papyrus, 1500 BC)

41.1 SUB-UNGUAL HAEMATOMA

This is extremely painful due to the pressure of trapped blood underneath the nail. Release of the blood results in an immediate relief of pain. One of the simplest methods is to rest the electrocautery V tip against the nail, switch on the current, and allow the wire to burn a small hole through the nail. As the nail itself is devoid of any nerve endings, the procedure is totally painless, provided undue pressure is not applied to the nail by the cautery. Once all the blood is released, the hole may be sealed with collodion or clear nail varnish, and allowed to grow out (Figs 41.1, 41.2 and 41.3).

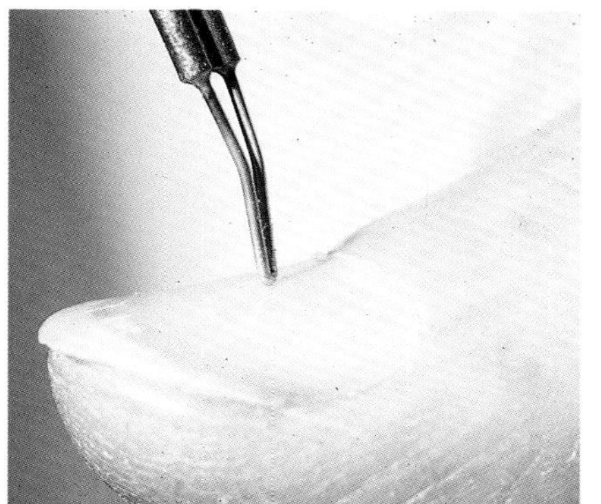

Fig. 41.2 The electrocautery burner is rested against the finger nail.

41.2 HORMONE IMPLANTS

Crystalline pellets of the hormones oestradiol and testosterone may be implanted subcutaneously by means of a special wide-bore trocar and cannula under local anaesthesia. Treatment is simple and effective and only takes a few minutes.

The usual implant site is the anterior abdominal wall 5 cm above and parallel to the inguinal ligament. The overlying skin is painted with Betadine alcoholic solution and infiltrated with 2–5 ml 1% lignocaine. A 5 mm incision is made with a No 11 scalpel blade and the trocar and cannula pushed through this incision into the subcutaneous fat layer, avoiding the rectus sheath. The trocar is removed and the implant pellet placed in the cannula using sterile forceps. (A sterile gallipot should be underneath the cannula in case the pellet drops out.) The obturator is then inserted in the cannula and the implant pushed into the fat layer. The cannula and obturator are now withdrawn while maintaining pressure over the site for one minute to minimize bruising. One suture or just a sterile adhesive strip and dressing is all that is needed to close the wound. Patients who have previously had a hysterectomy may be given just the implant – those with a uterus should have a course of oral norethisterone 5 mgm daily from days 17–28 to prevent endometrial hyperplasia.

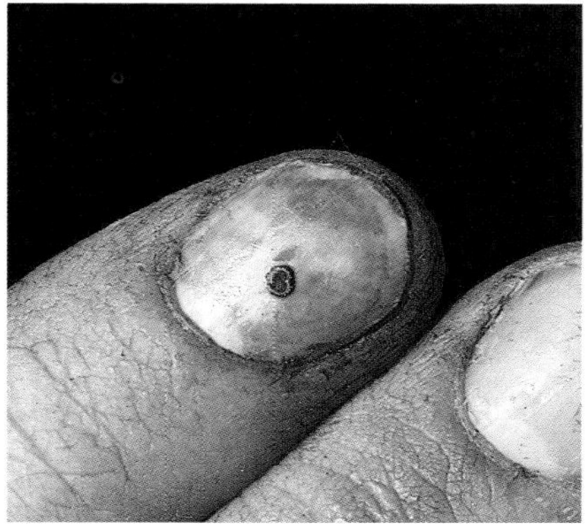

Fig. 41.3 A small hole is burned through the nail, releasing the blood.

41.3 REMOVAL OF SUB-UNGUAL SPLINTERS

These can be extremely painful, as can any attempts at removal. It may help to leave the splinter alone for two days, during which time slight suppuration will occur, loosening the splinter, and making subsequent removal easier. Except for very superficial splinters, it is more comfortable for the patient to anaesthetize the digit, either by a ring block or local infiltration, together with the application of a small tourniquet. The splinter may now be grasped firmly with straight Halstead's mosquito artery forceps, or splinter forceps and removed. Very deep, embedded splinters may sometimes be removed by using a 21 SWG (0.8 mm) needle which has had its point bent backwards to form a hooked barb.

41.4 SMALL SCALP LESIONS

Where a suture is judged inappropriate, small scalp lacerations can be closed by twisting a few hairs on either side of the wound, and knotting them together over the centre of the laceration. To prevent the knots slipping undone, they should be sprayed with tinct. benz. co. Whitehead's varnish, collodion or nabecutane. Thereafter the knot is left to grow out, or cut out after 10 days (see Fig. 9.1).

41.5 XANTHELASMATA

These may be treated with topical applications of monochloroacetic acid or pure liquefied phenol BPC. Great care is needed to avoid accidental burns to the eye or surrounding skin, and repeated small applications are preferred.

Other treatments include cauterization using the unipolar diathermy (Hyfrecator) electrocautery, or freezing with the cryoprobe, or infra-red coagulation with a sapphire interface.

41.6 REMOVAL OF FOREIGN BODIES IN EARS AND NOSES

Young children frequently insert small pieces of rubber, paper, plastic, peas and nuts etc., in nostrils and ears. If not noticed at the time, the first symptom may be a unilateral, offensive, blood-stained discharge. Examination of the nose or ear with an auriscope reveals the cause, and the offending object may usually be removed with a pair of Tilley's aural forceps. Foreign bodies in ears may be difficult to grasp, and may be more conveniently syringed out using an ear-syringe and warm water. Steel ball-bearings may need a powerful ophthalmic electromagnet for removal.

41.7 STONE IN THE SALIVARY DUCT

Obstruction to a salivary gland by a calculus in the duct gives a classical picture of intermittent swelling of the gland whenever the patient attempts to eat. If the calculus can be felt with the examining finger, a small bleb of local anaesthetic is injected, and a suture placed deeply behind the stone, which serves to steady the duct and also prevents the stone slipping into the hilum of the gland. An incision in the long axes of the duct is made over the stone, which may then be easily lifted out. The suture is removed, and no further treatment is needed.

41.8 EAR-LOBE CYSTS

These are particularly common and troublesome, occurring more frequently in young male patients. Many of the cysts become infected and discharge spontaneously. Treatment consists of either dissecting the cyst free after infiltrating the area with local anaesthetic, or incising the cyst, expressing the contents and cauterizing the lining of the cyst with a small cotton wool swab applicator soaked in pure liquefied phenol.

If the doctor possesses a pair of chalazion ring forceps, these are ideal for holding the ear-lobe and fixing the cyst. The introduction of fucidic acid gel (Fucidin Caviject) into the cavity before closure enables healing by primary intention to occur.

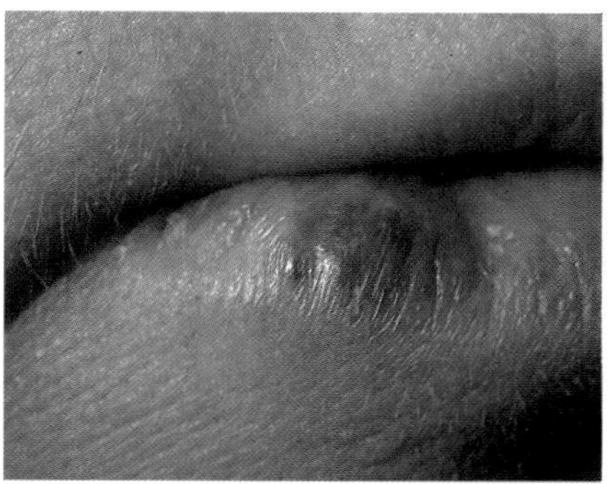

Fig. 41.4 Haemangioma on lower lip. Ideal for treating with electrocautery or Hyfrecator.

41.9 HAEMANGIOMA OF THE LIP

These lesions are relatively common, and may be readily treated by electrocautery, diathermy, cryotherapy or photocoagulation. After preliminary infiltration with local anaesthetic, the needle of the hyfrecator or electrocautery is inserted into the centre of the haemangioma; more than one treatment may be necessary to obtain a good cosmetic result (Fig. 41.4).

41.10 SKIN GRAFTING

Small skin grafts may be performed in the general practitioner's surgery, usually to treat skin loss following accidents. Tips of fingers are the commonest site; if only a small piece of skin has been lost, grafting is unnecessary, but if the complete tip of the digit has been removed, a pinch-skin graft may be attempted.

A donor site is chosen, usually the thigh or arm, and after preliminary infiltration, the chosen piece of skin excised. This is then carefully sutured in place over the injured digit, a tulle-gras dressing applied, and a firm, dry sterile gauze dressing applied and left in place for at least a week.

41.11 NASAL POLYPI

These may be removed with a wire snare; often they are multiple, and are situated in inaccessible sites, but if the doctor is fortunate enough to see a solitary nasal polyp, situated near the entrance, it may be snared off after preliminary topical local anaesthesia. Bleeding can be brisk, but usually stops spontaneously. Good illumination, preferably a spotlight and a head-mirror is essential.

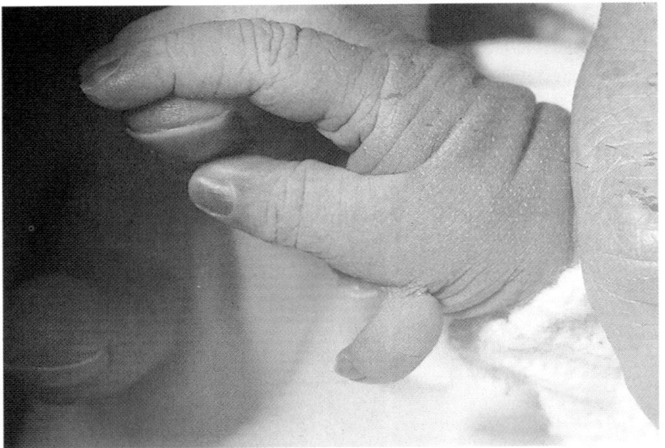

Fig. 41.5 Baby with extra 'thumb'.

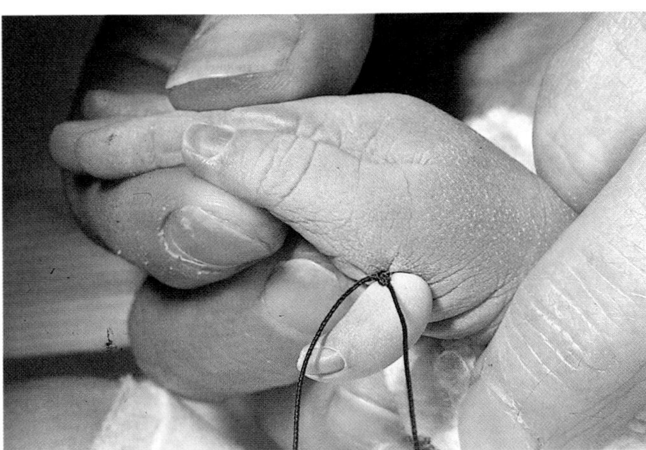

Fig. 41.6 Thread may be tied around the base, or alternatively the digit may be removed immediately with the electrocautery.

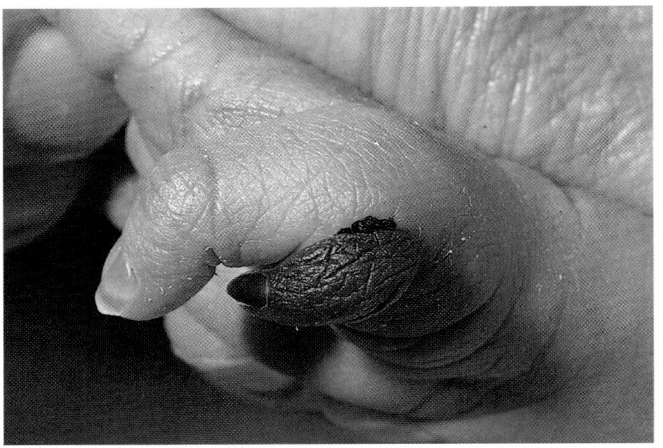

Fig. 41.7 After two weeks, the extra digit begins to separate.

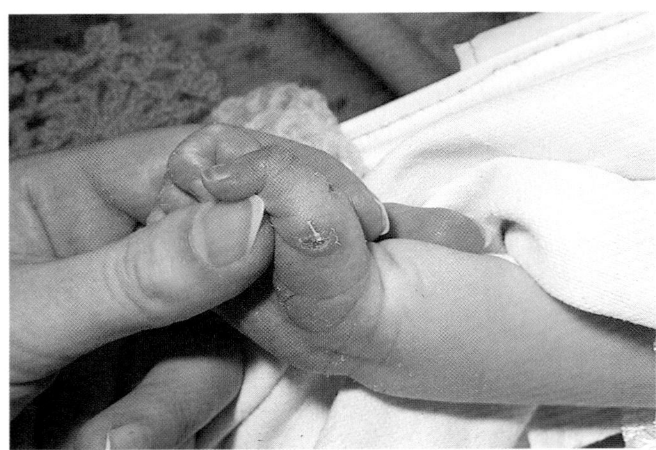

Fig. 41.8 The end result, four weeks later.

41.12 CONGENITAL EXTRA DIGITS

The majority of extra digits are inherited, and may be removed easily at birth either by tying a braided silk suture around the base, or preferably using the electrocautery (Figs 41.5, 41.6, 41.7 and 41.8).

41.13 ACCESSORY AURICLES

Accessory auricles or pre-auricular skin tags or polypi may be removed either by tying a braided silk suture around the base, or by excision and suturing; occasionally by the use of the electrocautery (Figs 41.9 and 41.10).

41.14 SUPERNUMERARY NIPPLES

Many patient suffer considerable embarrassment by the presence of supernumerary nipples and feel their problem is too trivial to consider

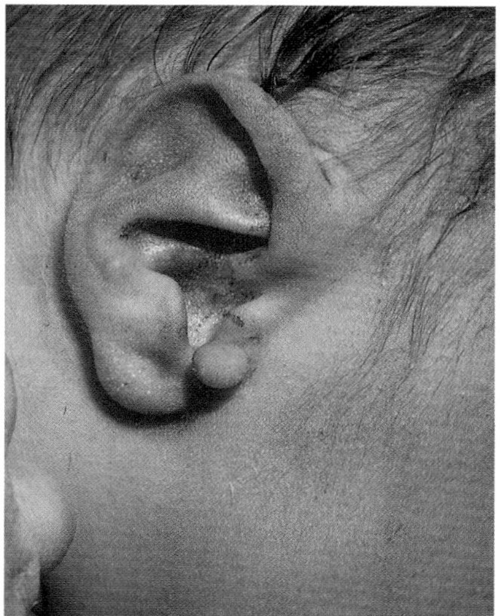

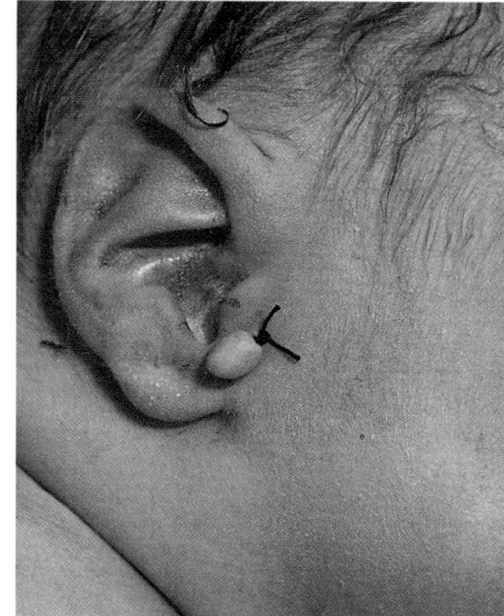

Fig. 41.9 An accessory auricle.

Fig. 41.10 Thread may be tied around the base, or alternatively the papilloma may be removed immediately with the electrocautery.

treatment. Excision is simple, effective and quick, and may be performed under local infiltration anaesthesia. (See Intradermal lesions Chapter 17 and Incisions Chapter 8) paying particular attention to the direction of the ultimate scar.

41.15 REMOVAL OF FOREIGN BODIES IN EYES

Good illumination and magnification are essential. The standard ophthalmoscope with the +20 D lens gives good vision. The application of one drop of local anaesthetic eye-drops makes the whole procedure comfortable for the patient and easier for the operator.

If the object can be seen on the front of the eye-ball, it can usually be removed with a wisp of cotton wool wrapped around the end of a thin wooden applicator.

Failing this, an eye-spud may be used, or even a 19 SWG (1.1 mm) needle provided great care is taken. The possibility of a penetrating injury to the eye-ball should always be borne in mind, particularly if there is a history of high-speed grinding or the use of cold chisels.

It may be necessary to evert the upper eye-lid: this can be done by grasping the eye-lashes with finger and thumb of one hand and gently pressing down on the lid with a blunt round rod.

41.16 ENTROPION (Fig. 41.11)

In the elderly, spasm of the orbicularis muscle results in inversion of the lower eye-lid which turns the eye-lashes so that they irritate the conjuctiva. This can be corrected by a simple 'skin and muscle' operation as follows: the conjunctiva is anaesthetized with topical 4% Lignocaine or similar local anaesthetic. The skin over the lower eye-lid is next infiltrated using 1% Lignocaine with 1:200 000 adrenalin and a pair of T-shaped forceps applied. A thin strip of skin, approximately 6 mm wide is excised, exposing the

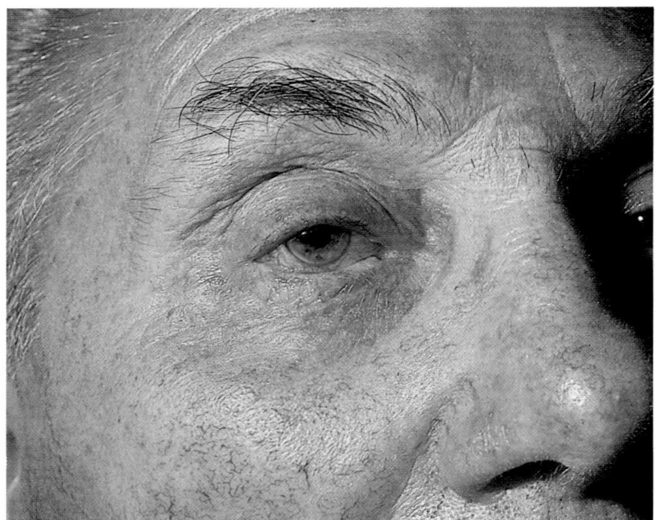

Fig. 41.11 Entropion.

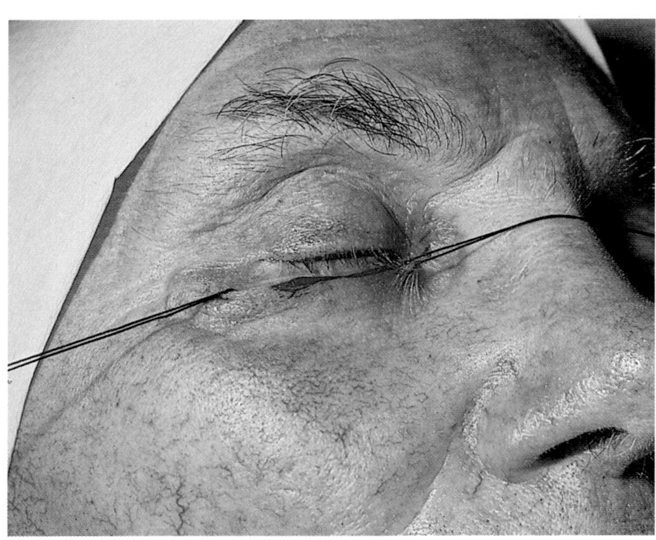

Fig. 41.12 A strip of skin is removed from the lower eye-lid.

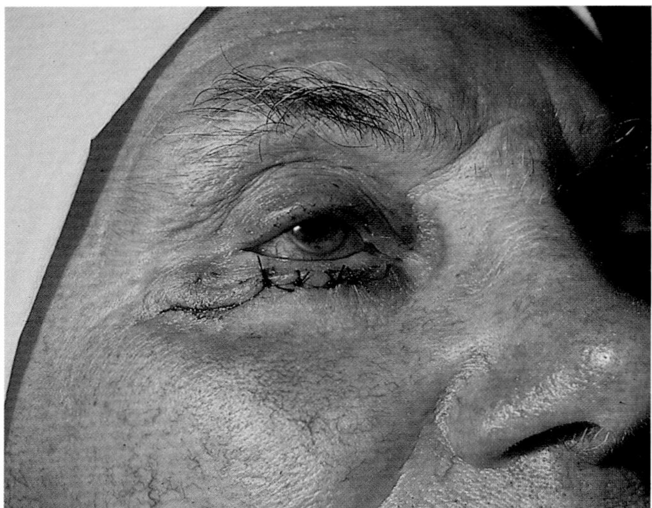

Fig. 41.13 After giving spot-burns to the underlying muscle, the skin is sutured.

underlying muscle, a portion of which is also excised (Fig. 41.12). Any bleeding is controlled with the electrocautery. Equidistant spot burns are now placed along the margin to create scarring, fibrosis and ultimate contracture, and the skin edges sutured with interrupted braided silk sutures 4/0 (metric gauge 1.5) (Fig. 41.13).

41.17 REMOVAL OF PACE-MAKER

One pre-requisite before cremation can be authorized is the removal of any cardiac pace-makers or implants, and the general practitioner may be asked to do this by the undertaker or relatives (Fig. 41.14).

A simple suture pack is all that is required (Chapter 2), an incision is made over the pace-maker which may be easily removed, together with the flexible wire electrode. The skin is then closed with interrupted sutures or adhesive tape.

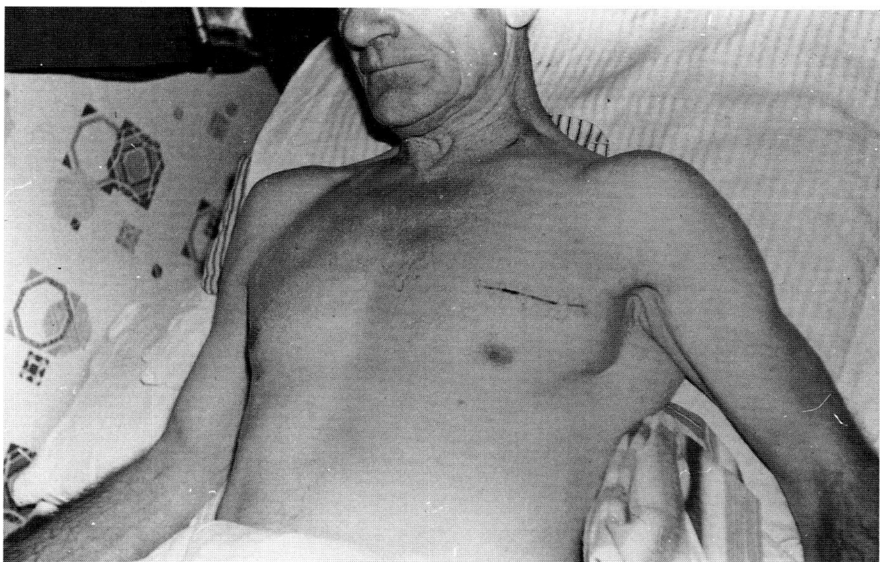

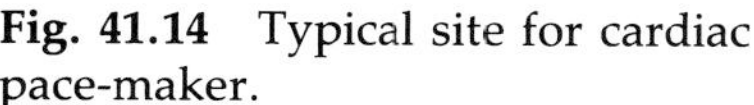

Fig. 41.14 Typical site for cardiac pace-maker.

41.18 FOREIGN BODY REMOVAL UTILIZING A BLOODLESS FIELD

The removal of small pieces of glass or metal can be extremely difficult if the operating field is covered with blood. Attempts to locate or remove such objects usually provoke further bleeding. It tends to be forgotten that a bloodless operating area can be obtained in any limb or digit by the use of a rubber tourniquet.

Any injection of local anaesthetic, either infiltration, digital nerve block or ring-block should be given first and the injured site then covered with a dry dressing or small ring pad if fragments of glass are likely to be embedded A rubber strip or Esmarch bandage may then be applied to exsanguinate the part, and a tourniquet applied. In the case of digits, this can be a thin rubber tube and artery forceps; limbs should have a pneumatic tourniquet applied. The absence of bleeding then enables the doctor to locate and remove any fragments of glass or metal more easily.

41.19 SYRINGING OF THE LACRIMAL DUCT

Blockage of the naso-lacrimal duct is now relatively uncommon, but the patency can readily be checked by syringing. Two instruments are needed: a Nettleship's dilator for enlarging the lacrimal puncta, and a lacrimal cannula and syringe. First, pressure should be applied over the lacrimal sac on the side of the nose to see if any pus or mucus discharges through the punctum; then 4% Lignocaine eye-drops are applied to the conjunctiva. Next the lower lid is everted to expose the inferior punctum which is dilated with the point of the Nettleship's dilator. It should now be possible to insert the lacrimal cannula and syringe the duct using sterile normal saline.

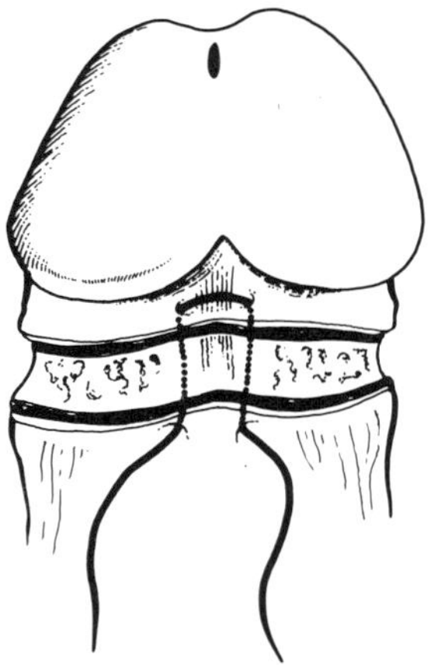

Fig. 41.15 The 'three-in-one' fraenal stitch.

41.20 CIRCUMCISION

In children and infants a general anaesthetic is preferable, but in adults the operation may be done under local anaesthesia. Infiltration with plain Lignocaine 1% is adequate. Two pairs of haemostats are applied to the edges of the prepuce and a dorsal slit performed to within 6 mm of the corona. Another haemostat is applied to the fraenum, and the requisite amount of prepuce excised. The skin edges and mucosa are sutured together with fine 3/0 dexon interrupted stitches. It is important to include the fraenal artery in a three-in-one stitch as shown (Fig. 41.15). A dressing of ribbon gauze and tinct. benz. co. completes the operation.

41.21 REMOVAL OF FISH-HOOKS

During the fishing season, a number of patients are always seen with fish-hooks embedded in various parts of their anatomy. Attempts by the patient to remove the hook usually fail due to the barb. If a pair of strong wire-cutters are available, the eye of the hook should be cut off, and then with a needle holder or artery forceps, the hook pushed through the skin and removed (Figs 41.16, 41.17 and 41.18).

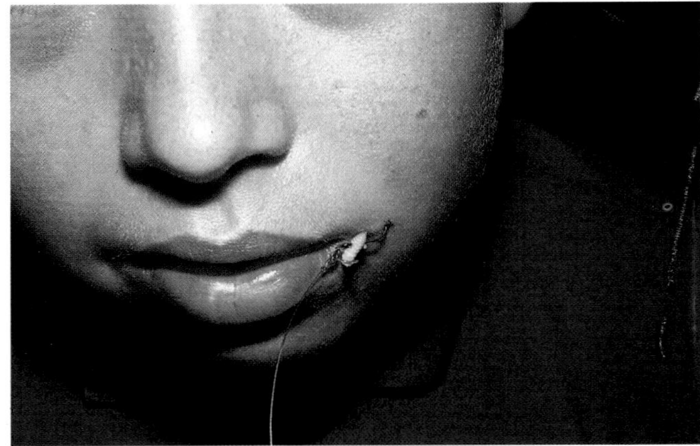

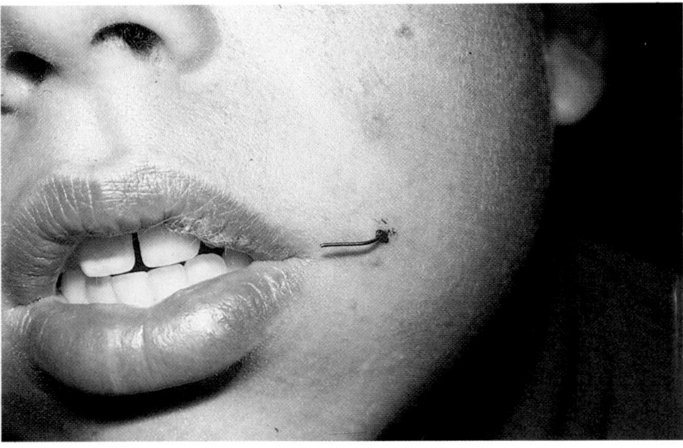

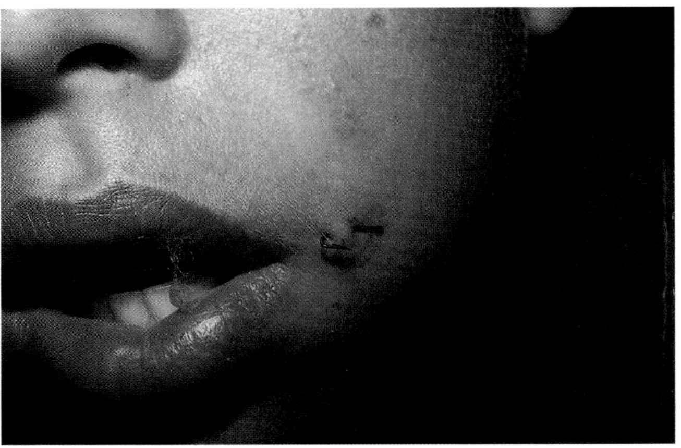

Fig. 41.16 A fish-hook embedded in the cheek.

Fig. 41.17 One end of the hook is cut off with wirecutters.

Fig. 41.18 The hook may now be pushed through, and removed.

FORTY-TWO

Resuscitation

'How is the surgeon transported, to discover motion returning to the lips and eyelids of a man apparently dead and when he perceives that the heart palpates and respiration is restored!'

(Dominique-Jean Larrey, 1766–1842)

Every hospital and doctor's surgery should have facilities for giving emergency resuscitation for the 'collapsed' patient, and a basic knowledge of first aid and cardiopulmonary resuscitation is essential for members of the staff working in these premises.

The combined manual of first aid produced by the St John Ambulance Association, the St Andrew's Ambulance Association and British Red Cross Society is excellent.

A patient who has 'collapsed' at the surgery may be suffering from any of the following:

1. A vasovagal attack (faint)
2. Profound vasovagal attack leading to a convulsion
3. Epileptic attack
4. Myocardial infarction
5. Allergic reaction to drugs administered
6. Anaphylactic reaction to drugs administered
7. Pulmonary embolism
8. Concealed haemorrhage
9. Cerebro-vascular attack (stroke)
10. Acute psychiatric crisis
11. Cardiac arrest.

It is helpful to keep all resuscitation equipment together in one place, known to all members of the staff. The exact contents of any 'resuscitation kit' will vary depending on the preference of the doctors, but the following will provide a nucleus which can be supplemented with additional equipment if needed:

1. A selection of plastic airways
2. Endotracheal tubes
3. Laryngoscope
4. Intravenous cannulae
5. Giving sets for intravenous fluids
6. Oxygen cylinders and giving sets
7. Suction apparatus
8. Positive-pressure inflator (Ambu)
9. Sphygmomanometer
10. Electrocardiogram machine or monitor
11. Cardiac defibrillator
12. Large selection syringes and needles
13. Emergency drugs, intravenous fluids and plasma expanders.

42.1 THE VASOVAGAL ATTACK

These are undoubtedly the commonest causes of 'collapse' seen by the doctor. The patient may complain of not feeling well, becomes pale, sweaty, anxious, with cold, clammy skin and a slow imperceptible pulse. The patient is usually sitting or standing at the time, and if left in this position, will lose consciousness due to cerebral ischaemia secondary to hypotension. It is a common accompaniment to injections or painful or unpleasant experiences and is usually self-limiting as consciousness returns as soon as the patient falls to the ground.

First aid treatment consists of lying the patient on the floor and elevating the lower limbs to increase the venous return to the heart, watching the airway at the same time. Recovery is normally rapid. Because vasovagal attacks can occur in the most unexpected patients it is a good rule always to insist that the patient lies on the couch or operating theatre table rather than be seated in a chair for any minor surgical procedure.

42.2 PROFOUND VASOVAGAL ATTACK LEADING TO CONVULSION

In this, the patient appears to faint, but then has a short epileptiform convulsion. Unlike a major epileptic fit, the patient recovers consciousness quickly and is able to resume his or her activities without any impairment. Treatment consists of lying the patient down and placing in the recovery position. If the airway can be guarded, the patient may be placed on his or her back and the lower limbs elevated to hasten recovery of consciousness.

42.3 MAJOR EPILEPTIC CONVULSION

This may arise in a patient known to suffer from epilepsy, or may occur without any previous history of attacks. If a solitary fit occurs, the patient should be placed in the recovery position and the airway guarded. Should multiple fits occur (status epilepticus) intravenous Diazepam should be given, and oxygen administered via a high concentration mask.

42.4 MYOCARDIAL INFARCTION

A patient may suffer a myocardial infarction while in the doctor's surgery; immediate resuscitation may be life-saving. Nitrites given immediately may reduce the severity of the infarction, oxygen should be given via a high-concentration face-mask, pain relieved by diamorphine or morphine, nausea by cyclizine, bradycardia by intravenous atropine, and arrhythmias by intravenous Lignocaine. The early insertion of an intravenous cannula is valuable as it gives access to the circulation should subsequent collapse occur. Arrangements to transfer the patient to hospital should be made, and if possible electrocardiographic monitoring done, with cardiac defibrillation available should cardiac arrest occur.

42.5 ALLERGIC REACTION TO DRUGS ADMINISTERED

It is always wise to enquire from the patient whether he or she has any allergies or drug sensitivities, and beware of any interreactions with drugs to be administered. Should a reaction occur, intravenous antihistamines and steroids should be administered; an intravenous cannula inserted, regular blood-pressure checks made, and any shock corrected.

42.6 ANAPHYLACTIC REACTION

These are extremely rare, but very frightening when they occur. Sudden circulatory collapse occurs. The patient should be immediately placed on the floor or a couch; legs elevated and adrenalin administered, together with intravenous steroids, antihistamines and fluid replacement. Oxygen and ventilation may be necessary.

42.7 PULMONARY EMBOLISM

This may be very difficult to diagnose outside hospital. First aid treatment consists of maintaining an airway, the administration of oxygen, the introduction of an intravenous cannula, and urgent admission to hospital.

42.8 CONCEALED HAEMORRHAGE

This may arise from a bleeding duodenal ulcer, ruptured ectopic pregnancy, or following trauma from a ruptured liver, kidney or spleen. The patient will be shocked, with a rising, rapid, feeble pulse, and falling blood pressure. First aid treatment aims to restore the blood volume by the insertion of an intravenous cannula and administration of plasma expanders after first taking blood for grouping and cross matching.

42.9 CEREBRO-VASCULAR ATTACK

As with a myocardial infarction, any patient may suddenly develop a cerebro-vascular attack while attending the doctor. The patient with a cerebral haemorrhage suddenly loses consciousness, may have localizing signs, and may die within 48 hours. The only first aid treatment is the maintenance of an adequate airway and oxygen if necessary, with transfer to hospital. Occlusion of a cerebral artery from thrombosis or embolus may respond initially to re-breathing via a polythene bag. In this, a large polythene bag is placed over the nose and mouth and the patient requested to re-breathe until they find it uncomfortable. This allows the carbon dioxide levels in the lung to rise – giving cerebral vasodilation. Additionally, intravenous dexamethasone has been used to reduce intracranial oedema.

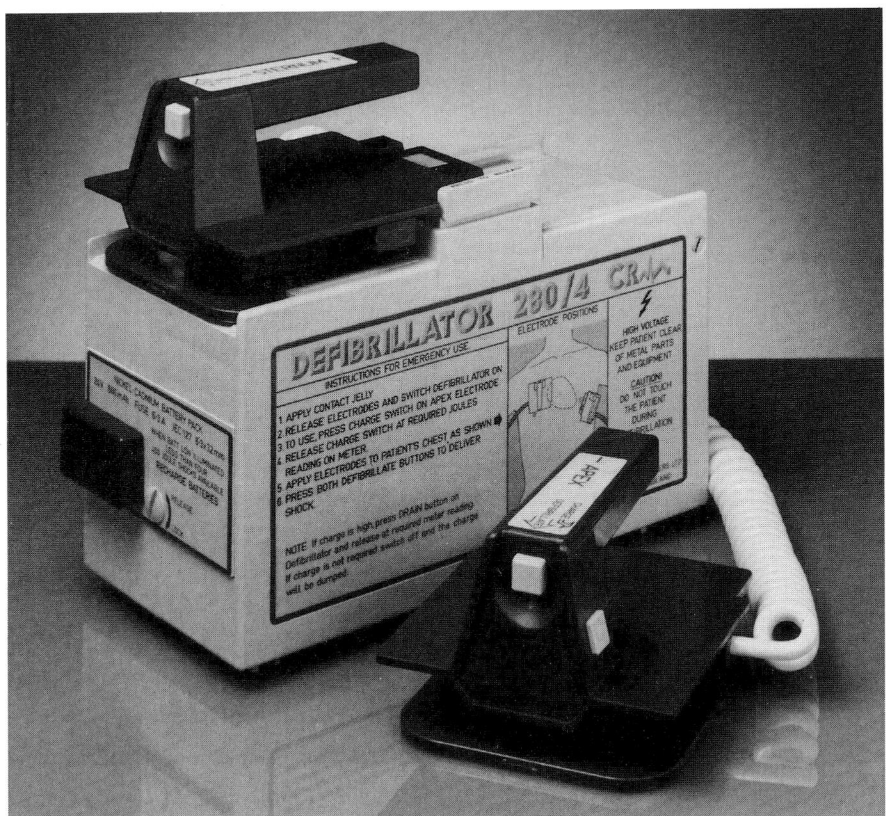

Fig. 42.1 Cardiac defibrillator. 280/4 (Cardiac Recorders Ltd).

42.10 THE ACUTE PSYCHIATRIC CRISIS

This may manifest itself as hypo-mania, excitability, confusion, delusions, or violence. There is usually a preceding history of psychiatric disturbance. First aid treatment consists of reassurance, and if necessary intravenous Chlorpromazine or Diazepam.

42.11 CARDIAC ARREST

This is the most serious of all 'collapses'. It may arise following a myocardial infarction, following fright, or spontaneously with no obvious cause. It is diagnosed by an unconscious patient with absent pulses, and irregular, infrequent respirations which eventually stop. Following this, the pupils become widely dilated and fixed.

42.11.1 First-aid treatment

If an ECG monitor is immediately available, and the cause is shown to be ventricular fibrillation, immediate cardiac defibrillation should be performed, giving a DC shock of up to 400 Joules, repeating if necessary. Oxygen and endotracheal intubation should be instituted, together with the insertion of an intravenous cannula. Following successful defibrillation, intravenous Lignocaine 100 mg and Dexamethasone 5 mg should be given.

Severe bradycardia should be treated with intravenous atropine 300–

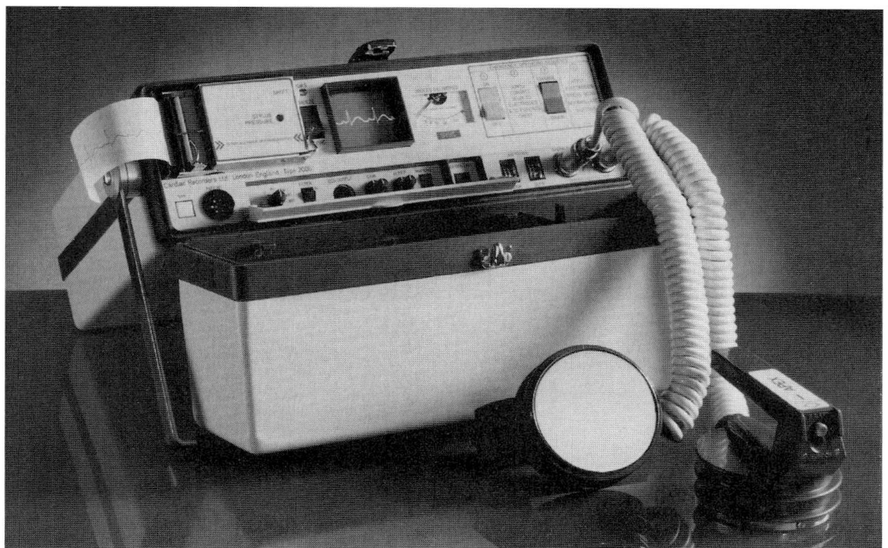

Fig. 42.2 Cardiac defibrillator monitor and ECG machine (Cardiac Recorders Type 2006).

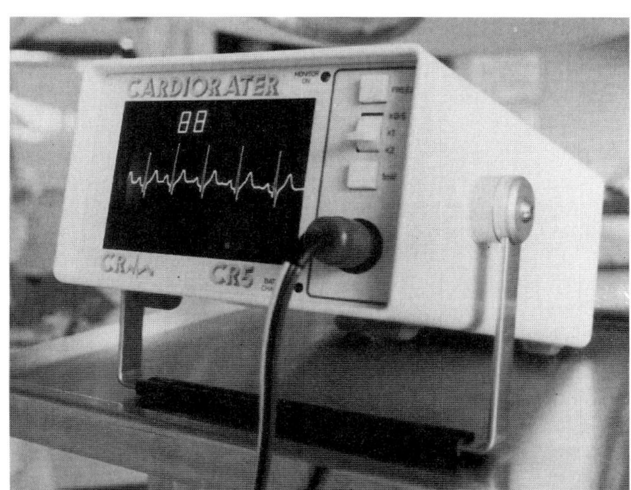

Fig. 42.3 The CR5 cardiorater (Cardiac Recorders Ltd).

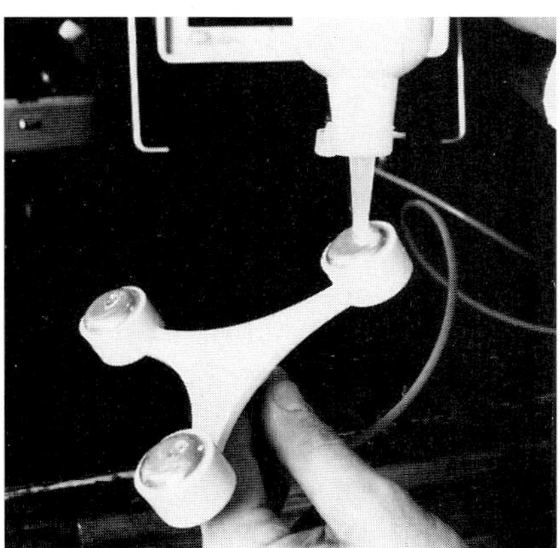

Fig. 42.4 A tripod chest electrode gives immediate tracings (Cardiac Recorders Ltd).

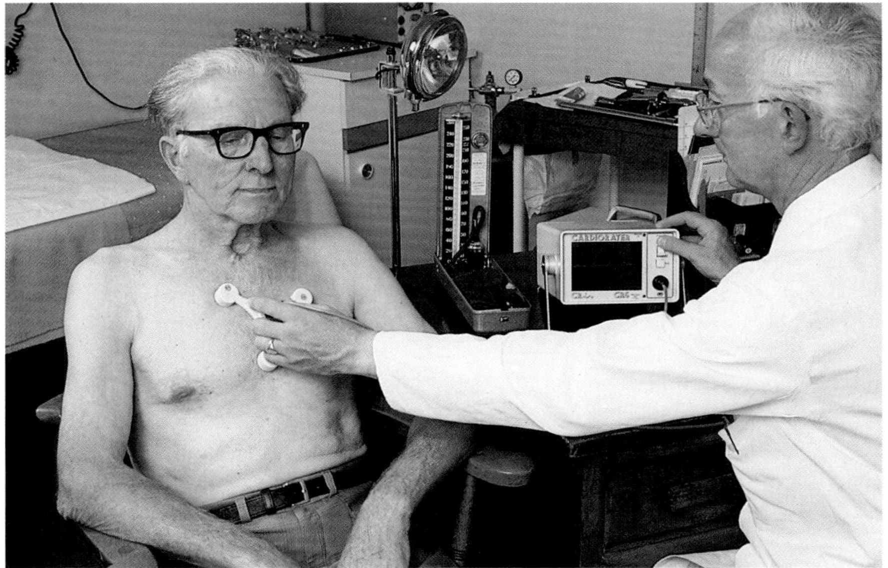

Fig. 42.5 The use of the tripod electrode with the CR5 cardiac monitor (Cardiac Recorders Ltd).

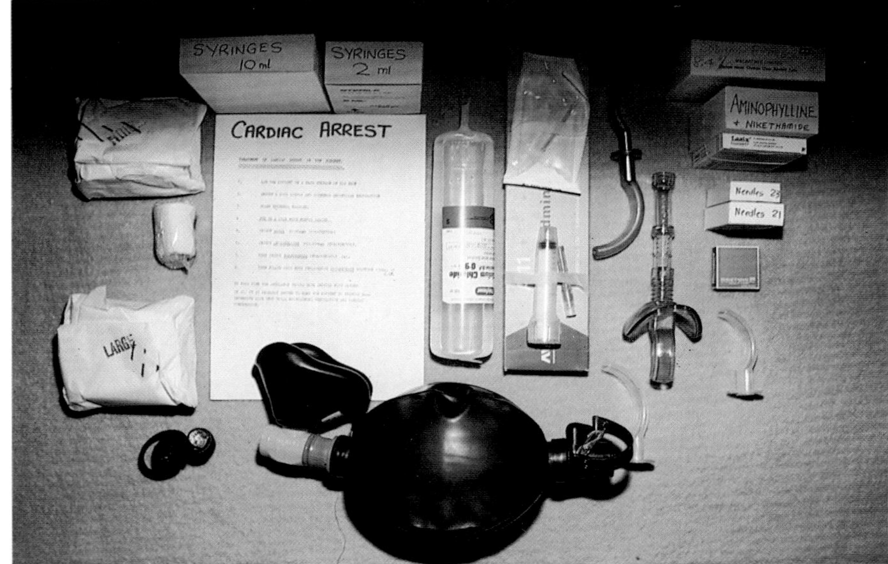

Fig. 42.6 Contents of a simple 'cardiac arrest' box.

600 μg while asystole should be treated with intravenous adrenalin 1:1000 1 ml to induce ventricular fibrillation which can be converted to sinus rhythm by DC defibrillation.

Acidosis is treated by intravenous sodium bicarbonate 8.4% 50–150 ml and cardiac failure by intravenous frusemide 20–40 mg.

Throughout all these procedures, cardiopulmonary resuscitation by mouth-to-mouth artificial respiration and external cardiac compression should be maintained.

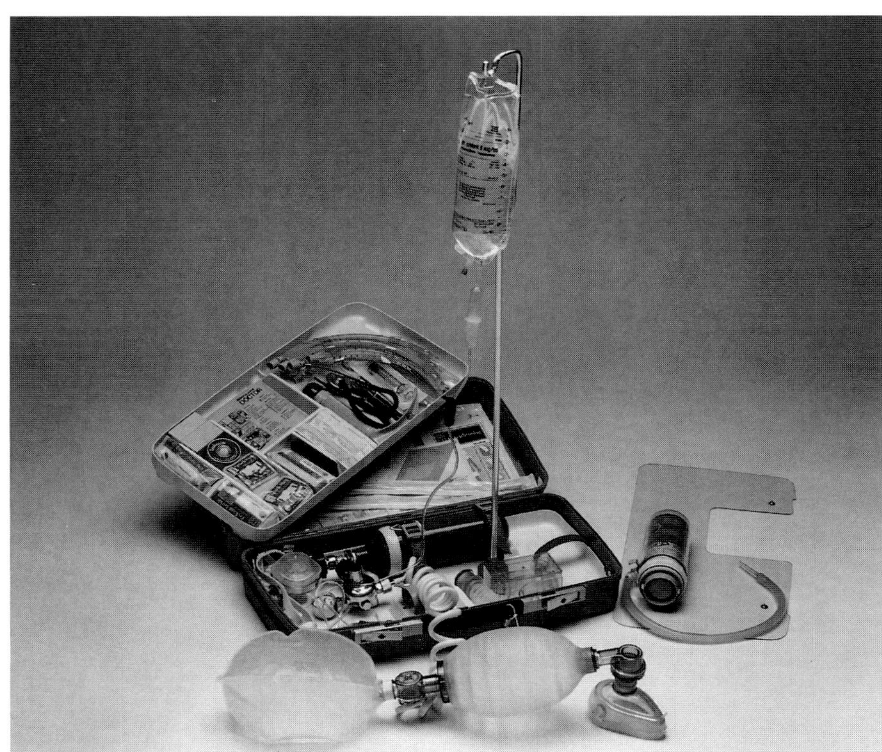

Fig. 42.7 A comprehensive resuscitation kit which may be kept in the treatment room, or kept in the boot of the doctor's car for immediate use both at road traffic accidents and in the patient's home. (Laerdal Modulaide 'Doctor' complete (Laerdal Medical Ltd)).

FORTY-THREE

The general practitioner and the National Health Service

'I hope the House will not hesitate to tell the British Medical Association that we look forward to this act starting on 5th July 1948 and that we expect the Medical Profession to take their proper part in it because we are satisfied that there is nothing in it that any doctor should be otherwise than proud to acknowledge'

(Aneurin Bevan, 1897–1960)

The remuneration of a general medical practitioner working within the National Health Service is derived from the number of patients registered on his or her 'list' together with additional item-of-service payments and allowances as follows [54].

1. Standard capitation fees (Para 21)
2. Standard capitation fees for patients aged 65–74
3. Standard capitation fees for patients aged over 75
4. Supplementary capitation fees (Para 23)
5. Basic practice allowance (Para 12)
6. Supplementary practice allowance (Para 22)
7. An allowance for group practice (Para 15)
8. An allowance for an assistant (Para 18)
9. Fees for temporary residents (Para 32)
10. Fees for maternity medical services (Para 31)
11. Emergency treatment fee (Para 33)
12. Payment for the administration of a general anaesthetic (Para 34)
13. Rural practice payments (Para 43)
14. Night visit fees (Para 24)
15. Fees for providing contraceptive services (Para 29)
16. Fee for immediately necessary treatment (Para 36)
17. Items of service fees: immunizations (Para 27) and cervical cytology (Para 28)
18. Prolonged treatment and expensive drugs (Para 44)
19. Special list drugs (Para 44)
20. Tariff basis drugs (Para 44)
21. Seniority payments (Para 16)
22. Vocational training allowance (Para 17)
23. Post-graduate training allowance (Para 37)

Despite the complexity of the above 23 groups, there is no provision for paying an item-of-service fee for those general practitioners who wish to undertake minor surgery for their NHS patients even though fees have been negotiated for such services as contraception, cervical cytology and immunizations. The general practitioner is expected to provide minor surgery within his or her contract at no additional remuneration, and this probably explains why so few general practitioners undertake any surgical procedures, and why so many patients with minor surgical conditions are referred to hospital. Far from providing any incentives for general practitioners to undertake minor surgery, there are positive *disincentives* as the doctor will have to purchase all the equipment and instruments personally, without being able to reclaim any part of it, neither will he or she be able to claim a fee from the Government, or be allowed to charge the patient a fee.

However, certain paragraphs within the Statement of Fees and Allowances are applicable to minor surgery, and careful utilization of these paragraphs will enable the doctor to marginally increase his or her income.

Before considering these paragraphs, it is important to clarify when a doctor may charge a fee. Under their terms of service, general practitioners are expressly forbidden from asking for, *or receiving*, payment for, or token in lieu of, the provision of any medical service for any patient registered with them under the National Health Service [55]. The only exceptions which are allowed are for certain documents, private certificates and vaccination certificates. A GP is allowed to accept private fee-paying patients, provided they are not already registered with the GP or his or her partners under the National Health Service, and charges may be made to such patients for all medical services rendered.

In the past it was suggested that a general practitioner could request the removal of a NHS patient from his or her list for three months and treat the patient privately, in which case the charging of a fee, is allowable. Although this is perfectly legal, most doctors would not be happy to do it, and it cannot be recommended.

An item-of-service fee is payable for a minor surgical operation performed on a patient receiving emergency medical treatment who is not registered with that general practitioner, nor any of his or her partners. In this case, form FP 32 is completed, provided the emergency was not caused by the use of a motor vehicle on the road! What constitutes a minor surgical operation is not defined in this section of the regulations, but it does show that the Government recognizes that in certain situations, an item-of-service payment for a minor surgical procedure is appropriate.

Likewise, a separate item-of-service fee is payable for the administration of a general anaesthetic, provided a second qualified doctor (not a trainee general practitioner) is in attendance and personally administers the anaesthetic. This is claimed on form FP 31. Thus, although the numbers of general anaesthetics given in general practice outside hospital is decreasing, nevertheless, there is a recognition by the Department of Health that the administration of a general anaesthetic qualifies for an additional payment. No such item-of-service payments exist for the administration of any local anaesthetic, be it infiltration, nerve block or epidural. It is possible, however, to obtain indirect re-imbursement by careful use of the 'Red Book' utilizing paragraph 44.13 for *all* injections, anaesthetics, suture materials, intra-uterine contraceptive devices, and skin closure strips, as follows:

1. The doctor personally purchases all injections, anaesthetics, sutures, coils and skin closure strips.
2. For each patient where any of the above are used, and which the doctor or their nurse personally administers, the doctor writes the items on a standard FP 10 prescription form.

3. The patient pays *no* prescription charge, irrespective of age or exemption category.
4. Once per month, all prescriptions are sent to the Central Prescription Pricing Bureau together with a claim form FP 34 duly signed.
5. The doctor is subsequently refunded as follows:
   (a) The basic price of the item used.
   (b) An 'on-cost' allowance.
   (c) A 'container' allowance.
   (d) A dispensing fee

This results in a very small profit on each item prescribed. As an example, for the excision of a sebaceous cyst, the practitioner could submit prescriptions for three items used, viz., local anaesthetic, suture materials and Steri-strips. Although somewhat cumbersome, nevertheless it provides a small additional income, and at least helps the practitioner from making a loss, and at present is the only method available for claiming any fee.

In addition to utilizing paragraph 44.13 savings may be achieved by writing a prescription for certain drugs, dressings and appliances used for any surgical procedure, giving it to the patient, who then brings it back for use by the doctor on that particular patient. However, it must not be overlooked that the general medical practitioner already receives a few pence each year included in the patient's capitation fee to take account of the occasional bandage and dressing.

Items which may be obtained on prescription include the following:

All bandages, whatever type and size,
Elastoplast bandages,
Eye pad and bandage,
Triangular bandages,
Cotton wool, lint, gamgee, gauze,
Catheters, drainage bags,
Self adhesive tapes,
Povidone-iodine alcoholic solution,
Any drugs, ointments, creams, drops,
Injections and insufflations used.

43.1 OBTAINING HELP FROM HEALTH AUTHORITIES

The majority of health authorities will welcome general practitioners undertaking their own minor surgery, and if approached, will generally be very willing to offer help. Advice about the choice and variety of surgical instruments can always be obtained by approaching the District Supplies Officer, the Operating Theatre Sisters or the Central Sterile Supplies Department manager. The hospital will usually have favourable arrangements for bulk buying surgical instruments and will often be able to include the general practitioner in their scheme.

Similarly, the Hospital Supplies Officer may know of obsolete items such as operating theatre tables, lights, trolleys, and other such equipment which may be purchased by the general practitioner for a nominal sum.

If the practitioner intends using CSSD instrument packs, it is worth discussing with the hospital the possibility of using their autoclaves, particularly if the hospital is near the general practitioner's surgery. Some Health Districts make a small service charge for CSSD facilities – others waive this charge in recognition of the considerable financial savings resulting from the general practitioner undertaking minor surgery. Either way, pre-packed pre-sterilized instrument sets are invaluable and greatly increase the scope and safety of what can be done. Where the doctor is well known to the hospital, certain less-used instrument packs such as abdominal paracentesis, lumbar puncture or chest aspiration sets may be loaned to save the practitioner having to purchase instruments.

43.2 COLLABORATION WITH CONSULTANT COLLEAGUES

It is always a good policy to obtain the support of local consultant surgeons should advice or help be required. Generally this is willingly given and improves relationships; assuming that general practitioners only tackle what they feel they can safely complete, the need for help seldom arises, but it is reassuring to know that it is there if required.

43.3 THE PRIVATE PATIENT

General practitioners are entitled to treat private patients as well as to accept National Health Service patients. Where a doctor has an exclusively private practice, and no NHS patients, arrangements are straightforward – the doctor charges for all medical services rendered, and included in these may be fees for minor surgical operations; there is no set scale of fees – this is left entirely to the discretion of the doctor. Where a general practitioner has a predominantly National Health Service list of patients, he or she is still entitled to accept fee-paying patients but the overall earnings from private practice should not exceed 10% of the total practice income otherwise the GP will be liable to forfeit certain allowances.

If a patient is treated privately, he or she cannot be registered as a National Health Service patient with that doctor or any of his or her partners, neither can the patient be given a National Health Service prescription and the doctor cannot utilize paragaph 44.13 of the Statement of Fees and Allowances. Thus the fee for the operation must include the cost of all drugs, anaesthetics, suture materials, service charges and dressings used.

APPENDIX 1

Surgical instrument and equipment suppliers

UK Suppliers

Abbot Laboratories Ltd: Queenborough, Kent, ME11 5EL, Tel: 07956 63371, Telex 96347.

Arterial Medical Ltd: 313, Chase Road, Southgate, London N14 6JB, Tel: 01 882 1971 (General equipment).

Ash Instruments Division – Dentsply Ltd: 9, Madleaze Estate, Bristol Road, Gloucester GL1 5SG (Dental needles and syringes).

Astra Pharmaceuticals Ltd: Home Park Estate, Kings Langley, Herts WD4 8DH, Tel: 09277 66191 (Local anaesthetics).

Baxter Dental Ltd: Unit 6 and 7, The Crystal Centre, Elmgrove Road, Harrow, Middlesex, Tel: 01 863 2361.

BCB: 2, Moorland Road, Cardiff, CF2 2YL, Tel: 0222 464464.

John Bell and Croyden: 52–54, Wigmore Street, London W1H 0AU, Tel: 01 935 5555, Telex: 8955447 (Surgical instruments).

Bridge Medical Direct: 57, Grenfell Road, Maidenhead, Berks SL6 1ES, Tel: 0628 73721 (General instruments).

British Oxygen Company Ltd: Tunnel Avenue, East Greenwich, London SE10 0JN, Tel: 01 858 3255 (Entonox and nitrous oxide).

Becton Dickenson Ltd: Between Towns Road, Cowley, Oxford OX4 3LY (Hypodermic needles).

Cardiac Recorders Ltd: 34, Scarborough Road, London N4 4LU, Tel: 01 272 9212, Telex 297352 (ECG and de-fibrillators).

Cardiokinetics Ltd: 2, Kansas Avenue, Salford, M5 2GL, Tel: 061 872 8287, Telex 665271 (Disposable cauteries).

Chilworth Medical Ltd: 31, Dorking Road, Chilworth, Guildford, Surrey GU4 8NW, Tel: 0483 64706 (Infra-red coagulator).

Clement Clark Ltd: 15, Wigmore Street, London W1H 0DH, Tel: 01 580 8053, Telex 298626 (Perkins tonometer).

Doctors' Shop: Morgan Grampian House, 30, Calderwood Street, London SE18 6QH, Tel: 01 855 7777 (General equipment).

Doctor Surgery Shop: Russell House, 137, High Street, Guildford GU1 3AD, Tel: 0483 502125 (General equipment).

Doherty Medical Hospital Equipment: Eedee House, Charlton Road, London N9 8HS, Tel: 01 804 1244.

Downs Surgical PLC: Church Path, Mitcham, Surrey CR4 3UE, Tel: 01 648 6291, Telex 927045 (Surgical instruments).

Duncan Flockhart Ltd: 114–116 Curtain Road, London EC2A 3AH, Tel: 01 739 3451 (Local anaesthetics).

Eschmann Bros and Walsh Ltd: Peter Road, Lancing, West Sussex BN15 8TJ, Tel: 0903 761122, Telex 877075 (Theatre equipment).

Ethicon Sutures Ltd: PO Box 408, Bankhead Avenue, Edinburgh EH11 4HE, Scotland, Tel: 031 453 5555, Telex 727222.

Gallops Trolleys: Rock-a-Nore Road, Hastings, East Sussex TN34 3DW, Tel: 0424 421485, Telex 897076.

George Gill and Sons (Surgical) Ltd: Surgill House, Holbrook Industrial Estate, Halfway, Sheffield S19 5GZ, Tel: 0742 482111.

Philip Harris Medical Ltd: Freepost, Hazelwell Lane, Stirchley, Birmingham B30 2PS, Tel: 021 458 2020.

Holborn Surgical Instrument Co Ltd: Dolphin Works, Margate Road, Broadstairs, Kent CT10 2QQ, Tel: 0843 61418.

Keeler Instruments Ltd: Clewer Hill Road, Windsor, Berks SL4 4AA Tel: 07535 57177, Telex 847565 (Ophthalmic Instruments).

Key-Med Ltd: Key-Med House, Stock Road, Southend-on-Sea, SS2 5QH, Tel: 0702 616333, Telex 995283 (Endoscopes and cryoprobes).

Kimberley Clark Ltd: Larkfield, Maidstone, Kent ME20 7PS, Tel: Maidstone (0622) 77700, Telex 93356 (Paper towels and sheets).

Laerdal Medical Ltd: 2, Vinson Close, Orpington, Kent BR6 0EG, Tel: 0689 76634 (Resuscitation kit).

Ledu Lamps Ltd: Unit 6, Kennet Road, Crayford, Kent DA1 4QN, Tel: 0322 57529, Telex 8956592 (Lights).

Macarthy's Surgical: Selinas Lane, Dagenham, Essex RM8 1QD, Tel: 01 593 7511 (Instruments).

Medequip: Pembroke House, 36/37, Pembroke Street, Oxford OX1 1BL, Tel: 0865 724631 (General equipment).

Millbrook Medical: 16, The Grove, Radlett, Herts WD7 7NF, Tel: 09276 3695 (General equipment).

3-M United Kingdom: 3-M House, PO Box 1, Bracknell, Berks RG12 1JU, Tel: 0344 426726 (Steri-strips, skin staplers, tapes).

Nova Instruments Ltd (Chiropody) Mill House, 127, Newgatestreet Road, Goffs Oak, Herts EN7 5RX, Tel: 0707 875600 (Chiropody).

OEC Orthopaedic Ltd: Waterson Industrial Estate, Bridgend, South Glam. CF31 3YN, Tel: 0656 55221, Telex 497920 (Tourniquet).

One Thousand and One Lamps Ltd: 4, Barmeston Road, London SE6 2UX Tel: 01 698 7328 (Lights).

Rimmer Bros Ltd: 18/19, Aylesbury Street, Clerkenwell, London EC1R 0DD, Tel: 01 251 6494 (Electrocauteries).

Rocket of London: Imperial Way, Watford, Herts WD2 4XX, Tel: 0923 39791, Telex 922531 (Surgical Instruments).

Schuco International London Ltd: Lyndhurst Avenue, Woodhouse Road, London N12 0NE, Tel: 01 368 1642, Telex 893312 (Hyfrecator).

Seward Medical Ltd: UAC House, Blackfriars Road, London SE1 9UG, Tel: 01 928 9431, Telex 919021 (Surgical instruments).

Spembly Medical Ltd: Newbury Road, Andover, Hampshire SP10 4DR, Tel: 0264 65741, Telex 47403.

STD Pharmaceuticals Ltd: 6–7, Broad Street, Hereford HR4 9AE, Tel: 0432 272152, Telex 35421 (STD for sclerotherapy).

Stiefel Laboratories (UK) Ltd: Holtspur Lane, Wooburn Green, High Wycombe, Bucks HP10 0AU, Tel: 06285 24966, Telex 849312 (Disposable skin biopsy punches).

Surgical Equipment Supplies Ltd: Westfields Road, London W3 0RB, Tel: 01 992 3212, Telex 8954919, SESCOG (Sterilizers).

Chas Thackray Ltd: PO Box HP 171, 1 Shire Oak Street, Leeds LS6 2DP, Tel: 0532 744711 (Theatre equipment and instruments).

Thames Valley Medical: Chatham Street, Reading, Berks RG1 7HT, Tel: 0734 595835.

Travenol Laboratories Ltd, Thorpe Lea Manor, Thorpe Lea Road, Egham, Surrey TW20 8HW, Tel 0784 34388 (Tru-cut biopsy needles).

Warecrest Ltd: Unit D4, Cowdray Centre, Cowdray Avenue, Colchester, Essex CO1 1BW Tel: 0206 561404 (C28 Rechargeable electrocautery).

John Weiss and Son Ltd: 11, Wigmore Street, London W1H 0DN, Tel: 01 636 5893 (Ophthalmic instruments and equipment).

North America and Canada suppliers

Aaron Medical Industries PO Box 261196, Tampa, Florida 33685 (Disposable electrocauteries).

American Hospital Services: 7080 River Road, Suite 131, Richmond, BC V6X 1X5.

Amsco Canada: 77, Hale Road, Brampton, Ontario L6W 3J9.

Bard Canada Inc: 2345 Stanfield Road, Mississauga, Ontario L4Y 3Y3.

Birtcher Corporation: 4501 N. Arden Drive, El Monte, CA 91731, PO Box 4399 El Monte, CA 91734 (213) 575 8144 TWX9105873446 (Hyfrecator).

Clement Clarke Inc: 6947 Americana Parkway, Reynoldsburg, Columbus, Ohio 43068, USA.

Cyanamid Canada Inc/Davis and Geck: 2255 Shepherd Avenue, Willowdale, Ontario M2J 4Y5.

Downs Surgical Inc: 2500 Park Central Boulevard, Decatur GA, 30035 USA.

Downs Surgical Canada: 5715 McAdam Road, Mississauga, Ontario, L4Z 1PG Canada.

Electro-Med: 3278 Oak Street, Victoria, BC V8X 1P7.

Ethicon Inc: Route no. 22, Somerville, New Jersey 08876 USA, Tel: 201 524 0400, Telex 833487.

Frigitronics of Connecticut Inc: 770, River Road, Shelton CT 06484, Tel: 203 929 6321.

Johnson and Johnson Inc: 2155 Pie IX Boulevard, Montreal, Quebec H1V 2E4.

Keeler Instruments Ltd: 456 Parkway, Lawrence Park Industrial District, Broomhall P.A. 19008 USA, 215 353 4350, Telex 831370.

Kimberley Clark Co.: 1400 Holcomb Bridge Road, Roswell, Georgia 30076, USA.

Laerdal Medical Corporation: 1 Labriola Court, Armonk, NY 10504.

Ledu Corporation: 25, Lindeman Drive, PO Box 358, Trumbull CT 06611, USA, Tel: 203 371 5500 (Lamps).

3-M: 3-M Centre, St Paul, MN 55101.

Omnis Surgical Inc: 1425 Lake Cook Road, Deerfield, Illinois 60015, 312 480 5600.

Roboz Surgical Instrument: 810, 18th St. N.W. Washington DC 20006.

Chas. F. Thackray (USA) Inc: 175-X New Boston Street, Woburn, Massachusetts 01801, Tel: (617) 935 6831.

APPENDIX 2

Corresponding trade names for drugs named in the book

Drug	United Kingdom	Canada	United States of America
Lignocaine	Xylocaine	Xylocaine	Octocaine
Prilocaine	Citanest	Unavailable	Xylonest
Bupivicaine	Marcain	Marcaine	Marcain
Chlorhexidine	Hibitane	Hibitane	Hibiclens
Povidone iodine	Betadine	Betadine	Isodine
Diazepam	Valium	Valium	Valium
Sodium tetradecyl	STD	Trombovar	Sotradecol
Glutaraldehyde	Cidex	Cidex	
Atropine	Atropine	Atropine	Atropine
Ethyl Chloride	Ethyl Chloride	Ethyl Chloride	Ethyl Chloride
Pethidine	Pethidine	Demerol	Demerol
Entonox	Entonox	Entonox	
Methylprednisolone	Depo-medrone	Depo-Medrol	
Triamcinolone	Lederspan	Aristocort	
Chloramphenicol	Chloromycetin	Chloromycetin	Chloromycetin
Adrenalin	Adrenalin	Epinephrine	Epinephrine

References

1. Brown, John Stuart (1979) Minor Operations in General Practice. *British Medical Journal* **1,** 1609.
2. Robertson, Brian (1982) Minor Surgery in General Practice saves Resources *B.M.A. News Review*, November, iv.
3. St John Ambulance, St Andrew's Ambulance Association. First Aid Manual (4th edn), The British Red Cross Society.
4. Bier, August (1908) Uber einen neuer weg Localanaesthesie an den Gliedmassen zu erzeugen. *Arch. Klin. Chir.* **86,** 1007.
5. Holmes, C. McK. (1963) Intravenous regional analgesia: a useful method of producing analgesia of the limbs. *Lancet*, **1,** 245.
6. Thorn-Alquist, A. M. (1971) Intravenous regional anaesthesia: a seven year survey. *Acta Anaesthesiol, Scand.* Supplement 40.
7. Ware, R. J. (1975) *Anaesthesia* **30,** 817.
8. Ware, R. J. (1979) Intra-venous regional anaesthesia using bupivicaine. *Anaesthesia*, **34,** 231.
9. Pattison, Charles W. (1984) A review of the Bier's block technique. *The Practitioner*,**228,** 235.
10. Mason, M. Andrew (1983) Regional anaesthesia with bupivicaine. *Lancet*, November 5th, 1085.
11. Langer, K. (1861) Ueber die Spaltbarkeit der Cutis. *Sitzungsb. d., K. Akad. d. Wissensch Matt.-naturw.* C1, **43,** 23.
12. Fomon, Samuel (1939) *The Surgery of Injury and Plastic Repair.* Williams and Wilkins Co, Baltimore Md. p. 50.
13. Berson, Morton (1948) *Atlas of Plastic Surgery.* Grune & Stratton, New York p. 3.
14. Barsky, Arthur (1950) *Principles and Practice of Plastic Surgery.* Williams and Wilkins Co., Baltimore Md. p. 38.
15. Smith, F. (1950) *Plastic and Reconstructive Surgery – A Manual of Management.* W. B. Saunders and Co., London p. 213.
16. Kraissl, Cornelius (1951) The selection of appropriate lines for elective surgical incisions. *Plastic and Reconstructive Surgery*, **8,** 1.
17. Nash, J. R. (1979) Sclerotherapy for hydrocele and epididymal cysts. *British Journal of Surgery*, **66,** 289.
18. Haye, K. R. and Maiti, H. (1985) Self treatment of condylomata acuminata using 0.5% podophyllin resin, *The Practitioner*, **229,** 37.
19. Fegan, W. G. (1983) Continuous compression technique of injecting varicose veins. *The Lancet*, **ii,** 109.
20. Fegan, W. G. (1967) *Varicose Veins, Compression Sclerotherapy*, London, Heinemann.
21. Feathers, R. S. (1981) Varicose Veins in Women, *Maternal and Child Health*, 318.
22. Maiti, H. and Haye, K. R. (1985) Self treatment of condylomata acuminata using 0.5% podophyllin resin topically for three days. *The Practitioner*, **229,** 37.
23. Dagnall, J. Colin M.Chs. (1981) The history, development and current status of nail matrix phenolisation, *The Chiropodist*, p. 315.
24. Boll, O. F. (1945) Surgical correction of ingrowing toe-nails, *Journal of the National Association of Chiropodists*, **35**(4) 8.
25. Suppan, R. J. and Ritchilin, J. D. (1962) A non-debilitating procedure for ingrown toe-nail, *Journal of the American Podiatry Association*, **52,** 900.
26. Barrish, S. J. (1909) The phenol-alcohol technique, *Current Podiatry*, **18**(7) 18.
27. Swerdlow, M. (1973) The relief of pain in terminal illness. Symposium on terminal care, *Modern Geriatrics*, 137.

28. Morton, E. R. (1969) The treatment of naevi and other cutaneous lesions by electrolysis, cautery, and refrigeration *Lancet*, **ii,** 1658.
29. Morton, E. R. (1910) The use of solid carbon dioxide, *Lancet*, **ii,** 1268–70.
30. White, A. C. (1899) Liquid air in medicine and surgery, *Med. Rec.* 2899, **56,** 109.
31. Lloyd Williams, K. and Holden, H. B. (1975) Cryosurgery in general and ENT surgery, *British Journal of Hospital Medicine*, 14.
32. Chamberlain, Geoffrey (1975) Cryosurgery in gynaecology, *British Journal of Hospital Medicine* 26.
33. Hopkins, Philip (1982) *Proceedings of the fifth annual meeting of the American College of Cryosurgery*, New Orleans, USA, p. 12.
34. Hopkins, Philip (1983) Cryosurgery by the general practitioner, *The Practitioner*, **227,** 1861.
35. Eberhart, Noble M. (1911) *A Working Manual of High Frequency Currents*, Chicago, New Medicine Publishing Co.
36. Ellis, Professor Harold (1984) Sigmoidoscopy, *Update 1*, p. 981.
37. Ellis, Professor Harold (1984) Rectal bleeding and the general practitioner, *Cancer Care* **1,** (4), 4.
38. Brown, John Stuart (1983) Sigmoidoscopy in general practice, *Journal of the Royal College of General Practitioners*, **33,** 822.
39. Goligher, J. C. (1967) *Surgery of the Anus, Rectum and Colon*, Bailliere Tindall and Cassell, London, pp. 120.
40. Gabriel, W. B. (1956) Minor Ano-rectal Operations in *Pye's Surgical Handcraft*, John Wright and Sons Ltd, Bristol), pp. 426.
41. Lewis, M. I. (1972) Cryosurgical haemorrhoidectomy, *Diseases Colon and Rectum*, p. 128.
42. Alexander-Williams, J. (1982) The management of piles, *British Medical Journal*, **285,** 1137.
43. Barron, J. (1963) Office ligation of internal haemorrhoids, *American Journal of Surgery*, **105,** 563.
44. Steinberg, D. M., Liegois, H. and Alexander-Williams, J. (1975) Long term review of the results of rubber band ligation of haemorrhoids, *British Journal of Surgery*, **62,** 144.
45. Panda, A. P. et al (1975) Treatment of haemorrhoids by rubber band ligation, *Digestion*, **12,** 85.
46. Lord, P. H. (1975) Conservative management of haemorrhoids 2 – dilation treatment, *Clinical Gastroenterology*, **4,** 601.
47. Yeates, W. Keith (1984) Vasectomy, *Update*, 1229.
48. McEvedy, B. V. (1962) Simple ganglia, *British Journal of Surgery*, **49**(218), 584.
49. Brett, M. S. (1977) Operations for ganglion in *Operative Surgery – The Hand* (eds Robb and Smith), Butterworth, London, p. 369.
50. Woltman, H. W. (1941) Neuritis associated with acromegaly, *Archives of Neurology and Psychiatry*, **45,** 680.
51. Pulvertaft, R. Guy (1977) Decompresion of the median nerve in *Operative Surgery – The Hand*, 3rd edn, Butterworth, London p. 271.
52. Fansa, M. R. and Helal, B. (1976) Carpal tunnel – surgical treatment, *Nursing Mirror*, p. 47.
53. Pulvertaft, R. Guy (1977) Tenosynovitis stenosans and de Quervain's syndrome in *Operative Surgery – The Hand* (eds Robb and Smith) 3rd edn, Butterworth, London, p. 363.
54. Statement of Fees and Allowances payable to general medical practitioners in England and Wales (The 'Red Book') National Health Service General Medical Services.
55. The National Health Service (General Medical and Pharmaceutical Services) Regulations 1974 (SI 1974 no 160) as amended by SI 1982 no 1283, Schedule I, Part I, Paragraphs 32–34.
56. Studd, John (1986) A Practical Guide to HRT, *MIMS Magazine*, **1,** 21–22.

Index